PHARMACOLOGY
FOR THE **SURGICAL**
TECHNOLOGIST

SIXTH EDITION

PHARMACOLOGY FOR THE SURGICAL TECHNOLOGIST

Tiffany Howe, CST, CSFA, FAST, MBA

Vice President for Teaching and Learning,
Western Dakota Technical College,
Rapid City, South Dakota

Angela Burton, CST, FAST

General Clinical Resource,
Black Hills Surgical Hospital,
Rapid City, South Dakota

ELSEVIER

Elsevier
3251 Riverport Lane
St. Louis, Missouri 63043

Pharmacology for the Surgical Technologist, SIXTH EDITION   ISBN: 978-0-443-10909-6

Notice

Practitioners and researchers must always rely on their own experience and knowledge in evaluating and using any information, methods, compounds or experiments described herein. Because of rapid advances in the medical sciences, in particular, independent verification of diagnoses and drug dosages should be made. To the fullest extent of the law, no responsibility is assumed by Elsevier, authors, editors, or contributors for any injury and/or damage to persons or property as a matter of products liability, negligence or otherwise, or from any use or operation of any methods, products, instructions, or ideas contained in the material herein.

Previous editions copyrighted 2021, 2017, 2012, 2006, 1999

Content Strategist: Kelly Skelton
Content Development Specialist: Priyadarshini Pandey
Publishing Services Manager: Deepthi Unni
Project Manager: Sindhuraj Thulasingam
Design Direction: Ryan Cook

Printed in India

Last digit is the print number: 9   8   7   6   5   4   3   2   1

Working together
to grow libraries in
developing countries

www.elsevier.com • www.bookaid.org

This edition of the textbook is dedicated to our friends, mentors, and colleagues Kathy Snyder and the late Chris Keegan for their commitment to the advancement of the surgical technology profession and their passion for educating future surgical technologists and surgical first assistants.

REVIEWERS

Stephanie E. Austin, CST, FAST, AAS, BAS, MA
Assistant Professor/Director of Surgical Technology
Walters State Community College
Sevierville, Tennessee

Marcene Elwell, BSN, RN, CNOR, CST
Surgical Technology Program Director
Western Nebraska Community College
Scottsbluff, Nebraska

Rhonda R. Green
Clinical Coordinator
Collin College
McKinney, Texas

Janice Grewatz, BS, CST/CSFA, CSPDT, FAST
Program Director and Associate Professor
Parkland College
Champaign, Illinois

Dr. Yvette Jackson, EdD, RN, MSN, CNOR, CST
Surgical Technology Director/Educator
Coastal Alabama Community College
Minette, Alabama

Jessica Lynn Lemmon, BSCHA, CST
Certified Surgical Technologist/Program Director of Surgical
Technology
Pima Medical Institute—Tucson Campus
Tucson, Arizona

James J. Mizner, Jr, RPh, MBA
Founder and President
Panacea Solutions Consulting
Reston, Virginia

Lori Giordano O'Leary, MSN, RN, CST, CNOR
Adjunct Faculty, Professional Development Specialist
Gateway Community College
New Haven, Connecticut
Middlesex Hospital
Middlesex, Connecticut

Mark Wilms, CST, CRCST, CHL, M.Ed.
Surgical Technology Program Director
Pima Medical Institute
Denver, Colorado

More than 25 years ago, a committee of instructors met to work on revisions to the *Core Curriculum for Surgical Technology*. During the meeting, the topic of textbooks surfaced—in particular, pharmacology textbooks. It was generally agreed that no adequate pharmacology textbook for surgical technologists existed. As the discussion progressed and we complained about the situation, a question was posed: "Well, are you going to be part of the problem or part of the solution?" This sixth edition of *Pharmacology for the Surgical Technologist* is our continuing response to that question and aligns with the most recent edition of the *Core Curriculum for Surgical Technology*. It offers a distinct combination of subject matter. The text is organized into three units, each focusing on information specific to the surgical environment. Students learn a framework of pharmacologic principles to apply the information in surgical situations; review basic math skills; learn commonly used medications by category, with frequent descriptions of actual applications; and learn basic anesthesia concepts, not previously presented at this level, to function more effectively as a surgical team member.

Special learning tools used in this text include the following:

- Learning Objectives, which are stated at the beginning of each chapter
- Key Terms, which are boldfaced in the chapters
- Insight boxes, which offer additional information on the subjects
- Quick Questions, which encourage students to review materials and apply previous knowledge
- Illustrations, including surgical photographs, which are designed to familiarize the student with the surgical environment
- Tables and Boxes, which condense information to enhance learning
- Tech Tips, Caution, and Make It Simple features, which aid in understanding and applying information
- Chapter Key Concept summaries and Chapter Review questions, which emphasize critical content
- Advanced Practices sections, which emphasize the role of the surgical first assistant
- Drug Category Index by surgical specialty
- Glossary of terms

These features have been developed to assist the student in learning new and often unfamiliar material. Key terms are bolded in the text and included in the glossary. Students should be encouraged to use a medical dictionary, as needed, for routine medical terminology used throughout the text. Learning objectives are used to guide the students through the material, emphasizing important concepts. Additional learning activities available on the Evolve website are designed to help students think about concepts from a broader perspective and apply content at a more personal level, particularly at their local clinical facilities.

ACKNOWLEDGMENTS

We would like to acknowledge and sincerely thank Kathy Snyder and the late Chris Keegan for their commitment of 20-plus years developing and revising the first four editions of this textbook. We are honored to have been asked to move forward with future revisions of this textbook, and are humbled by your confidence to continue your vision for educating future surgical technologists/surgical first assistants and advocating for all surgical patients. We would also like to thank all students, instructors, and practitioners who have been involved in the creation and revisions of all editions. We are grateful to Elsevier staff for their expertise and guidance through this edition. Thank you to the Western Dakota Technical College Surgical Technology Program for use of their laboratory and supplies for textbook photos. Thank you to our family, friends, and colleagues for their continued support and patience while we collaborated on this textbook revision.

CONTENTS

Introduction to Pharmacology

As a surgical technologist, you will mix and measure medications and deliver them to and from the sterile field. This means you will be dealing with pharmacology—the science of drugs. In this unit, we look at general pharmacological information, including how medications are measured, what kinds of medications are used, the laws that pertain to them, how they are labeled, and how they are administered to the surgical patient. We look at the medications themselves—their sources, names, classifications, routes by which they are administered, and their forms. This unit provides a framework of pharmacological terms, concepts, and principles, ones that help you understand current information about medications and prepare you to assimilate new information effectively. We then focus on laws, regulations, and medication labels. You will see the importance of laws to regulate medications and the information found on medication labels, what types of laws exist, and which government agencies enforce the laws. You will also learn what acts govern your scope of practice in regard to medications. Next, we address precision because it is critical to deliver exactly the right quantity and strength of any medication. Thus we review mathematics that you need to do the job. We include an initial mathematics quiz, so you can determine your skills and what areas you need to review. There is a refresher on basic computation techniques and a review of measurement systems used in medicine, especially the metric system and basic conversions. Patient safety depends on accuracy, and the surgical technologist is the last line of defense against medication errors in the sterile field. Finally, we concentrate on methods you will use when handling medications, including aseptic technique, the steps for proper medication identification, and clear labeling of all medications on the sterile field.

Basic Pharmacology

OBJECTIVES

After completing this chapter, you should be able to do the following:

1. Define terms and abbreviations related to pharmacology.
2. State sources of drugs and list examples of drugs from each source.
3. List and describe several classes of drugs relevant to surgical practice.
4. Explain medication orders used both in prescriptions and in surgery.
5. List the parts of a medication order used in surgery.
6. Identify drug distribution systems used in hospitals.
7. List and describe types of drug forms.
8. Compare and contrast medication administration routes used in surgery.
9. Explain the four processes of pharmacokinetics.
10. Identify and discuss aspects of pharmacodynamics.

The science of pharmacology is a diverse study of the interactions between chemicals and biological systems. In the broadest sense, it includes toxicology, food science, agriculture, and medicine. When chemicals are used to treat diseases, we call them drugs or medications. Medical pharmacology is a rapidly expanding field of study because new drugs are being developed nearly every day. An understanding of basic principles in pharmacology can help the surgical technologist deal with such constant developments. Students should seek to build a framework of principles so they can incorporate new information more easily. When a new drug is introduced into surgical practice, the surgical technologist should be able to understand information about the drug by applying the principles of pharmacology. This chapter presents an introduction to the foundations of pharmacology that can be applied throughout a professional career in surgical technology.

DRUG SOURCES

Drugs in use today come from three main sources: natural sources, chemical synthesis, and biotechnology. Natural sources include plants, animals, and minerals. The study of drugs derived from natural sources is called *pharmacognosy*.

At one time, plants were nearly the only source of medicines available. Today, only a few prescription drugs relevant to surgical practice are still derived directly from plant sources. Examples of current drugs made from plants include atropine from the roots of the belladonna plant (*Atropa belladonna*; deadly nightshade; Fig. 1.1), digitalis from the leaves of the purple foxglove, and morphine from the seeds of the opium poppy (Table 1.1). The trend toward alternative medicines has initiated a closer look at plants as sources of important and helpful chemicals in the natural state (Insight 1.1). Chemicals produced by plants also hold great promise in the development of drugs to treat cancer. One such drug is paclitaxel (Taxol), which is derived from *Taxus baccata* and is used to treat breast cancer.

Animals provide a source for some drugs, particularly hormones. Cattle and hog endocrine glands were the best available source of hormones before the advent of biotechnology. We describe drugs derived from hogs as *porcine* and those from cattle as *bovine*. Thus thyroglobulin (Proloid)—a purified extract of hog thyroid gland—is porcine in origin, whereas thrombin—a topical hemostatic—is bovine in origin. The early form of insulin is both bovine and porcine because it was obtained from the pancreas of cattle and hogs. Estrogen was another hormone obtained

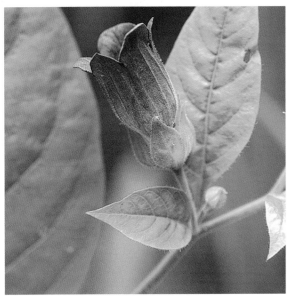

Fig. 1.1 Atropa belladonna. Courtesy Martin Wall Botanical Services. (From Ulbrich C: *Natural standard herbal pharmacotherapy*, ed 1, St Louis, 2010, Elsevier.)

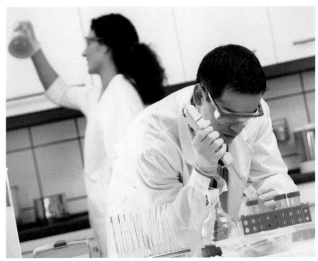

Fig. 1.2 A pharmaceutical laboratory. iStock.com/LajosRepasi

TABLE 1.1   Examples of Plant-Derived Drugs Relevant to Surgical Practice

Drug	Category	Plant
Atropine	Anticholinergic	Atropa belladonna
Cocaine	Local anesthetic	Erythroxylum coca
Digoxin	Cardiac agent	Digitalis purpurea
Ephedrine	Sympathomimetic	Ephedra sinica
Morphine	Analgesic	Papaver somniferum
Papaverine	Smooth muscle relaxant	Papaver somniferum
Pilocarpine	Parasympathomimetic	Pilocarpus jaborandi

INSIGHT 1.1   In Search of New Drugs

Sometimes the quest for new drugs involves some very old sources. It has long been said that a glass of wine is good for you, and archaeologists know the ancient Egyptians thought the same. When the 5100-year-old tomb of Pharaoh Scorpion I was excavated, more than 700 jars were discovered in one of the chambers. Some of the jars contained wine residue with medicinal additives. These additives might have come from a relative of the present-day wormwood (*Artemisia sieberi*), blue tansy, herbs, and tree resins. The jars were imported from several sites in the ancient world, in what we know today as Israel and Palestine. These jars demonstrate how humans from thousands of years ago had turned to their natural environments for effective plant remedies. It will take our modern technology using biomolecular analysis to isolate these active components. Scientists are working with physicians to see whether any of these compounds might be useful today—perhaps in the fight against cancer.

from an animal source. Conjugated estrogen (Premarin) was obtained from the urine of pregnant horses and so is referred to as *equine* in nature.

Minerals, such as calcium, magnesium, and silver salts in several forms, are used in some pharmacological agents. For example,

Tums and Mylanta are antacids that contain calcium (Tums) and magnesium (Mylanta) hydroxides. Silver sulfadiazine (Silvadene cream) is an antimicrobial agent used in dressings for burn patients that contains silver salts (see Chapter 5). Even gold is used, for example in aurothioglucose (Solganal), an antiarthritic agent.

The second major source of drugs is chemical synthesis in the laboratory (Fig. 1.2). There are two ways for drugs to be *synthesized*, that is, put together. *Synthetic drugs* are drugs that are synthesized from laboratory chemicals. *Semisynthetic drugs* are drugs that start with a natural substance that is extracted, purified, and altered by chemical processes. The vast majority of modern drugs are either synthetic or semisynthetic. Meperidine (Demerol) is an example of a synthetic drug; it is made from chemicals, yet its pain-relieving effects are similar to those of opium. Many types of penicillin, such as amoxicillin, are semisynthetic drugs. The penicillin group of drugs was originally derived from a natural mold (*Penicillium*), the active substance of which is extracted and purified in the chemical laboratory. Another example of semisynthetic drugs is the aminoglycoside group of antibiotics, the active substance of which is obtained from the bacterial species *Streptomyces*.

An increasing source of drugs has been provided by the science of biotechnology. The term biotechnology is used to refer to the concepts of genetic engineering and recombinant deoxyribonucleic acid (DNA) technology. The science of biotechnology has many applications in pharmacology and has provided significant improvements in the treatment of various conditions. Biotechnology is a process that allows scientists to produce proteins from bacteria—proteins that were previously available only from animals. Molecular biologists use bacteria as tiny factories to produce the proteins they need to make drugs. They do this by altering the DNA of bacteria, such as *Escherichia coli* (*E. coli*). How? By physically inserting a gene into the DNA of a single *E. coli* cell—a gene that *codes for* (tells the cell to make) a certain protein (Fig. 1.3). When the bacterial cell has this gene incorporated into its DNA, it becomes a miniature copying machine, producing daughter cells that have daughter cells that have daughter cells—each with the new gene and each producing the desired protein. Because this reproduction process occurs very rapidly, large volumes of the desired protein can be obtained quickly. The specific protein is extracted and purified in the laboratory and prepared for administration to a patient. Molecular biologists also use cultures of mammalian cell lines, such as genetically altered Chinese hamster ovary (CHO) cells, to produce various therapeutic proteins. Adalimumab (Humira) is an example of a drug developed with recombinant DNA technology and mammalian cell lines. In general, CHO cells provide more stable gene expression and higher volumes of the desired proteins than bacterial cells and are becoming the primary choice of cell lines for pharmacological use.

Among the drugs produced by biotechnology are human insulin (Humulin), human growth hormone (Nutropin), human thyroid-stimulating hormone (Thyrogen), and the thrombolytic agent alteplase (Activase). Drugs such as these are always administered by injection; they cannot be taken orally because they are proteins, which are digested when consumed. Genetically engineered proteins do not cause the adverse side effects—for example, immune or allergic reactions—often seen in the long-term use of drugs from animal sources. The hepatitis B vaccine (Engerix-B, Recombivax HB) is another product of biotechnology. This vaccine is of particular interest to surgical technologists because it is one of the required vaccinations for healthcare providers.

DRUG CLASSIFICATIONS

Drug classifications are used to group drugs that are used for similar purposes (Table 1.2). Learning the drug classification of common medications is particularly helpful to the surgical technologist in practice because many classification titles will provide clues to the use or purpose of a medication. For example, a vasoconstrictor will cause contraction of the walls of blood vessels and restrict blood flow. An ophthalmic agent is specially formulated for use in the eye only, and an otic medication is specially formulated for use in the ear.

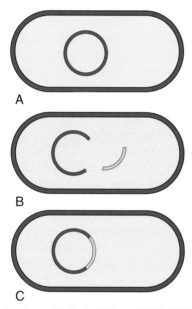

Fig. 1.3 Biotechnology. (A) *Escherichia coli* DNA. (B) Desired gene is inserted into bacterial DNA. (C) Bacterial DNA with recombinant gene.

> **? MAKE IT SIMPLE**
>
> Use of medical terminology word-building techniques to define the drug class will help in the understanding of a medication's purpose—for example, *anesthetic:* "an-" means without and "-esthesia" means sensation. Thus, an anesthetic agent causes a loss of sensation. Another example, *thrombolytic:* "thrombo-" means blood clot, "-lysis" is to break down, and "-tic" is a suffix meaning pertaining to. Thus, a thrombolytic is a medication given to break down a blood clot.

Some drugs can be listed in multiple classes. For example, aspirin relieves pain, fever, and inflammation, so it is classified as an analgesic, an antipyretic, and an antiinflammatory agent.

We can also classify drugs in broader categories by what they do, what they affect, and what they are; thus classification categories may include the following:

• *Therapeutic action:* what they do for a patient; for example, analgesics relieve pain.

TABLE 1.2   Drug Classifications

Therapeutic Action	Physiologic Action	Body System	Chemical Type
Analgesic	α-adrenergic blocker	Cardiovascular agent	Barbiturate
Anticoagulant	Cholinergic	Dermatologic agent	Benzodiazepine
Antiemetic	Diuretic	Ophthalmic preparation	Hormone
Antihistamine	Hemostatic	Urinary tract agent	Narcotic
Antihypertensive	Histamine receptor antagonist		Oxytocic
Antiinflammatory	Muscle relaxant antagonist		Steroid
Antineoplastic	Narcotic antagonist		
Antipyretic	Tranquilizer		
Antispasmodic	Vasoconstrictor		
Sedative			
Thrombolytic			

- *Physiological action:* what they do in the body; for example, histamine receptor antagonists block histamine production.
- *Affected body system:* what they affect; for example, cardiovascular agents affect the heart and circulatory system.
- *Chemical type:* what they are; for example, barbiturates are a class of chemical compounds derived from barbituric acid.

📌 TECH TIP

Classes of drugs frequently used from the sterile back table include antibiotics, anticoagulants, antiinflammatory agents, and local anesthetics.

Drugs are also classified by how they may be obtained. The distinction between prescription and nonprescription, or over-the-counter (OTC), drugs is a legal classification. In addition, some prescription medications are classified as controlled substances. Legal classifications are discussed in Chapter 2.

MEDICATION ORDERS

Prescriptions

When treatment requires a specific drug, a licensed physician or designee, such as a physician assistant or nurse practitioner, writes a prescription for the drug. State governments have the power to regulate which medical professionals write prescriptions, so there may be variations in practice from state to state. Fig. 1.4 shows a typical written prescription form. As shown, prescriptions must include the date, name of the patient, name of the drug, dosage, route of administration, and frequency or time of administration. It must also bear the prescriber's signature. Notice that the printed form contains the name, address, telephone number, and Drug Enforcement Administration (DEA) number of the prescriber. The DEA requires that this number be listed on any prescription for a controlled substance (see Chapter 2). A written prescription usually designates the drug by trade name, but may indicate that a generic substitution is permissible. When writing prescriptions, physicians (or their designees) use abbreviations and symbols (Table 1.3) for directions, dosages, frequency, and administration routes. Pharmacists interpret these symbols and give the drugs to the patient, along with instructions for proper use. Many pharmacies use computer database systems that provide specific, detailed printouts to the patient of such important drug information as side effects, precautions, normal usage, and storage. Prescriptions such as the one shown are not generally used during a patient's hospitalization, so they have little or no use during surgery.

Written prescriptions occasionally present difficulties in interpreting handwriting. The introduction of electronic prescribing, or *e-prescribing*, may significantly reduce medication errors that are due to misinterpretation of poorly handwritten prescriptions. E-prescribing is the process of generating, transmitting, and filing prescriptions through a computer-based system (Fig. 1.5). These systems also provide ready access to important prescriber safety information, such as patient medication history and allergies. In the hospital setting, any medications to be administered to the patient must be ordered by

Fig. 1.4 A typical prescription form.

TABLE 1.3 Abbreviations for Medication Directions, Dosages, Frequency and Administration

Abbreviation	Meaning
aa	Of each
ad lib	As desired
amt	Amount
c̄	With
KVO, TKO	Keep vein open, to keep open
npo, NPO	Nothing by mouth (nil per os)
per	By means of, by
Rx	Take
s̄	Without
sig	Label
sos	Once if necessary
stat	Immediately

a licensed physician or designee and written on a physician's order sheet or entered into the electronic prescribing system.

Medication Orders in Surgery

In surgery, the medication order may be one of several types, such as standing orders, verbal orders, 'immediately' (STAT) orders, and 'as needed' (PRN) orders.

A standing order, or *protocol*, is used for common situations requiring a standard treatment. For example, institutions participating in the Surgical Care Improvement Project may have

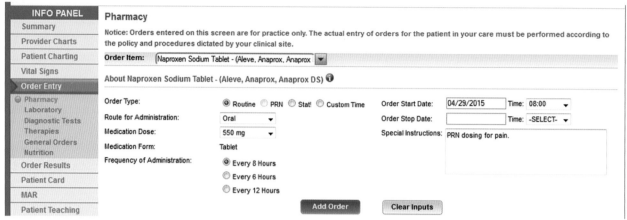

Fig. 1.5 An example screenshot of e-prescribing. (Courtesy SimChart for the Medical Office, Elsevier, Inc., 2016.)

INSIGHT 1.2 Practical Math—Calculating Drug Dosages at the Sterile Back Table

Some drugs are available in various strengths, such as lidocaine. How much of the drug is given (dose) depends on the strength *and* the volume. The same dosage of lidocaine can be given in different ways. For example, 30 mL of 1% lidocaine delivers the same dosage as 15 mL of 2% lidocaine or 60 mL of 0.5% lidocaine.

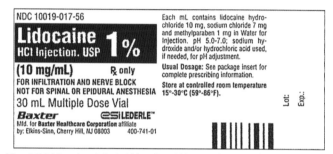

Fig. 1.6 Lidocaine label. Lidocaine 1% contains 1 g of medication per 100 mL solution and 10 mg per mL. (From Morris DG: *Calculate with confidence*, ed 6, St Louis, 2014, Elsevier.)

---

a standing order in place stating that all patients undergoing specified surgical procedures are to receive a particular prophylactic antibiotic 1 hour before the incision. In the operating room, surgeons' preference cards contain standing orders for specific surgical procedures. For example, Dr. Vigil's preference card for abdominal aortic aneurysm repair may include a standing order for 5000 units of heparin (a systemic anticoagulant; see Chapter 9) in 1000 mL of sodium chloride solution (saline, 0.9% NaCl) for topical irrigation. A standing order of this type informs the operating room team that the indicated medication should be ready on the sterile back table as a standard part of the setup for that procedure.

Verbal orders are commonplace in surgery because a surgeon may request a particular drug to be administered either from the sterile field or by the anesthesia care provider. For example, during a carotid endarterectomy (approximately 3 minutes before the application of vascular clamps to the carotid artery), Dr. Vigil may give a verbal order to the anesthesia care provider to administer 5000 units of heparin intravenously (IV). Verbal orders in surgery are usually for a one-time single administration of a medication. The verbal order is documented in the patient's record.

Usually given verbally, STAT orders indicate that a drug is to be administered immediately and one time only. The most common use of STAT orders in surgery is during cardiac arrest resuscitation or other emergent situations.

PRN stands for pro re nata, which means that the drug may be given as needed. For example, during septoplasty performed with the patient under local anesthesia, the analgesic meperidine (Demerol) may be administered PRN to reduce patient discomfort.

In surgery, medications routinely needed during a procedure are listed on the surgeon's preference card (see Fig. 10.4). The preference card should list all pertinent information, such as drug strength and quantity. Surgical medication orders on preference cards usually contain the drug name, strength, and volume. For example, when a radiopaque contrast medium (see Chapter 6) is needed, the preference card might state "Omnipaque 300—10 mL." Unlike medication orders given in nursing care units, the surgeon administers all medications in the sterile field, so route of administration and frequency are not usually stated on surgeons' preference cards.

Many abbreviations are used to represent drug forms, dosages, routes, and timing of administration. Dosages are stated in a particular unit of measure, usually in the metric system, and abbreviated, such as 300 mg or 10 mL. The dosage of a medication is the medication strength (usually expressed as a percentage) multiplied by the volume administered (Insight 1.2).

For example, lidocaine (Xylocaine) may be injected for local anesthesia (see Chapter 13) and therefore is listed on the preference card as "lidocaine plain 1%—30 mL." This indicates that a 30-mL vial of a 1% solution of lidocaine without epinephrine should be delivered to the sterile back table and prepared for use (Fig. 1.6). It may not be necessary to use the entire 30 mL during the procedure, so the surgical technologist in the scrub role reports the final amount (volume) and strength used to the circulator and anesthesia care provider, who record the dose.

TABLE 1.4   Abbreviations for Frequency of Medication Administration

Abbreviation	Meaning
bid	Twice a day
h, hr	Hour
prn, PRN	As necessary (pro re nata)
q	Every
qh	Every hour
q2h	Every 2 hours
qid	Four times a day
tid	Three times a day
stat	Immediately

For regular hospital medication orders, the route of administration is usually abbreviated; for example, if a drug is to be given intravenously, it is designated as IV. The frequency or time of administration is also clearly stated and often abbreviated; for example, if the drug is to be taken twice a day, it is designated bid. Table 1.4 lists common abbreviations used to represent frequency of drug administration. Again, most surgeons' preference cards do not list the route or frequency because the surgeon is administering all medications given at the surgical site.

> ### ! CAUTION
> Some abbreviations have been associated with an increased risk of misinterpretation and possible medication errors. The Joint Commission, which accredits hospitals and other healthcare institutions, requires accredited facilities to publish a "do not use" list for potentially dangerous abbreviations, acronyms, and symbols (see Table 2.2). Before using what you may think are standard abbreviations, consult this list at your facility.

DRUG DISTRIBUTION SYSTEMS

Dispensing prescription drugs is the responsibility of a licensed pharmacist; that is, pharmacists must *release* drugs, either directly to patients or to the physician or surgeon who orders them. In hospitals, drugs are often released for secure storage in various patient care areas so they can be distributed as necessary.

> **NOTE:** In all medical facilities, controlled substances (such as morphine) must be stored in a secure location once they have been released from the pharmacy. Individual institutional policies are put in place to account for and document the use of controlled substances.

Distribution systems for drugs used in surgery vary among institutions. In large hospitals with many operating rooms, a satellite pharmacy within the surgical suite may dispense drugs as needed for each procedure. Other, often smaller, facilities may maintain a medication room or cabinet where they store

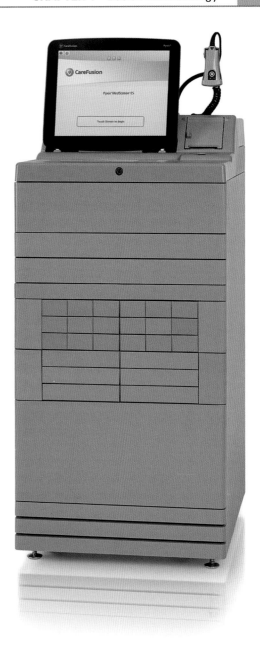

Fig. 1.7 A computer-automated drug dispensing system. (Reproduced with permission from CareFusion.)

frequently used drugs, such as antibiotics and local anesthetics. In addition, some hospitals use a system of mobile drug carts, which must be exchanged for restocking after the drugs are used. For example, emergency-response drug carts, known as *crash carts*, are used for cardiac arrest and other emergency situations (see Fig. 15.2). Such carts may be restocked on an exchange basis to ensure the immediate availability of all necessary drugs.

Computer-automated dispensing systems are frequently used for medication distribution in surgery (Fig. 1.7). These systems have been developed to minimize medication administration errors. A barcode-scanning system allows an approved user access to particular medications ordered for a particular patient.

TABLE 1.5	Abbreviations for Drug Forms or Preparations
Abbreviation	**Meaning**
cap	Capsule
gtts	Drops
soln	Solution
susp	Suspension
tab	Tablet
ung	Ointment

DRUG FORMS OR PREPARATIONS

Drugs are available in several different forms or preparations. Drugs may be in solid, semisolid, liquid, or gas form. The form of drug administered affects both the onset of drug actions and the intensity of the body's response to the drug. Liquids, for example, tend to act more quickly than solids, and gases or vapors tend to act even faster. Drug form also dictates route of administration. For example, the antibiotic Neosporin Original comes in ointment (semisolid) form, which must be applied topically only. Some drugs are available in more than one form. For example, 2% lidocaine (Xylocaine), a local anesthetic agent, is available in jelly for topical application and in solutions of various strengths for injection. The names of drug forms are often abbreviated in drug orders. Table 1.5 lists several common abbreviations for drug forms.

Solids

Many drugs come prepared in solid form. These drugs may be in capsule (cap) or tablet (tab) form and are administered orally. Capsules are gelatin cases containing a drug in powder or granule form; tablets are a compressed form of the drug, usually combined with inert ingredients. Capsules and tablets are rarely used in surgery because oral administration is required. In most cases surgical patients must be kept NPO (from the Latin *nil per os*, nothing by mouth), or they may be under a general anesthesia and unable to swallow.

Some drugs come in powder form and are contained in glass vials. Such powders must be mixed with a liquid (reconstituted) to form a solution that can be administered by injection (Fig. 1.8). For example, several antibiotics administered in surgery are powders that must be reconstituted with sterile water or a sodium chloride solution (saline, 0.9% NaCl) to make an injectable solution. Other drugs, such as dantrolene (Dantrium), an infrequently used yet important skeletal muscle relaxant, also come in powder form and must be reconstituted before use (see Chapter 15).

Semisolids

Semisolid preparations include creams, foams, gels, and ointments. Creams consist of active ingredients in a water base, whereas ointments contain active ingredients in an oil, lanolin, or petroleum base. Gels (such as K-Y Jelly) are thicker than creams but are still water based. Examples of semisolid drugs used in surgery include lidocaine (Xylocaine) jelly for topical anesthesia, Silvadene cream 1% for burns, estrogen cream for vaginal packing, and Neosporin Original ointment for wound dressing.

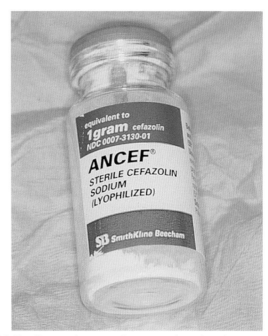

Fig. 1.8 Sterile powder must be reconstituted to form a solution that can be administered by injection. (From Misch CE: *Contemporary implant dentistry*, ed 3, St Louis, 2008, Elsevier.)

Liquids

Several types of liquid drug preparations are available. Many liquid medications are available in solution. A solution is a mixture of drug particles (called the solute) fully dissolved in a liquid medium (called the solvent, such as water or saline). Several common solutions are used from the sterile back table, including sodium chloride solution (saline, 0.9% NaCl) irrigation, antibiotic irrigation solutions, and heparin irrigation solution. Liquid nasal sprays, such as oxymetazoline (Afrin), may also be used from the sterile back table.

Drugs may also be in suspension. A suspension is a form in which solid, undissolved particles float (are suspended) in a liquid. Suspensions should be shaken before administration to evenly distribute particles throughout the liquid. Cortisporin otic, used in ear surgery, is an example of a medication in suspension form used from the sterile back table.

> **TECH TIP**
>
> Just before handing a medication in suspension to the surgeon, simply roll the syringe or vial between your fingers or palms to mix the suspended particles evenly.

Another type of liquid medication form is an emulsion, in which the medication is contained in a mixture of water and oil bound together with an emulsifier. An emulsifier is used to bind together two substances that do not normally mix. A household example of an emulsion is mayonnaise, in which lecithin (contained in egg yolks) binds egg yolks and oil together and keeps the substances from separating. Medication emulsions are usually either water in oil or oil in water, depending on the medication's solubility. The most common emulsion used in surgery is propofol (Diprivan), an intravenous sedative-hypnotic agent used for induction of general anesthesia (see Chapter 14). Lecithin is also the emulsifier in propofol, so it is contraindicated in patients with an allergy to eggs.

Drugs in liquid form may also be administered orally, as *elixirs* (sweetened solutions of alcohol) or *syrups* (sweetened aqueous solutions); however, elixirs and syrups are rarely, if ever, used in surgery because of the NPO status for surgical patients.

Gases

The only common medication available in gas form is nitrous oxide, an inhalation anesthetic agent. Other inhalation anesthetic agents, such as desflurane (Suprane) (see Chapter 14), are known as volatile liquids. Volatile liquid agents are vaporized through an apparatus on the anesthesia machine into gas form for administration.

DRUG ADMINISTRATION ROUTES

Medications are formulated for administration by a specific route. In addition to the drug form, the route by which a drug is given can affect onset time and body response. Drugs may be administered by several different routes, only a few of which are used commonly in surgery. There are two categories of medication administration routes: enteral and parenteral. The enteral route indicates that the medication is taken into the gastrointestinal (GI) tract, primarily by mouth (orally). The term *parenteral* indicates any route other than the digestive tract, the most common of which are topical, subcutaneous, intramuscular, and intravenous.

? MAKE IT SIMPLE

Use medical terminology word-building techniques to help you understand the terms *enteral* and *parenteral*. The root word or combining form "enter/o-" means intestines, and the adjective ending "-al" means pertaining to. The combining form "/o" is not used when the suffix begins with a vowel, so the word *enteral* means pertaining to the intestines or intestinal tract. The prefix "para-" indicates beside or beyond (the "a" is dropped when the root word begins with a vowel), so the term *parenteral* means outside, or *not within*, the intestinal tract.

The oral route (PO, from the Latin *per os*, "by mouth") is the simplest and most common way to administer many drugs. Tablets or capsules are swallowed and readily absorbed through the lining (mucosa) of the GI tract. Certain drugs may irritate the GI mucosa and should therefore be given with food. Other drugs may be inactivated by increased amounts of digestive enzymes and so are best taken between meals. When drugs are administered orally, onset of action is usually slower and duration of effect is usually longer than with other routes. However, some drugs are completely inactivated by the digestive process and therefore must not be given orally. Insulin, a hormone, and heparin, an anticoagulant, are not effective when administered orally.

The oral route is rarely used in surgery because the patient must be kept NPO before surgery and because many patients are under general anesthesia during surgery and so are unable to swallow. Standard medication orders, such as prescriptions and hospital orders, state the route of administration, usually in abbreviated form (Table 1.6, Fig. 1.9).

TABLE 1.6 Abbreviations for Drug Administration Routes

Abbreviation	Meaning
buc	Buccal
ID	Intradermal
IM	Intramuscular
IV	Intravenous
PO, po	Orally (per os)
pr	Per rectum
pv	Per vagina
subcut, SubQ	Subcutaneous
sl	Sublingual
top	Topical

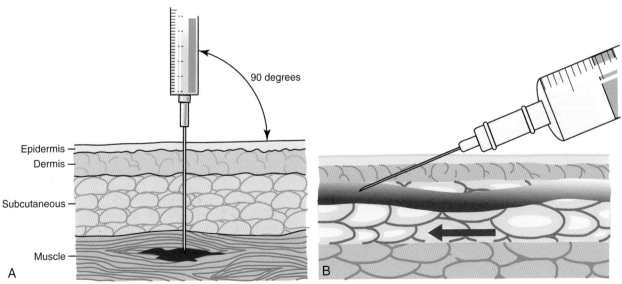

Fig. 1.9 (A) Intramuscular injection (IM). (B) Intravenous injection (IV). (From Workman ML: *Understanding pharmacology*, St Louis, 2011, Elsevier.)

The vast majority of medications used in surgery are administered parenterally. The most common parenteral routes are topical, subcutaneous, intramuscular, and intravenous. Some medications are available in topical preparations, which are intended for application to the skin or a mucous membrane–lined cavity. Some topical agents work at the site of application; this is called a *local effect*. Some topical medications exert a systemic effect, that is, throughout the entire body. Examples of topical medications with local effect include steroid creams for rashes and antibiotic ointment for cuts. Applied to the affected area, these agents work directly on the immediate site. Topical medications delivered through transdermal patches, such as those for hormone replacement therapy (estradiol), nicotine cessation (Nicoderm), and motion sickness (scopolamine), exert a systemic effect. Even though these types of agents are applied to an area of the skin, once absorbed, the agents will have an effect on the entire body. Blood supply to the topical administration area affects the speed of absorption. Topical medications are absorbed slowly through the skin but are absorbed rapidly when applied to blood supply-rich mucous membranes.

> **NOTE:** Some medications, though taken orally, are actually topical in that the tablet (pill) is held in the mouth, either in the cheek (buccal) or under the tongue (sublingual) and allowed to dissolve. The medication is absorbed through the mucous membrane of the mouth and does not pass directly into the GI tract.

Several topical medications are used in surgery. Antibiotic ointments, such as Neosporin Original, may be used on the surgical incision as part of the postoperative wound dressing. Topical hemostatic agents (see Chapter 9) are used almost exclusively in surgery. Agents, such as Avitene, may be applied to bleeding surfaces of the liver or spleen during trauma surgery to enhance coagulation.

Topical antibiotic irrigation is common in surgery, in which case an antibiotic solution is poured or squirted into the surgical site (Fig. 1.10). In many vascular procedures, a solution of heparin (an anticoagulant; see Chapter 9) is used as a topical irrigation to help prevent the formation of blood clots in operative vessels during surgery.

> **NOTE:** Vascular procedures may also involve using intravenous heparin for systemic effect. But when used as a topical irrigation, heparin exerts a more significant local effect because the operative vessel is usually clamped off, preventing systemic absorption of the agent.

Instillation of a medication into a mucous membrane–lined cavity, such as the eye, nose, or urethra, may also be considered a topical route or application. A number of medications are instilled into body cavities intraoperatively in situations unique to surgery. For example, tetracaine drops may be instilled into the eye for local anesthesia for cataract extraction (see Chapter 10), oxymetazoline (Afrin) may be instilled into the nasal cavity for vasoconstriction during sinusoscopy, or lidocaine (Xylocaine) jelly may be instilled into the urethra as topical anesthesia for cystoscopy. During diagnostic gynecologic

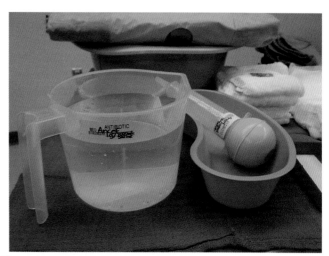

Fig. 1.10 Antibiotic irrigation used during surgery is an example of a topical application of a medication.

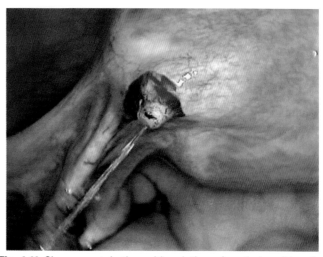

Fig. 1.11 Chromopertubation with solution of methylene blue dye indicates the patency of the proximal tubal portion. Note that in this photo, the uterine tube has been excised and the methylene blue solution is exiting the remaining tubal stump. (From Falcone T: *Clinical reproductive medicine and surgery*, St Louis, 2007, Elsevier.)

laparoscopy, a methylene blue solution may be instilled via a cervical cannula into the uterus. This procedure is known as a tubal dye study or chromotubation and is used to assess tubal patency in patients with infertility. Methylene blue solution fills the uterus and exits through the uterine tubes into the pelvic cavity when the tubes are patent (open) (Fig. 1.11). The laparoscope is used to observe the blue solution exiting the tubal fimbria. If the tubes are blocked by scarring, the solution cannot enter the pelvic cavity. Another example of medication instillation occurs during operative cholangiography. Although not as frequently performed currently because of the availability of endoscopic retrograde cholangiopancreatography, intraoperative cholangiography involves the instillation of radiopaque contrast media (ROCM) into the common bile duct to detect gallstones under X-ray. If present, common bile duct stones will be evident on radiograph as shadows in the ROCM. For additional information on diagnostic agents, see Chapter 6.

Inhalation is a means of medication administration that can be considered topical. Some asthmatic drugs are administered through a respiratory inhaler or through a nebulizer—a device that converts liquid drugs into an inhalable mist. The drug is absorbed in the bronchi of the lungs, providing local relief of bronchoconstriction. In surgery, anesthetic gases are administered via inhalation, but these drugs exert systemic rather than local effects.

Subcutaneous injections are given beneath the skin into the subcutaneous tissue layer. Common sites for subcutaneous injections are the upper lateral aspect of the arm, the anterior thigh, and the abdomen. Depending on blood supply, absorption from subcutaneous tissue is fairly rapid. Only a few drugs are administered subcutaneously in surgery; for example, heparin may be injected subcutaneously, preoperatively, in cardiothoracic surgery to help prevent pulmonary embolism when working near the great vessels.

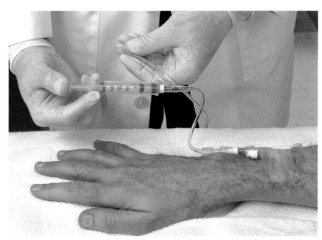

Fig. 1.12 A drug may be administered by intravenous injection. (From Lilley LL: *Pharmacology for Canadian health care practice*, ed 2, St Louis, 2011, Elsevier.)

> **! CAUTION**
>
> The Institute for Safe Medication Practices (ISMP) has identified that the abbreviations for subcutaneous administration, including "SC," "SQ," and "sub q" are frequently mistaken for other meanings. The ISMP recommends using "subcut" or "subcutaneously" to indicate this intended route of administration.

A few drugs used in surgery are administered intramuscularly (IM). Intramuscular injections are usually given into a large muscle mass, such as the deltoid, gluteal, or vastus lateralis. Intramuscular absorption is usually rapid because of the large absorbing surface and good blood supply. An example of a drug given IM in surgery is ketorolac, a nonsteroidal antiinflammatory drug used for postoperative pain relief.

Probably the most common example of the parenteral route used at the surgical site is the administration (injection) of a local anesthetic agent for intraoperative pain control. Local anesthesia during a surgical procedure may be accomplished with an agent such as lidocaine (Xylocaine), which is injected into multiple tissue layers as needed. Frequently, a longer-acting local anesthetic (such as bupivacaine) is used to inject the surgical site for postoperative pain control. For a more detailed discussion of local anesthetics, see Chapter 13.

Most medications administered parenterally during surgery are given IV, that is, within a vein, as shown in Fig. 1.12. A small catheter is inserted into a vein and connected to tubing called an *infusion set*. The infusion set is attached to a bag of intravenous fluid for administration. Drugs may then be injected, as needed, into port sites located along the tubing. Drugs may be given all at once, as a bolus, or by slow infusion. Absorption is immediate for medications administered IV because the agent goes directly into the bloodstream.

Other parenteral routes are used less frequently. *Intradermal* injections are given between layers of skin, as seen in tuberculin skin testing and allergy testing. A local anesthetic may be injected intradermally before placing an intravenous catheter, thereby reducing discomfort at the insertion site. *Intraarticular* injections (into the joint space) of antiinflammatory agents or local anesthetics may be given after arthroscopy. *Intrathecal* injection of an anesthetic agent is administered into the spinal subarachnoid space to diffuse into cerebral spinal fluid. During cardiac arrest resuscitation, a drug such as epinephrine may be injected directly into the heart; this is called an *intracardiac* injection.

PHARMACOKINETICS

The study of pharmacokinetics focuses on how the body processes drugs, and the science of pharmacodynamics examines how the action of the drug affects the body (Fig. 1.13). The science of pharmacokinetics studies a medication from administration through four basic physiological processes: absorption, distribution, biotransformation, and excretion (Table 1.7). The patient's general health has a significant effect on how the body processes drugs. For example, if the patient's blood supply, liver function, or kidney function is compromised, the ability to process medications is also compromised.

Absorption

To be effective, a drug must first be absorbed into the body. Absorption is the process by which a drug is taken into the body and moves from the site of administration into the blood. Drugs are absorbed from the site of administration into the bloodstream and enter systemic circulation. Speed of absorption, or absorption rate, varies by administration route and by blood supply to the area. Solubility of the drug (its ability to be dissolved) also affects the absorption rate. If a drug is in solid form, it must dissolve before it can be absorbed. Drugs in suspensions absorb faster than solid drugs, and solutions absorb faster than suspensions. For example, a solution instilled in the conjunctiva will absorb more quickly than an ointment applied to the conjunctiva.

Oral absorption varies depending on the drug's chemical structure and the pH (acidity) and motility of the GI tract. If the digestive tract is highly motile, as in patients with diarrhea, ingested drugs may not be adequately absorbed. Conversely, if the patient is constipated, drugs may be fully absorbed, sometimes to toxic levels. Intramuscular absorption is rapid if water-based drug solutions are injected and is slower if the solution is an oil-based

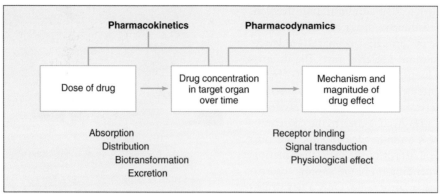

Fig. 1.13 Relationship between pharmacokinetics and pharmacodynamics. (From Brenner GM, Stevens CW: *Pharmacology*, ed 4, St Louis, 2012, Elsevier.)

TABLE 1.7 Four Processes of Pharmacokinetics

Process	Primary Body System
Absorption	Body system varies by administration route (e.g., integumentary, GI, respiratory)
Distribution	Circulatory system
Biotransformation	Biliary system (liver)
Excretion	Urinary system (kidney)

emulsion. The amount and vascularization of muscle mass also affect the rate of absorption of medications given IM. Intravenous absorption is immediate because drugs are injected directly into the bloodstream. The absorption rate of drugs given subcutaneously depends on blood supply to the area of injection.

NOTE: Rapid drug absorption can be undesirable in surgery when local anesthetics are used. The anesthetic agent must stay in the desired area to exert its desired effect. Thus, a vasoconstrictor, usually epinephrine, may be added to the anesthetic agent to narrow the small blood vessels in the local area and delay absorption of the anesthetic agent into systemic circulation. Local vasoconstriction will prolong the anesthetic agent's effect (see Chapter 13).

Absorption of drugs given by inhalation, especially inhalation anesthetics, is rapid because of the huge numbers of capillaries in the alveoli of the lungs. Some drugs administered by inhalation (such as steroids for asthma) are specifically formulated for local effect and so do not absorb rapidly. Mucosal tissues provide excellent absorption for some drugs because of the number of capillaries just under the mucosal surface. Common mucosal administration sites include the respiratory tract, oral cavity, and the conjunctiva.

Although most drugs are not absorbed easily through skin, some are specifically formulated to overcome the skin barrier. Such drugs are administered transdermally from patches. For example, scopolamine patches are used to treat motion sickness; they release the drug slowly so it may be absorbed through skin over a period of hours.

Thus, absorption of a medication depends on the formulation of the drug, the route of administration, and the extent of blood supply to the site of administration.

Distribution

Once a drug has been absorbed into the bloodstream, the process called *distribution* begins. The circulatory system transports the drug throughout the body and drug molecules eventually diffuse out of the bloodstream to the site of action. The term bioavailability indicates the degree to which the drug molecule reaches the site of action to exert its effects. Several factors affect a drug's bioavailability, including the acid-base balance (Insight 1.3). Because drug molecules are carried to all parts of the body, their effects can be seen in locations other than the intended area. The amount of drug reaching the site of action depends on the general condition of the patient's circulatory system, on the effective blood flow to the intended area (tissue perfusion), and on the extent of plasma protein binding. Areas with high blood flow include the heart, liver, and kidneys, and tissues with low blood flow include bone, fat, and skin. For example, because bone has very limited blood flow, intravenous antibiotics often have little effect in treating bone infections. In addition, two barriers exist that limit the distribution of certain drug molecules to particular sites. The placental barrier allows some molecules to pass to the fetus, while restricting others. The blood-brain barrier also limits passage of certain molecules into brain tissue.

INSIGHT 1.3 Bioavailability and Acid-Base Balance

A number of factors affect the bioavailability of a drug, including the size of the drug molecule (smaller molecules pass more easily through plasma membranes), lipid solubility (lipophilic molecules pass easier than hydrophilic molecules), and ionization of the drug molecule. Nonionized molecules pass through plasma membranes easier than ionized molecules. Acid-base balance also plays a role in drug bioavailability. An example of this concept in surgery occurs when a local anesthetic (a weak base) is injected into an infected wound (an acidic environment). The local anesthetic agent becomes ionized (a basic pH in an acidic condition) and cannot easily enter the lipid membrane of nerves to reach the site of action. If the agent does not readily enter the membrane, its intended effect may be delayed or reduced.

PLASMA PROTEIN BINDING

Not all drug molecules in the bloodstream are available to bind at the site of action. Some drug molecules bind to proteins (albumins and globulins) contained in plasma—the liquid portion of blood—through a process known as plasma protein binding. Both the amount of plasma protein in the blood and the binding characteristics of the drug determine the extent to which a drug is bound. Some drugs are highly bound (up to 99%), some are only minimally bound, and others are not bound at all. Highly bound drug molecules have a longer duration of action because they stay in the body longer and a lower distribution to the site of action. The only drug molecules available to exert effects on the body are unbound molecules. Unbound drug molecules are considered *bioactive*.

Plasma protein binding is usually nonspecific; that is, plasma proteins can bind with many different drug molecules. It is also competitive in that drug molecules compete with other drug molecules for protein-binding sites, significantly changing the amount of available drug. Potential hazards arise if patients are taking different drugs that compete for the same binding sites. For instance, if a patient taking warfarin sodium, a highly bound anticoagulant, takes aspirin, the aspirin will bind with the same plasma protein sites, making more warfarin available than is needed (Fig. 1.14). If more than the expected amount of warfarin is available, overmedication and excessive anticoagulation may occur. Highly bound drugs used in surgery include propofol (Diprivan), fentanyl, and diazepam.

Plasma protein binding is reversible. When the concentration of unbound drug in blood is lowered, either by metabolism or by excretion, bound molecules are released from binding sites. The extent of plasma protein binding can prolong a drug's effects and contribute to drug-drug interactions.

Biotransformation

The circulatory system also distributes drugs to the liver, the major structure of the biliary system. In the liver, the chemical composition of a drug is changed by a process called *metabolism* or *biotransformation*. The goal of biotransformation is to change lipid-soluble drug molecules into water-soluble molecules that can be more easily excreted. The liver is the primary site for biotransformation, but for some drug molecules, this process may take place in other locations, such as plasma, lungs, GI tract, or kidneys. Biliary biotransformation takes place when liver cells (hepatocytes) containing enzymes break down some drug molecules into other molecules called *metabolites*. The effectiveness of liver enzymes depends on several factors, including patient age, concurrent drug therapy, organ disease (e.g., cirrhosis), and nutritional status. Only unbound (bioactive) drug molecules can be biotransformed. Some drugs are completely broken down and some are not broken down at all, but most drugs are at least partially biotransformed.

Some drugs are actually *prodrugs;* this means they are administered in an inactive form, which is biotransformed into an active drug to produce the needed effect. Examples of prodrugs include the antiglaucoma agent dipivefrin (Propine, see Chapter 10) and the proton-pump inhibitor (see Chapter 12) omeprazole (Prilosec). Dipivefrin is also an example of a drug that is not broken down by the liver, but at the site of administration (the eye). Dipivefrin is a prodrug that is biotransformed into epinephrine in the eye by enzyme hydrolysis. Hydrolysis is the addition of water to break chemical bonds of a larger molecule to form two smaller molecules (in this case into epinephrine and pivalic acid).

All drugs taken *orally* enter the liver through the hepatic portal circulation (Fig. 1.15) before entering systemic circulation.

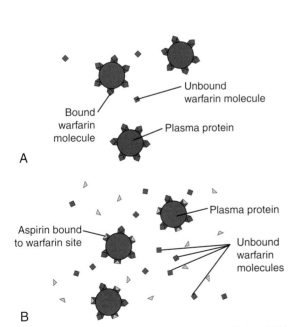

Fig. 1.14 Plasma protein binding of aspirin and warfarin. (A) Warfarin binds to specific receptor sites on plasma proteins. (B) Aspirin binds to the same receptor sites, making more warfarin available.

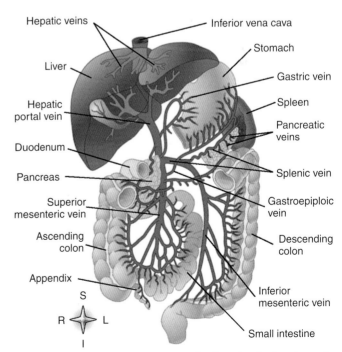

Fig. 1.15 Drugs administered orally are distributed to the liver for metabolism by the hepatic portal circulation. (From Huether SE, McCance KL: *Understanding pathophysiology*, ed 5, St Louis, 2011, Elsevier.)

The hepatic portal circulatory system is the venous drainage of the upper GI tract, carrying molecules absorbed by the gut into veins leading to the liver. Many drugs undergo a first-pass effect, which means they may be altered or nearly inactivated when passing through the liver, potentially reducing the drug's effectiveness. Once liver enzymes begin to transform drug molecules though, the enzymes are less able to break down additional amounts of the drug; thus repeated dosing may be used to overcome the first-pass effect. Drugs administered parenterally or sublingually are not subject to the first-pass effect.

Excretion

Medications taken into the body are eliminated in the process called *excretion*. Some drug molecules are eliminated in the bile, feces, or skin, but most unchanged drugs and metabolites are excreted by the kidneys and eliminated in urine (Fig. 1.16). Notable exceptions to urinary excretion are volatile anesthetic agents, which are excreted by the lungs. The circulatory system carries blood to the kidneys, where it is filtered and returned to general circulation. Two renal processes remove drug molecules and metabolites from the body: glomerular filtration and tubular secretion. Only drug molecules *not* bound to plasma proteins (i.e., *bioactive* molecules) will be filtered out of blood plasma reaching the glomerulus. How much unbound drug is filtered out depends on the glomerular filtration rate, which depends on blood pressure and blood flow to the kidneys. Tubular secretion uses cellular energy to force drugs and their metabolites from the bloodstream for elimination. Some drugs, depending on their characteristics and the pH of urine, may be reabsorbed and returned to circulation by tubular reabsorption. Factors influencing renal elimination of drug molecules include presence of kidney disease, such as renal failure, the pH of urine, and the concentration of drug molecules in the plasma.

PHARMACODYNAMICS

As stated previously, pharmacodynamics is the study of how drugs exert their effects on the body, at both the molecular and physiological levels. The human body responds to different drugs in varying degrees and at various rates. Drugs may also have more than one effect on the body and this is taken into consideration when prescribing medications.

❓ MAKE IT SIMPLE

Pharmacokinetics is the study of what the body does to drugs (how the body processes drugs).

Pharmacodynamics is the study of what drugs do to the body (how drugs affect the body).

Drugs must be able to reach the site of action and interact with cells to produce therapeutic effects. In most cases, drugs bind to specialized proteins, or receptors, on cell membranes. Some drugs are specific in action and some are nonspecific. Interaction with the target site produces the intended effect, whereas interaction with other cells may produce what are called side effects.

Drug molecules with specific mechanisms interact with specific receptors' sites on cell membranes. This specificity has been described by the lock-and-key analogy: the lock is the receptor site on the cell membrane (usually a protein complex), and the drug molecule is the key that fits in that specific lock. Very few

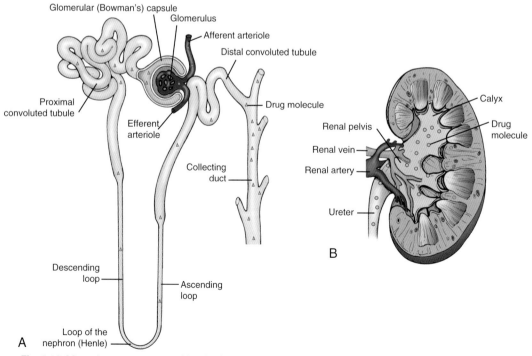

Fig. 1.16 Most drugs are excreted by the kidneys. Drugs are removed in the nephrons (A) and eliminated by the kidneys (B).

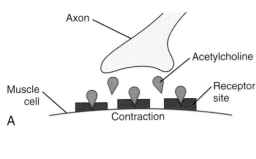

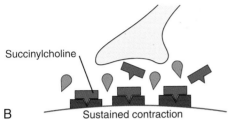

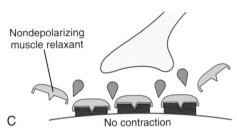

Fig. 1.17 Receptor site agonist and antagonist action. (A) Acetylcholine is a natural agonist. (B) Succinylcholine is a chemical agonist. (C) Nondepolarizing muscle relaxants act as antagonists.

drugs are exactly specific to a certain receptor; instead, most drug molecules will react with several types of receptors.

Agonists are drugs that bind to or have an affinity for (attraction to) a receptor and cause a particular response (Fig. 1.17). This can be compared with the analogy of a key opening a lock. Natural agonists include neurotransmitters, such as acetylcholine, and hormones. Some drugs, such as succinylcholine, act as chemical agonists. Drugs that bind to a receptor and prevent a response are called *antagonists* (see Fig. 1.17). Antagonists are also called *receptor blockers*. Following the lock-and-key analogy, an antagonist can be thought of as a key that fits the lock but cannot open it (cause a response). Antagonists may be competitive, that is, bind to sites and prevent the agonist from reaching the site, or noncompetitive, in that the antagonist alters the target site, preventing the agonist from causing the intended effect.

Drug antagonism is responsible for many drug interactions, some of which are not desired. Many patients receive multiple drug therapies so potential exists for several drug-drug interactions. Multiple drugs may cancel each other out or reduce each other's effects. Vitamin K is given as an antidote for warfarin if the patient has been overanticoagulated because additional amounts of vitamin K in the body can overcome the effect of warfarin. An example of a drug that reduces the effect of another drug is the antibiotic amoxicillin. When it is given to a patient taking oral contraceptives, the effectiveness of the contraceptive may be reduced.

A drug that enhances the effect of another drug is called a *synergist*. Some drug-drug interactions may cause a dramatic increase in the intended effect of the primary drug, as seen in aspirin-warfarin interactions.

In addition to interacting with another drug, some drugs may also interact with vitamins, minerals, and/or herbal supplements. For example, the effect of tetracycline is compromised when it is taken with dairy products containing calcium. However, it is important to keep in mind that most drugs do not interact with foods or other drugs.

Not all drug actions are receptor-type interactions. For example, antibiotics may interfere quite specifically with certain aspects of bacterial cell metabolism, such as penicillin inhibiting the formation of bacterial cell wall (see Chapter 5). Some drugs interact specifically with certain enzymes rather than receptor sites on a cell. A drug molecule may bind with a particular enzyme and either inhibit or stimulate the enzyme's activity to produce the desired effect.

An example of a nonspecific (i.e., not a drug-receptor complex) interaction is a drug molecule's ability to change the chemical environment surrounding the target cell. For example, mannitol—an osmotic diuretic—increases the osmotic pressure of urine; this means it reduces the reabsorption of water and produces large amounts of dilute urine. Antacids, such as sodium bicarbonate, chemically neutralize acid in the stomach.

Several terms are used to clarify aspects of pharmacodynamics, and the surgical technologist should become familiar with the common terms as applied to the surgical patient. The reason or purpose for giving a medication is called the *indication*, whereas reasons against giving a particular drug are called *contraindications*. For example, a particular antibiotic may be indicated for a bacterial infection, but is contraindicated when the patient has a known hypersensitivity to that antibiotic.

Some important terms should be understood regarding the timing of expected drug effects. The time between administration of a drug and the first appearance of effects is called the *onset*. A drug's onset can be affected by the administration route, absorption rate, and efficiency of distribution to the site of action. The time between administration and maximum effect is called the *time to peak effect*. Steady state, or equilibrium, is achieved when the amount of drug entering the body is equal to the amount of drug being eliminated. The time between onset and disappearance of drug effects is called the *duration*. A drug's duration of action, or drug half-life, refers to the length of time the drug concentration is in the therapeutic range. Some drugs have a very short duration of action, such as propofol (6–8 minutes), whereas other drugs have a long duration of action, such as warfarin (a single dose is active for 2–5 days).

A number of terms are used to describe the body's response or reaction to medications. A side effect is a predictable, but unintended, effect of a drug. Side effects are rarely serious but usually unavoidable. An example of a side effect is the drowsiness that often occurs when antihistamines are used.

Adverse effects are undesired, potentially harmful side effects of drugs. Adverse effects include nausea and vomiting, drug toxicity, hypersensitivity, and idiosyncratic (unusual) reactions. Drug toxicity may be the result of accidental overdosing or failure of the body to process the drug properly, as seen in patients with kidney or liver dysfunction. In cases of drug toxicity, the primary effect of the drug may be exaggerated, such as excessive anticoagulation when taking warfarin. Some drugs may be particularly toxic (usually in high doses) to a specific organ, such as the liver, kidney, or even the ear. For example, some antibiotics are known to be ototoxic in high doses; that is, they have the potential to damage the hearing mechanism (see Chapter 5). Acetaminophen can cause hepatotoxicity, and ibuprofen can cause nephrotoxicity.

> ### ? MAKE IT SIMPLE
>
> Use medical terminology word-building techniques to help you learn the meaning of terms used in pharmacodynamics. The suffix "-toxic" means poisonous or damaging; the root word for the liver is "hepat/o"; a root word for kidney is "nephr/o"; and a root word for ear is "oto." Thus, hepatotoxic means damaging to the liver, nephrotoxic means damaging to the kidney, and ototoxic means damaging to the (inner) ear. In addition, the root word "idi/o" means "unknown," indicating that the cause of idiosyncratic drug reactions (IDRs) is not known at this time.

Drug hypersensitivity is an adverse effect resulting from previous exposure to the drug or a similar drug. A patient may become sensitized to a drug after one or more doses, then exhibit an allergic response on subsequent administration of the drug. An allergic response may be immediate, with symptoms ranging from mild to severe. Mild allergy symptoms include the appearance of raised patches on the skin (wheals) with itching, commonly known as hives (Fig. 1.18). A severe allergic reaction, called *anaphylaxis*, can result in swollen bronchial passages and possible circulatory collapse (see Chapter 15). Delayed allergic reactions can occur days or weeks after a drug is taken and can include fever and joint swelling.

When the exact mechanism of an adverse drug effect is not known, the term *idiosyncratic drug reaction* (IDR) is used. IDRs are rare and unpredictable adverse effects of some drugs on individuals. Some IDRs are thought to be related to a type of allergic response, but many of these reactions are unique to specific patients and particular drugs. One type of IDR that may occur in surgery is malignant hyperthermia (see Chapter 15), which is a life-threatening response to certain drugs attributable to a genetic defect. The emerging science of pharmacogenetics (see Chapter 2) may someday help identify and prevent some idiosyncratic drug effects.

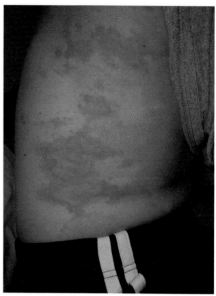

Fig. 1.18 Urticaria (hives). (From Amar SM, Dreskin SC: Urticaria, *Primary Care* 35(1):141–157, 2008.)

In the fascinating science of pharmacodynamics, some specific mechanisms of drug actions are known, but much remains to be discovered regarding many physiological interactions involved in drug therapy.

> ### KEY CONCEPTS
>
> - Knowledge of basic principles of pharmacology can provide the surgical technologist with a solid foundation on which to build an understanding of the many drugs used in surgery.
> - Drugs can be sourced from natural sources, such as plants, animals, and minerals, or be developed in chemistry and molecular biology laboratories.
> - Drug classifications are often helpful in identifying the purpose or use of a drug.
> - Medication orders may be in various forms in surgery and must be interpreted precisely.
> - Drugs come in several forms or preparations, and surgical technologists must be able to recognize the form needed for the intended purpose.
> - Pharmacokinetics is the study of the four basic steps the body uses to process drugs: absorption, distribution, metabolism, and excretion.
> - The study of how drugs exert their effects is called *pharmacodynamics*. Most drugs interact with receptors on target cell membranes to produce the desired effect.
> - Many important terms are used to describe aspects of pharmacodynamics.

▌ LEARNING THE LANGUAGE (KEY TERMS)

Using your textbook or a standard medical dictionary, look up and write the definitions of each term.

absorption	emulsion	plasma protein binding
adverse effect	enteral	reconstituted
agonist	excretion	side effect
antagonist	hypersensitivity	solubility
bioavailability	idiosyncratic drug reaction	solution
biotechnology	indication	suspension
biotransformation	local effect	synergist
bolus	onset	systemic effect
contraindication	parenteral	topical
distribution	pharmacodynamics	
duration	pharmacokinetics	

REVIEW QUESTIONS

1. What are the sources of drugs used today? State examples.
2. Why is understanding the drug classification helpful to the surgical technologist?
3. What types of medication orders are used in surgery?
4. If you are assigned to a clinical facility, what type of drug distribution system is used there?
5. Which types of drug forms do you have in your home medicine cabinet?
6. What is the most common medication administration route used in surgery?
7. Describe each of the four processes of pharmacokinetics.
8. How is a side effect different from an adverse effect?

CRITICAL THINKING

Scenario 1

Mr. Dhang is a 75-year-old man taking warfarin for recurrent deep vein thrombosis. He recently began experiencing frequent, almost daily, headaches, but has not consulted his physician. He has started taking aspirin to treat his headaches.

1. Why is taking aspirin, while also taking warfarin, a problem?
2. How does the presence of aspirin alter the effect of warfarin?
3. What adverse effects might you expect to see?

Scenario 2

Dr. Smith has a standing order for 1 g of Ancef mixed with 1000 mL of saline on the back table for total knee procedures. His patient, Mrs. Brown, has an allergy to penicillin and is scheduled for surgery tomorrow.

1. Where would the surgical technologist find this standing order?
2. Are any changes needed to the standing order? If so, why?

BIBLIOGRAPHY

Bardal S, Waechter J, Martin D: *Applied pharmacology*, St Louis, 2011, Saunders/Elsevier.

Fulcher E, Fulcher R, Soto C: *Pharmacology principles and applications*, ed 3, St Louis, 2012, Saunders/Elsevier.

Indiana University, Bloomington, Information About Drugs: Adapted from Engs, R.C. Alcohol and Other Drugs: Self-Responsibility, Bloomington, IN, 1987, Tichenor Publishing Company. © Copyright Ruth C. Engs, Bloomington, IN, 1996: www.indiana.edu/~engs/rbook/drug.html.

Institute for Safe Medication Practices, ISMP's list of error-prone abbreviations, symbols, and dose designations: https://www.drugs.com/article/prescription-abbreviations.html#table1.

Taylor L., Plant based drugs and medicines, Raintree Nutrition, Inc.: www.rain-tree.com/plantdrugs.htm#.VcBy77Upqf5.

The Joint Commission, Do not use list fact sheet: www.jointcommission.org/resources/news-and-multimedia/fact-sheets/facts-about-do-not-use-list/.

The Joint Commission, Surgical Care Improvement Project.

U.S. Food and Drug Administration: www.fda.gov

INTERNET RESOURCES

Drugs.com, Professionals, Cortisporin otic suspension prescribing information: www.drugs.com/pro/cortisporin-otic-suspension.html.

Advanced Practices for the Surgical First Assistant
Chapter 1—Basic Pharmacology

KEY TERMS

drug dependence
H&P (history and physical)
potentiation

tachyphylaxis
therapeutic range
tolerance

MEDICATION ORDERS

As a physician extender, one of the surgical first assistant's duties may be to write out the physician's prescriptions and medication orders. Then the physician will clarify, verify, and sign them. It is imperative for the surgical first assistant to have a working knowledge of commonly accepted and approved medical abbreviations and the basic components of a medication order. (See abbreviations in this chapter, and refer to Chapter 2 for a listing of "do not use" abbreviations.) Other listings are also published, such as those under the ISMP. The surgical first assistant should never act outside the scope of practice in medication prescriptions or administration.

For some orders, usually those found in the clinical setting, the *time* the order was written must also be included, as well as any special notations. Notice the first six components of a medication order are essentially the six rights of medication administration. (See the "six rights" and additional information in Chapter 4.) These are closely checked and verified every time a medication is prepared and administered to assure patient safety. It is very important to include all components of the prescription or medication order; if any are omitted, the order is considered invalid and is not a legal order.

Safeguarding prescription pads is an important priority. Not only is this a safe practice, but also a legal consideration. Prescription pads may be a carbon-copy type, which will have a copy for the patient's record, or carbonless. In this case, a copy of the prescription can be made for the chart. If a multiple-line prescription pad is used, the surgical first assistant or physician can obliterate the unused lines to prevent any alteration of the original prescription. Prescription pads should never be used as notepads but only for writing prescriptions. Other orders, such as for laboratory tests, should be on a laboratory request form.

> **! CAUTION**
> All prescription pads must be secured in a safe location, no matter whether they are in the clinical or office setting. The physician should never sign prescription blanks in advance.

The surgical first assistant may be involved in routine preoperative, immediate postoperative, and dismissal orders and/or prescriptions. For example, preoperative orders may include shaving the operative site and verifying the patient has had prophylactic antibiotics. Immediate postoperative orders address monitoring vital signs, intravenous fluids, antibiotics, pain medications, and wound management, such as bleeding, drains, and tubes. Dismissal orders may include pain medications, antibiotics, follow-up appointments, and wound care at home.

> **ASSISTANT ADVICE**
> It is good practice to review the patient's **history and physical (H&P)** pre-operatively. Care must be taken to verify the patient's history to include any OTC or herbal medications. Many patients do not consider these medications as part of their medical history, yet they can cause serious complications and interactions with other drugs.

> **ASSISTANT ADVICE**
> Traditionally, there have been four clinically accepted vital signs: temperature, pulse, respirations, and blood pressure. Pain has been added to this group as a fifth vital sign to more accurately and efficiently assess the patient's needs.

> **! CAUTION**
> The international system of units (SI) abbreviations is used in this text. Note that milligrams are abbreviated as mg and milliliters as mL. These appear to be similar but are NOT interchangeable. Milligram (mg) is a unit of weight, whereas milliliter (mL) is a unit of volume. Confusing the two can have serious consequences in dosage calculations.

Medication Effects on the Patient

There are several factors that affect drug activity in the body. These include drug administration, disintegration, pharmacokinetics, pharmacodynamics, and individual differences among patients. Drug administration involves the route, the achievement of therapeutic range (also called *levels* or *index*) in the bloodstream, and medication errors. The therapeutic range of a drug is its plasma concentration between the minimum effective level for obtaining the desired result and the minimum level of its toxicity. If a drug's therapeutic range is narrow, its level in the blood should be closely monitored. For drugs that are not considered highly toxic, monitoring may not be required. Disintegration is how readily the drug is broken down or dissolved. Pharmacokinetics, as described in this chapter, refers to the way drugs are moved through the body, and pharmacodynamics is how a drug works or its mechanism of action. This involves the drug-receptor cell interaction. Finally, there are physiological and psychological differences to consider. These include age, sex, genetics, diet and nutrition, disease, and other medications the patient may be taking.

When two or more medications are administered to a patient, the drugs will have no effect on each other, increase each other's effect, or decrease each other's effect. Some medications are affected by food because food in the stomach can decrease absorption of drugs. Herbal preparations can also interact with medications, even though they are OTC. As discussed in this chapter, drugs may be agonists, synergists, or antagonists. Other terms that apply to these principles are potentiation, competitive antagonist, noncompetitive antagonist, and partial agonist. Potentiation occurs when two drugs are taken together and their effect is greater than the effect of either drug given alone. A competitive antagonist is an agent with an affinity for the same receptor site as the agonist; this competition inhibits the action of the agonist. A noncompetitive antagonist is an agent that combines with different parts of the receptor mechanism and inactivates the receptor so that the agonist cannot be effective, regardless of its concentration in the patient's system. A partial agonist is an agent that has an affinity, but may antagonize the action of other drugs that have greater ability to produce a specific result, regardless of dosage.

Remember that everyone reacts differently to the same medication, and some patients may have inadvertent responses.

Medication tolerance is a phenomenon in which the body has decreased responsiveness to a medication through repeated exposure to the agent. Many medications can produce tolerance, but it is most commonly seen in opiates and various other central nervous system depressants. being used, but also to a medication with similar pharmacological properties (particularly those that act on the same receptor sites). Tolerance levels will vary from person to person; to maintain therapeutic levels, the physician will order blood tests and may have to increase the dosage. Reversal of a medication tolerance can be achieved by discontinuing the agent.

ASSISTANT ADVICE

Use the blood levels and numbers as guidelines and listen to the patient for a full understanding of a medication's effects.

Another type of tolerance is termed *tachyphylaxis*. This is a unique situation in which tolerance may occur after only one or two doses. Tachyphylaxis can develop very quickly and the patient's initial response to the medication cannot be reproduced, even with a larger dose of the agent.

Drug Dependency

Through a suggestion from the World Health Organization, the terms *addiction* and *habituation* have been replaced with the term *drug dependence*. The general term of drug dependence avoids the social stigma associated with drug abuse. Drug dependency is defined as a physiological and psychological compulsion to take a drug periodically or continuously, despite its negative or dangerous effects. However, a physical dependence is not always an addiction. For example, some drugs (medications) are prescribed for high blood pressure or for their antiinflammatory actions. They can cause the body to physically depend on their effects, but this is not considered an addiction. Other drugs cause addiction without medication value, such as heroin. Tolerance to a drug is usually part of addiction.

ADVANCED PRACTICES: REVIEW QUESTIONS

1. When writing a medication order, a surgical assistant's duty is to:
   a. sign and initial the order for the physician
   b. have the physician verify, clarify, and sign it
   c. verify that the required components are present on the order
   d. have the physician sign it before checking the order
2. Prescription pads are:
   a. signed in advance by the physician
   b. kept in an area where they can be easily accessed
   c. used to order blood work
   d. kept in a secure place
3. Which of the following has been added to the four basic vital signs?
   a. Pain
   b. Heart rate

   c. Respirations
   d. Pupil reaction
4. If a prescription is written on a carbonless pad, it is good practice to:
   a. have the physician sign it ahead of time
   b. make a copy of the prescription for the chart
   c. obliterate the signature line to prevent forgery
   d. write two prescriptions and keep one for future use
5. Therapeutic range is verified by:
   a. checking the patient's reaction to the medications
   b. the patient's symptoms abating
   c. taking the patient's vital signs
   d. testing the patient's blood

ADVANCED PRACTICES: BIBLIOGRAPHY

Fulcher E, Fulcher R, Soto C: *Pharmacology principles and applications*, ed 3, St Louis, 2012, Saunders/Elsevier.
Kee JL, Hayes ER, McCuistion LE: *Pharmacology: a patient-centered nursing process approach*, ed 8, St Louis, 2015, Saunders/Elsevier.
Mosby's medical dictionary, ed 12, St Louis, 2012, Mosby/Elsevier.
Rothrock JC, Seifert PC: *Assisting in surgery: patient-centered care*, Denver, CO, 2010, Competency and Credentialing Institute.

ADVANCED PRACTICES: INTERNET RESOURCES

Boston University School of Medicine, Pharmacology & Experimental Therapeutics, Glossary of Terms and Symbols Used in Pharmacology: www.bumc.bu.edu/busm-pm/academics/resources/glossary/.

Institute for Safe Medication Practices, ISMP's list of error-prone abbreviations, symbols, and dose designations: https://www.drugs.com/article/prescription-abbreviations.html#table1.
The Free Medical Dictionary, Potentiation: http://medical-dictionary.thefreedictionary.com/potentiation.
U.S. Drug Enforcement Administration: www.dea.gov.

Medication Development, Regulation, and Resources

OBJECTIVES

After completing this chapter, you should be able to do the following:
1. Define terms and abbreviations related to medication development, regulation, and resources.
2. Describe international, federal, state, and local roles in regulating drugs.
3. Discuss The Joint Commission and the role it plays in drug regulation.
4. Describe medication development and testing, as well as the role of the US Food and Drug Administration.
5. Describe pharmacogenetics and pharmacogenomics.
6. Discuss medication labeling, and distinguish between brand, generic, and chemical medication names.
7. List and describe information found on medication labels.
8. Obtain and discuss medication information from various pharmacology resources.

OUTLINE

As a surgical technologist, you should be aware of federal, state, and local roles in regulating drugs and their administration. Thus, in this chapter, we present a broad overview of federal drug legislation and federal agencies and a general discussion of international, state, and local regulations. Because new medications are approved for use regularly, we also briefly consider the process that leads to this approval—testing, studies, and the use of genetic technology. Finally, we look at available medication references, which will help you to obtain information useful to your practice as a surgical technologist.

MEDICATION REGULATION

Throughout history, some individuals have misrepresented, misused, and abused medicinals, such as herbs, chemicals, and drugs. As societies progressed, their governments recognized the need to regulate or control the use of these substances. Before the 20th century, medications of all kinds were sold freely in the United States, both to physicians and consumers. Thus, neither physician nor consumer had any real proof of a medication's safety or effectiveness. Medicines were sold by "medicine men" in traveling shows, in stores, and even by mail order. There was no legal requirement for a physician's prescription. This situation began to change early in the 1900s, when the federal government stepped in to protect consumers and to regulate the pharmaceutical industry. The states also established

practice acts to regulate the dispensing and administration of medications (Insight 2.1).

International Laws

International regulation of medications is under the authority of the World Health Organization (WHO), a specialized agency of the United Nations. It acts as the coordinating authority on international public health, providing technical assistance in the drug field and promoting research on drug abuse. Its tasks include combating disease and promoting the general health of all people. The WHO (www.who.int/) publishes a report annually, *The World Health Statistics*, which combines expert assessment with a focus on a specific subject. This is to provide countries and all donor agencies with information to help them to make policies and funding decisions. The WHO does not enforce laws concerning drugs, so drug control is different from country to country. Some countries have more stringent laws than the United States, whereas some are less strict. As a result, drugs are often available in some countries before they have been approved for use in others. The WHO also publishes *Guidelines for Safe Surgery*, which includes such topics as antibiotic prophylaxis, types of adverse drug reactions and their treatment/prevention, causes of errors in delivery of perioperative medications, management of blood loss, and safe delivery of anesthesia. You may use the WHO's *Surgical Safety Checklist* in your facility. See Fig. 4.5 in Chapter 4.

INSIGHT 2.1   Complementary and Alternative Medications

Complementary and alternative medications, called CAM for short, are becoming very popular, with approximately 40% of adults reporting their use. Complementary medicine is used together with standard medical care. An example would be using acupuncture to help with the side effects of cancer treatments. Alternative medicine is used in place of standard medical care. An example would be to use mental healing for treating heart disease rather than traditional approaches. These are not part of standard care and may be defined as treatments that lack scientific evidence of safety and usefulness. The current medical system is based on the conventional approach of theory, knowledge, and research. This is centered around clinical medicine based upon principles of natural sciences, such as biology and chemistry. However, doctors are beginning to use these CAM therapies and often combine them with established medical therapies. The term for this practice is "integrative medicine." It was in the 1990s that consumers began to look outside the traditional approach toward alternative medicines. In 1992 the US Congress established the Office of Alternative Medicine (OAM) within the National Institutes of Health. In 1998 this office became the National Center for Complementary and Alternative Medicine (NCCAM), and in 2014 it became the National Center for Complementary and Integrative Health (NCCIH). Its mission is to define the usefulness and safety of CAM and their roles in improving healthcare. Consequently, more funding and research projects for information are possible. The NCCIH has categorized alternative healing and complementary medicines into five main areas: whole medical systems, mind-body medicine, biologically based practices, manipulative and body-based practices, and energy medicine.

An alternative medical system is a set of practices based on a philosophy different from Western biomedicine and includes Asian systems, folk healthcare, herbal medicines, massage, energy therapy, acupressure, acupuncture, and qigong. A traditional system from India is known as Ayurveda, which aspires to restore the individual's harmony of body, mind, and spirit. Native American, Middle Eastern, Tibetan, Central and South American, and African cultures have also developed traditional alternative medical systems. Other examples include naturopathic and homeopathic medicine. Naturopathic practices are based on the belief that the human body has an innate healing ability. These practices use diet, exercise, lifestyle changes, and natural therapies to enhance the body's ability to ward off and combat disease. Homeopathic medicine is based on the concept that "like cures like." Patients are treated with heavily diluted preparations that claim to cause effects similar to the symptoms presented. Homeopaths also use aspects of the patient's physical and psychological state in recommending remedies.

Mind-body explores the concept that the mind has an ability to affect the body (mental healing). These interventions include meditation, some types of hypnosis, music and art therapy, dance, and prayer. Biologically based practices include dietary supplements, such as herbs, and orthomolecular therapies. Herbs are considered as dietary supplements and so are regulated by the Department of Agriculture and the FDA. However, in this category, herbs are not subject to the strict regulations that apply to medications. Herbal medicine refers to the use of plant parts, such as seeds, berries, roots, leaves, bark, or flowers, for medicinal purposes. Although scientific study of herbs began in the United States approximately two centuries ago, herbs and other botanicals have been used in Asia for thousands of years. Orthomolecular therapies use different chemical concentrations to treat disease. These include magnesium, melatonin, and megadoses of vitamins. Manipulative and body-based practices include chiropractic methods, osteopathy, and massage. Finally, energy medicine includes biofield and electromagnetic field therapies. Biofield therapies are those that focus on fields that come from the body and include acupuncture, Reiki, qigong, and therapeutic touch. Electromagnetic fields come from sources other than the body and include magnetic fields, alternating current fields, or direct current fields. Although these fields have yet to be proven, the therapies are used with patients who have arthritis, cancer, or pain.

Federal Laws

Federal regulation of medications was initially intended to protect consumers from harmful, impure, untested, and unsafe medications. Thus, when the Pure Food and Drug Act was passed in 1906, it set standards for quality and required the proper labeling of medications. In 1938 the federal government began to address drug effectiveness. It passed the Food, Drug, and Cosmetic Act, which required animal testing of medications; before selling a new medication, pharmaceutical companies had to apply for approval to market the medication, and that approval was contingent on proof that the medication was effective on animals. The Durham-Humphrey Amendments to the Food, Drug, and Cosmetic Act were passed in 1952. These amendments required a physician's order to dispense certain medications, called *prescription drugs*, and established an over-the-counter (OTC) category of medications that did not require a prescription. However, even OTC drugs are studied to make sure they are safe for public use without a physician's guidance. Their labels must include sufficient warnings and instructions. Then in 1970 the Controlled Substances Act was passed. It designated certain medications as controlled substances. See Box 2.1 for a summary of these and other federal drug laws and their timelines.

The Controlled Substances Act of 1970 established classifications, known as schedules, of medications that had potential for abuse. These medications are specifically labeled to be easily identified. A large C signifies the drug as a controlled substance, and a Roman numeral designating its class (from I to V) appears with the C (Fig. 2.1). Five schedules (Table 2.1) were determined, based on the level of abuse and dependence potential and on appropriate medical uses for the medication. Drugs such as lysergic acid diethylamide are listed on the C-I schedule; they have high abuse potential and no accepted medical use. Controlled substances from the C-II schedule have high abuse potential but also have accepted medical uses, such as in the surgical setting. C-II controlled substances that are frequently used in surgery include alfentanil, cocaine, and morphine. Medications listed as C-III have moderate abuse potential, whereas medications on schedules C-IV and C-V have low abuse potential.

In 1973 the Drug Enforcement Administration (DEA) of the Department of Justice was established to enforce the Controlled Substances Act. It sets standards for handling controlled substances and has the legal authority to enforce those standards. Institutional policies and procedures for storing and handling controlled substances must comply with DEA standards, and documentation requirements must be strictly followed. For example, when hospitals administer narcotics, they must keep careful records of the amount of medication used as well as the date, patient, person administering the medication, and person obtaining it. Physicians or other health professionals who

BOX 2.1　Federal Drug Laws

Pure Food and Drug Act (1906)
- Required all drugs marketed in the United States to meet minimal standards of uniform strength, purity, and quality
- Required that preparations containing morphine be labeled
- Established two references of officially approved drugs: the USP and the NF (these two publications are combined and referred to as the USP-NF)

Federal Food, Drug, and Cosmetic Act (1938; amended in 1952 and 1965)
- Established the US FDA
- Established specific regulations regarding warning labels on preparations (e.g., cautions about a drug's capacity to cause drowsiness or become habit forming)
- Stated that both prescription and nonprescription drugs must be effective and safe
- Stated that all labels must be accurate and include the generic name
- Required FDA approval of all new drugs
- Designated which drugs could be sold OTC (i.e., without a prescription)

Controlled Substances Act (1970)
- Established the US DEA
- Set tighter controls on drugs capable of being abused (controlled substances) (e.g., depressants, stimulants, and narcotics)
- Required stricter security controls for anyone (physicians, pharmacists, hospitals) who dispenses, receives, sells, or destroys controlled substances
- Set limits on the use of prescriptions; established guidelines for the number of times a drug can be prescribed in a period of time and set rules on which preparations may be prescribed over the telephone to the pharmacy
- Required that each prescriber register with the DEA, obtaining a DEA number to be used on prescriptions
- Identified drugs that can be abused and that are addicting, classifying them into schedules according to the degree of danger

DEA, Drug Enforcement Administration; *FDA*, US Food and Drug Administration; *OTC*, over-the-counter; *USP-NF*, United States Pharmacopeia and National Formulary.

TABLE 2.1　Schedules of Controlled Substances

Schedule	Examples	Description
C-I	Heroin, LSD, PCP, marijuana[a]	Drugs with high abuse potential and severe physical and psychological dependence. No medicinal use, research only
C-II	Alfentanil, opium, cocaine, codeine, morphine	High potential for drug abuse. Accepted medical use but can lead to physical and psychological dependency. Specific restrictions
C-III	Anabolic steroids, products with low amounts of codeine	Potential for drug abuse less than in previous categories. Medically accepted for use. High psychological dependence, low physical dependence
C-IV	Diazepam, lorazepam, phenobarbital	Potential for dependency. Medically accepted for use. Limited psychological and physical dependence
C-V	Many antitussive and antidiarrheal agents	Very limited potential for dependence. Medically accepted for use. Many are OTC medications

Drugs may be moved from schedule to schedule on the list. A current schedule of all drugs controlled by the DEA can be obtained from that office at https://www.deadiversion.usdoj.gov/schedules/orangebook/c_cs_alpha.pdf.
LSD, Lysergic acid diethylamide; *PCP*, phencyclidine.
[a]Marijuana (cannabis) is currently legalized in some states for medicinal purposes. Please check individual state regulations.

Fig. 2.1 Symbol for a controlled substance with a schedule of II.

administer, dispense, or prescribe controlled substances are required to have a current state license and register with the DEA. The DEA assigns each a registration number, known as a DEA number, that is used to track controlled substances dispersed to patients.

Federal Agencies

There are two federal agencies that contribute policies for healthcare workers' (and public) safety, and these policies can influence drug regulation in the healthcare field. The Occupational Safety and Health Administration (OSHA) is an agency within the US Department of Labor. OSHA's mission is to ensure the safety and health of American workers by setting and enforcing standards. An example of how OSHA interacts with surgical technologists is the Occupational Exposure to Bloodborne Pathogens Standard, which was issued in 1991 and revised in 2001 in response to the Needlestick Safety and Prevention Act. OSHA estimates that 5.6 million workers in the healthcare industry and related occupations are at risk of occupational exposure to bloodborne pathogens. This group of people (including surgical technologists and surgical first assistants) is at risk for contracting hepatitis B, hepatitis C, and human immunodeficiency virus (HIV). The standard states that each employer must have a plan that ensures immediate and confidential postexposure treatment and follow-up procedures in accordance with current Centers for Disease Control and Prevention (CDC) guidelines. The CDC is an agency under the US Department of Health and Human Services. It is recognized as the leading federal agency for protecting the health and safety of people and for providing credible information to enhance health decisions. It serves as the national focus for developing and applying disease prevention and control. In 1995 the CDC issued a protocol for Emergency Needlestick Information recommending prophylactic medication treatment as soon as possible after a needlestick or sharps injury (<2 hours from the time of exposure). This treatment is known as *postexposure prophylaxis* (PEP) and is of importance to surgical technologists. Since the original report was published, it has been updated several times because of the approval of new antiretroviral drugs and the availability of new information on the treatment of HIV. PEP is the use of antiretroviral drugs as soon as possible after a significant occupational exposure to blood or other high-risk body fluids that are likely to be infected with HIV. Although these antiretroviral drugs are not found in the surgical setting, they should be familiar to those healthcare workers who are at risk. For current Preferred and Alternative HIV PEP Regimens, please refer to the updated CDC guidelines at https://www.cdc.gov/hiv/risk/pep/index.html.

> **NOTE:** You must be familiar with and strictly follow needlestick or sharps injuries protocol as set forth by your surgical technology program and also all policies relating to these incidents at your clinical sites.

State Practice Acts

State governments must comply with federal regulations. When federal and state laws concerning medications conflict, the stricter of the laws prevail. State laws known as *practice acts* govern the ordering, dispensing, and administration of medications. Such laws vary from state to state. For example, state laws regulate who—physicians, physician's assistants, or nurse practitioners—may prescribe drugs. They also regulate pharmacy practices, specifying how medications are to be dispensed and by whom (usually a licensed pharmacist). For example, drug substitution laws specify if a pharmacist may automatically substitute a generic equivalent for a prescribed medication if not indicated otherwise.

Physicians can "lend" or delegate some of their functions to others. For example, the surgical technologist functions as a "physician extender"—an extra pair of hands, so to speak. As such, surgical technologists perform medication-handling duties under the delegatory power of the physician. Each state controls the limits of this delegatory power through the Medical Licensing Board.

> **NOTE:** As a surgical technologist, you should be knowledgeable about the medication handling and administration laws in your state. State practice acts are public information; this means you can read these acts yourself to be correctly informed. This is important because the delegatory power and its interpretations differ from state to state. For example, many people believe that only nurses may administer medications to patients. However, in many states credentialed allied health professionals, such as perfusionists, respiratory therapists, and medical assistants, routinely administer medications legally. Surgical technologists must have direct knowledge of and function within the legal standards of medication administration determined by the state in which they practice.

Local Policies

When state laws do not specifically address the practice of surgical technology, published institutional policies should be used to determine the scope of practice. The role of the surgical technologist in drug handling is usually specified in institutional policies, which have local authority. The surgical technologist must be thoroughly familiar with medication administration policies and closely adhere to their stated limits. If current policies are outdated or do not reflect the scope of practice appropriate to the education and expertise of the surgical technologist, the institution should revise or update them as appropriate. The surgical technologist's job description may also contain relevant information regarding medication handling and administration.

> **! CAUTION**
>
> Under no circumstances should a surgical technologist exceed the limits of the facility's published job description. These job descriptions are subject to revision, as needed, to reflect current practice standards.

The Joint Commission

The Joint Commission evaluates and accredits more than 20,500 healthcare organizations and programs in the United States. These organizations include general and rehabilitation hospitals, critical access hospitals, ambulatory care providers (such as outpatient surgery centers), and office-based surgery facilities. The Joint Commission is the predominant standards-setting organization, and facilities that obtain its accreditation demonstrate their commitment to meeting certain performance standards.

Among The Joint Commission's standards are National Patient Safety Goals (NPSGs). These goals are established annually and address issues such as infection control; Universal Protocol for Preventing Wrong Site, Wrong Procedure, Wrong Person Surgery; and medical errors. In December 2013 an Implementation Guide for Surgical Site Infections was established. This free guide defines 23 effective practices and has statements from 17 participating hospitals. Beginning January 1, 2004, goals were expanded to include a list of "dangerous" abbreviations, acronyms, and symbols that should not be used in the clinical setting. This list was confirmed in May 2005 and is an effort to improve the effectiveness of communication among caregivers and to address the many inherent problems associated with misread abbreviations that contribute to medication errors. This list applies to all handwritten (including free-text computer entry) patient-specific documentation and preprinted forms. Accredited facilities are required to develop a "Do Not Use" list and must include terms as specified by The Joint Commission (Table 2.2). The Institute for Safe Medication Practices also publishes a list of error-prone abbreviations, symbols, and dosages. This can be found on its website at https://www.ismp.org/system/files/resources/2021-02/Error%20Prone%20Abbreviations%202021_0.pdf. Many facilities not only include these required terms, but have expanded their lists. It is important to check your facility's "Do Not Use" list. Currently, this list does not apply to health information technology preprogrammed systems (e.g., electronic medical records). However, this remains under consideration for the future, and facilities are being encouraged to eliminate, from any software, these items that are considered dangerous.

TABLE 2.2   "Do Not Use" Lists

THE JOINT COMMISSION'S OFFICIAL "DO NOT USE" LIST[a]

Do Not Use	Potential Problem	Use Instead
U, u (unit)	Mistaken for "0" (zero), the number "4" (four) or "cc"	Write "unit"
IU (International Unit)	Mistaken for IV (intravenous) or the number 10 (ten)	Write "International Unit"
Q.D., QD, q.d., qd (daily)	Mistaken for each other	Write "daily"
Q.O.D., QOD, q.o.d., qod (every other day)	Period after the Q mistaken for "I" and the "O" mistaken for "I"	Write "every other day"
Trailing zero (X.0 mg)[b]	10-fold overdose or underdose	Write "X mg"
Lack of leading zero (.X mg)		Write "0.X mg"
MS	Can mean morphine sulfate or magnesium sulfate	Write "morphine sulfate"
MSO_4 and $MgSO_4$	Confused for one another	Write "magnesium sulfate"

ADDITIONAL ABBREVIATIONS, ACRONYMS, AND SYMBOLS THAT COULD BE INCLUDED IN YOUR FACILITY'S OFFICIAL "DO NOT USE" LIST

Do Not Use	Potential Problem	Use Instead
> (greater than); < (less than)	Misinterpreted as the number "7" (seven) or the letter "L" Confused for one another	Write "greater than"; write "less than"
Abbreviations for drug names	Misinterpreted because of similar abbreviations for multiple drugs	Write drug names in full
Apothecary units	Unfamiliar to many practitioners Confused with metric units	Use metric units
@	Mistaken for the number "2" (two)	Write "at"
cc	Mistaken for U (units) when poorly written	Write "mL" or "milliliters" ("mL" is preferred)
μg	Mistaken for mg (milligrams) resulting in one thousand-fold overdose	Write "mcg" or "micrograms"

[a]Applies to all orders and all medication-related documentation that is handwritten (including free-text computer entry) or on preprinted forms.
[b]Exception: a "trailing zero" may be used only where required to demonstrate the level of precision of the value being reported, such as for laboratory results, imaging studies that report size of lesions, or catheter/tube sizes. It may not be used in medication orders or other medication-related documentation.
© "Do Not Use" Abbreviation List from http://www.jointcommission.org/facts_about_do_not_use_list/, The Joint Commission, 2018. Reprinted with permission.

DRUG DEVELOPMENT

Before legal regulation, drugs could be manufactured, sold, and administered without scientific proof of safety, quality, or effectiveness. At present all drugs must undergo stringent testing and provide proof of safety and effectiveness before release. This process can take as long as 15 years and cost more than $2.3 billion per drug. The US Food and Drug Administration (FDA) is an agency within the Department of Health and Human Services that consists of centers and offices (Insight 2.2). The Center for Drug Evaluation and Research (CDER) regulates the pharmaceutical industry, ensuring that basic standards are followed. These regulations include prescription drugs, OTC drugs, biological therapeutics, and generic drugs. The CDER evaluates all new drugs before they are sold and also monitors the more-than-10,000 existing drugs on the market. It observes television, radio, and printed drug advertisements for accuracy, as well as providing health professionals with information for consumers. To do this, the FDA inspects the facilities where drugs are made, reviews new drug applications, investigates and removes unsafe drugs from the market, and requires proper labeling of drugs. This extends to overseas facilities as well. As much as 80%

of prescription drugs used by American consumers come from India and China. In the past, the FDA has issued drug safety alerts for dozens of generic drugs from India and banned its exports of some generic versions of popular medicines. Investigators

INSIGHT 2.2   Orphan Drugs

There is another category of drugs called *orphan drugs*, which falls under the FDA Office of Orphan Products Development. This office's purpose is to advance development of drugs, biologics, devices, or medical foods that demonstrate promising results for the diagnosis and treatment of rare diseases and conditions. Although these drugs may be categorized more in the medical than the surgical realm of medicine, their purpose can affect the surgical team members and patients. The Orphan Drug Designation program assigns this status to drugs and biologics that are for the effective and safe treatment, diagnosis, or prevention of diseases or disorders that affect fewer than 200,000 people in the United States. This designation can also be applied to drugs that affect more than 200,000 people but are not expected to recover the costs for developing and marketing within 7 years following FDA approval. One such drug is RiVax, a vaccine that is intended for the prevention of ricin intoxication. Ricin toxin is thought to be a potential bioterror threat, and such a vaccine would act as a barrier for its use as a bioterrorism weapon.

continue to increase their scrutiny in overseas plants and fine these companies for not adhering to FDA standards.

> **NOTE:** The FDA permits physicians to prescribe approved medications for other than their intended purpose. This is called off-label use.

US Food and Drug Administration Pregnancy Categories

The FDA has developed a classification system related to medication effects on the unborn child, or fetus. This classification is useful for surgical medications in some medical situations: for example, a pregnant woman who has acute appendicitis and requires surgery. In medication literature and reference books, most medications have a pregnancy category listed. Categories A and B are considered to be within safe limits for medication use during pregnancy, with special attention given to the first trimester of the pregnancy (the first 3 months) (Table 2.3).

Pharmaceutical companies are continually developing new medications, and each must undergo required testing before FDA approval. This testing is an extensive process. Only five in 5000 drugs that enter preclinical testing progress to testing on humans. Then one of these five is approved. All new medications are first tested on animals to determine if they are safe to administer to humans. At least two species of mammals and of both sexes must be used for this initial stage of drug testing. During this process researchers look for toxic effects and determine safe dosage levels. Once the medication has proven safe in animals, the drug company applies to the FDA for permission to begin human testing, which consists of four primary phases (plus a phase for investigational new drug studies) (Insight 2.3).

Twenty-first-century technology is allowing scientists and pharmaceutical companies to test medications in a different way. Pharmacogenetics is the study of genetic factors in predicting a medication's action and how it could vary from its intended response. The term is the mixing of pharmaceuticals and

TABLE 2.3 US Food and Drug Administration Pregnancy Categories

Category	Description
A	No risk to fetus per studies
B	No risk in animal studies, and well-controlled studies in pregnant women not available. It is assumed there is little or no risk
C	Animal studies: a risk to the fetus. Controlled studies on pregnant women not available. Risk versus benefit of the drug must be determined
D	A risk to the human fetus has been proved. Risk versus benefit must be determined
X	A risk to the human fetus has been proved. Risk outweighs the benefit, and drug should be avoided during pregnancy

These categories are being reviewed for possible revision. Always check the FDA website for the most current information. From www.fda.gov.

INSIGHT 2.3 Phases of Human Medication Testing

Phase 0: This phase is a recent designation in accordance with the FDA's Guidance on Exploratory Investigational New Drug studies. It is also known as human microdosing and is designed to "speed up" development of promising drugs. This is a way to establish if the drug or agent has the expected outcome from preclinical studies. Phase 0 will be used for exploratory, first-in-human trials. It features the administration of a single small dose of the study drug to a limited number of subjects (usually 10–15) to gather preliminary data on the drug's pharmacokinetics and pharmacodynamics (see Chapter 1). Phase 0 testing is not designed to report on the safety or efficacy of a drug because the dose given is too low to cause any therapeutic effect. Drug development companies use these studies to decide which drugs have the best effects in humans to take forward for further development and testing. Some experts question the usefulness of this phase.

Phase I—Clinical Pharmacology: In the clinical pharmacology phase, the new medication is given to a small group (20–80) of healthy volunteers or those who have the problem that the drug manufacturer is hoping to treat. This group is usually males between the ages of 18 and 45 years. This phase is used to determine the dose level for symptoms of medication toxicity in humans and can take 1 to 2 years.

Phase II—Clinical Investigation: In the clinical investigation phase, the medication is given to a larger group (usually several hundred) of patients presenting with the disease or condition the medication was developed to treat. The clinical investigation phase is used to establish medication effectiveness and to determine optimum dosage and dose range. It can take 1 to 3 years.

Phase III—Clinical Trials: In the clinical trial phase, researchers continue to note medication effectiveness, safety, and side effects in large studies. In this phase, which begins only if no serious side effects occur in Phase II, the new medication is given to hundreds or thousands of patients, usually in large medical research facilities. The medication's effectiveness is verified, and its actions are characterized by various types of scientific studies. Several kinds of studies may be conducted. For example, in *double-blind studies* half of the testing group receives the medication and the other half receives an inactive substance called a placebo. Neither the subject patients nor the prescribing physicians know which group received the placebo until the study has been completed. The results of these and other studies must be thoroughly documented. This phase can take several years to complete.

Phase IV—Postmarketing Study: The postmarketing study phase occurs after the medication is released for use in treatment of the specified condition. In this phase the drug company continues to monitor the medication, gathering results from prescribing physicians. This continuing evaluation of the medication includes results from those patients excluded from the previous phases, such as pregnant patients and the elderly. These data must be gathered, analyzed, and reported to the FDA to document the medication's safety and effectiveness comprehensively. The time frame for this phase varies with the medication or with the study being performed.

genetics. Pharmacogenetics is vital technology because people have different genetic makeups and do not respond identically to medication dosage or intended therapy. Genetic factors can alter the metabolism of a medication and either enhance or diminish its action. Thus a patient can have a positive response, a negative response, or no response at all to a medication. Pharmacogenomics refers to the general study of all genes and genetic technology that determine medication behavior. However, the distinction between these two terms is so slight that they are used interchangeably. As technology allows scientists to create pharmacogenetic maps and catalog more genetic variations found within the human genome, pharmaceutical companies can create medications based on this knowledge. This could facilitate new medication discovery, develop "drug markers" to target specific diseases, revive previously failed medication candidates and match them with a specific population, and facilitate the medication approval process, which would lower the costs and risks of clinical trials. The drawbacks to pharmacogenetics are the complexity and cost of genetic research and educating healthcare providers in the use of this technology. For more information, go to the National Institutes of Health's website at www.nih.gov.

Marketing

During development, the drug company assigns a generic name to the new medication. Later, it selects a company trade name, which it uses for marketing purposes once the medication gains FDA approval. The US Pharmacopeia and National Formulary (USP-NF) assigns an official name to the new medication; this is usually the generic name. Once a drug has been approved for release, the pharmaceutical company responsible for the medication's development has exclusive rights to market that medication under its trade name for 20 years. This is called a *patent*. The process allows the drug company to recover development costs. However, this patent is issued before clinical trials begin, so the drug time of the patent may be from 7 to 12 years. After these exclusive rights have expired, other companies may begin to market a generic equivalent with a different trade name.

Medication Labeling

As previously mentioned, the federal Pure Food and Drug Act of 1906 established proper labeling of medications. It is important to correctly obtain (read) the information found on medication labels. It is recognized that surgical technologists do not directly administer medications to the patient. However, you will be obtaining medications for the sterile field and playing an important part in correct medication identification, labeling all medication containers, and avoiding medication errors. Medication labels display pertinent information that the surgical technologist must read and interpret accurately. Remember, you act as the last "checkpoint" before the surgeon administers the medication to the patient (Insight 2.4).

INSIGHT 2.4 Medications Under the Labels

The medications used as examples in the medication labeling section are the ones you will see used in the surgical setting or for the surgical patient. The first medication, Ancef, is an antibiotic. It may be used preoperatively, intraoperatively, or postoperatively to help fight infections. Refer to Chapter 5 for more on antibiotics. The next medication, Ciprodex Otic drops, is also an antibiotic with other medications mixed in (e.g., dexamethasone). Dexamethasone is a steroid used to decrease the body's inflammatory response. Refer to Chapters 5 and 8. The next, heparin sodium, is an anticoagulant that is used in vascular procedures. Refer to Chapter 9 for more on medications that affect the vascular system and the importance of correct heparin sodium strength and administration. The last medication mentioned is diazepam, a sedative. It is used preoperatively to help relieve the patient's anxiety. Refer to Chapter 12 for more information.

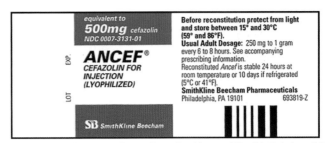

Fig. 2.2 Ancef label. (From Kee JL, Hayes ER, McCuistion LE: *Pharmacology: a patient-centered nursing process approach*, ed 8, St Louis, 2015, Saunders/Elsevier.)

Brand and Generic Names of the Medication

The manufacturer's name for a medication is called the *brand*, *trade*, or *proprietary name*. It is selected by the pharmaceutical manufacturer and used to market the medication. It is usually the most prominent word on the label. It may be in large or bold type, is always capitalized, and is very visible to promote the product. The name is followed by the ® sign, which means the name and the formula are registered. Directly under the brand name is the generic (nonproprietary) or official name in lowercase letters. The generic name is not owned by any one company, so it is not capitalized. On some labels the generic name may be placed inside parentheses. It is given to the medication by the USP, and by law the generic name must be identified on all medication labels. On the Ancef label (Fig. 2.2), the brand name appears in large, black letters. The generic name is cefazolin sodium and is printed underneath the brand name.

> **NOTE:** Each medication has several names—usually its brand or trade name, its generic name, and also its chemical name. The chemical name has meaning for chemists. It is a precise, systematic description of the chemical composition and molecular structure of the medication. Chemical names can be found in references, such as the *Physicians' Desk Reference* (PDR), but are not normally found on medication labels.

> **⚠ CAUTION**
> On some medication labels, only the generic name appears (as the diazepam label in Fig. 2.5). Be sure to cross-check medication names if you are unsure of their generic equivalents. Many generic spellings are very similar, yet the medications are vastly different, and an error could be fatal to the patient. It is important to also recognize that some variations may exist between generic medications produced by different manufacturers.

Manufacturer's name: This is also displayed on the label to advertise the company. See the SmithKline Beecham Pharmaceuticals on the Ancef label.

Dosage strength: This number on the label refers to dosage weight or the amount of the medication in a specific unit of measurement. On the Ancef label, the dosage strength of medication in the bottle is given as 500 mg.

Form: This identifies the composition of the medication. As discussed in Chapter 1, solid forms are tablets and capsules. Some are in powdered, or granular, form and can be combined with food or beverages. This is usually found in the medical rather than the surgical setting, such as for postoperative pain medications that the patient can take at home. Other medications must be reconstituted or liquefied by being dissolved in a solution, such as sterile water or sterile normal saline. These medications are then measured in an exact liquid volume, such as milliliters (mL) or cubic centimeters (cc). They may be crystalloid (a clear solution) or a suspension (solid particles in a liquid that separate in the container). On the Ciprodex Otic label (Fig. 2.3), the word *suspension* tells us the medication must be shaken to dilute the particles before it is administered to the patient (as discussed in Chapter 1). Other medication forms include creams, ointments, patches, and suppositories.

❓ QUICK QUESTION

Using medical terminology, what does the term *otic* tell you about where a medication is used? Read ahead to find the answer in the section of this chapter called Administration Route. So, to what does the term *ophthalmic* refer? See Chapter 10 for the answer.

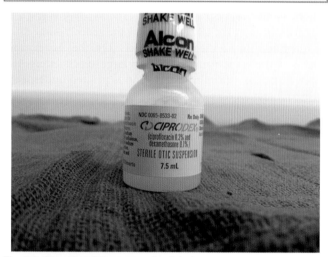

Fig. 2.3 Ciprodex Otic suspension label.

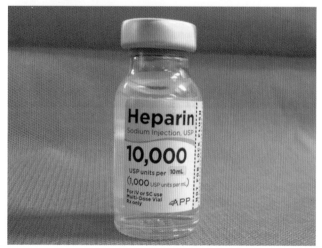

Fig. 2.4 Heparin sodium.

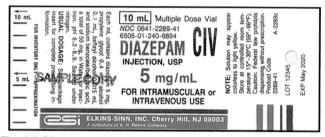

Fig. 2.5 Diazepam label. (From Kee JL, Hayes ER, McCuistion LE: *Pharmacology: a patient-centered nursing process approach*, ed 8, St Louis, 2015, Saunders/Elsevier.)

Supply dosage: This refers to dosage strength and medication form. Read it as "X measured units per quantity." For liquid medications, the supply dosage is the same as the medication's concentration. On the heparin sodium label (Fig. 2.4), there are 1000 units/1 mL of solution. Because of new product safety changes, the label also includes the total strength of the entire bottle, which is 10,000 units in 10 mL (see Insight 9.3 in Chapter 9). Note also that heparin sodium is the generic name of the medication and so has no registration mark.

Total volume: This is the full quantity contained in the bottle or vial, or its total fluid volume. For solids, it is the total number of individual items in the package. On the heparin label, there is a total volume of 10 mL because this medication is in liquid form.

Administration route: This refers to the method of medication delivery to the patient or body site. Refer to Chapter 4 for further information on medication administration. On the Ciprodex label, it states for otic use (in the ears only). The diazepam label states for intramuscular or intravenous (IV) injection, and the heparin label lists subcutaneous or IV use.

Label alerts: Manufacturers may print warnings on the packages, such as "refrigerate" or "protect from light." Suspension medications would carry the warning to "shake well," as seen on the Ciprodex container. Another example of an alert is red on the label of a local anesthetic agent, such as lidocaine. This would signify the presence of epinephrine (adrenaline) in the medication. Note the "CIV" on the diazepam label (Fig. 2.5). This alert signifies that the medication is a controlled substance and has been assigned the schedule of C-IV, meaning it has the potential for dependency. Refer to Table 2.1.

❓ MAKE IT SIMPLE

Red on the label of a *local anesthetic* agent means it contains epinephrine.

Expiration date: Medications should be used, discarded, or returned to the pharmacy by this date. This is very important information, and it is usually presented as a month/year (as May 2020 on the diazepam label, which would indicate the medication can be used until May 1, 2020). If any medication obtained from the pharmacy for a procedure shows a date already past, it should not be used because it is *outdated*. It should be returned to the pharmacy, and another should be obtained with a date that has not passed.

! CAUTION

If a medication is expired, it may have reduced potency or effectiveness. It can become chemically altered and provide a lethal effect to the patient.

Lot or control numbers: Federal law requires all medication packages to be identified with a lot or control number. If a medication is recalled, this number identifies the specific group of packages to be removed from shelves. The diazepam label gives the lot number as 12345.

Barcode symbols: These are used in sales, and they document medication dosing for record keeping. The FDA estimates once barcodes are used to automate medication documentation to the patient's bedside, there will be over 500,000 fewer adverse events over the next 20 years. You can see a barcode on the Ancef label.

National Drug Code (NDC): Federal law requires every prescription medication have an identifying number. It must appear on every manufacturer's label and is printed as NDC-•••••-•••-••. Note the code on the top of the Ancef label as NDC 00007-3131-01.

United States Pharmacopeia (USP) and National Formulary (NF): These codes are found on manufacturer-printed labels. These are two different official national lists of approved medications. Each manufacturer follows special guidelines that determine when to include these initials on the label. Initials are placed after the generic drug name. Note the initials "USP" on the heparin sodium and diazepam labels.

MEDICATION REFERENCES

When a medication has been approved for use, the pharmaceutical company must publish comprehensive information regarding it. This information must appear in package inserts and in compiled reference works. In addition, many medication information resources are available to medical, nursing, and allied health professionals. There are dozens of textbooks on pharmacology and various specialty areas within that science. Moreover, several pharmacology resources are expressly designed for use in clinical practice. Each surgery department should have such references readily available to the staff (Insight 2.5).

Prescribers' Digital Reference

One of the most frequently used pharmacology resources is the Prescribers' Digital Reference (PDR), formerly the Physicians' Desk Reference. It was first published in 1947 and was found in almost all physicians' offices, pharmacies, and clinics. It provides easy access to information on several thousand medications used in medical and surgical practice. The PDR is published annually and contains FDA-approved drug label information; brand and generic name indexes; warnings

and precautions; drug interactions, dosages, side effects, and safety information; pregnancy ratings; poison antidotes; and dietary supplements.

The Product Information section contains the manufacturer's information on approximately 3000 medications. Medications are listed alphabetically by manufacturer. Each entry includes data on indications (why it is used), effects, dosage, administration routes, methods, and frequency. It also includes warnings regarding side effects and contraindications. In addition, the Product Information section contains full-color, actual-size images of tablets, capsules, and other dosage forms and packages. The PDR also publishes separate references for nonprescription and ophthalmic medications. Its website offers readers information on a variety of topics, such as prescription medications, ITC medications, herbals and supplements, Health Information Centers, and clinical trials. There is a link on the homepage for healthcare professionals, which offers free www.pdr.net access (Fig. 2.6).

❓ QUICK QUESTION

Do you remember the definitions of indication and contraindication? If not, refer to the section on pharmacodynamics in Chapter 1.

NOTE: The information presented in the PDR is the same as that found in the manufacturer's package insert. Students may easily obtain package inserts for medications used in surgery. You can get them as medications are opened or from the pharmacy at your clinical site.

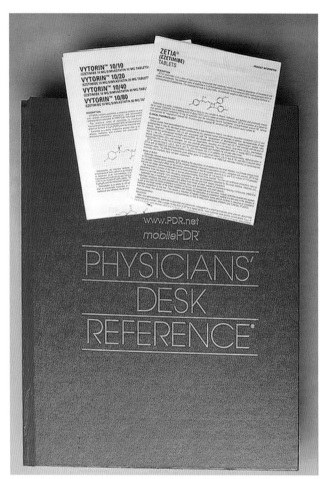

Fig. 2.6 Physicians' Desk Reference. Now known as the Prescribers' Digital Reference. (From Physicians' Desk Reference, PDR Network.)

United States Pharmacopeia and National Formulary

The USP-NF is the official medication list recognized by the US government. It is actually two publications—the Pharmacopeia and the Formulary—combined into three volumes. It is available in print and online at www.uspnf.com. The USP-NF lists standards for medication quality, safety, and effectiveness; it also contains information on the physical and chemical characteristics of listed medications. Used primarily by drug companies and pharmacists, the USP-NF is issued annually by the US Pharmacopeial Convention (a national committee of pharmacists, pharmacologists, physicians, chemists, biologists, and other scientific professionals). The US Pharmacopeia/Dispensing Information (USP-DI) is a related clinical reference divided into several sections, including one for healthcare professionals. This includes pharmacology, precautions to consider, side and adverse effects, and general dosing information. Another section gives medication information directed to the patient (client). It is written in understandable language and includes administration of medications, medication effects, indications, adverse reactions, guidelines for dosages, and what to do for missed doses. It should be noted there is also an *International Pharmacopeia*, which is revised every 5 years with supplements published in between. It

was first published in 1951 by the WHO and recently has focused on medications of public health importance. These include those that treat malaria, tuberculosis, HIV/acquired immunodeficiency syndrome, and medications for children. It appears in many languages and is available online.

American Hospital Formulary Service Drug Information

This reference is published annually and updated quarterly by the American Society of Health-System Pharmacists, Bethesda, Maryland. The American Hospital Formulary Service (AHFS) provides up-to-date information on most prescription medications marketed in the United States. It is considered to be unbiased because it does not contain information supplied only by the pharmaceutical manufacturers of the medications. Medications are listed according to therapeutic medication classification. The information includes chemistry and stability, pharmacological actions, pharmacokinetics, uses, cautions and precautions, contraindications, drug interactions, acute toxicity, dosage and administration, and medication preparation. It also contains information on OTC, ophthalmic, dermatologic, and orphan drugs. It is available for purchase online and can be accessed via the website www.ahfsdruginformation.com.

The Medical Letter

The *Medical Letter* on medications and therapeutics is published biweekly by the Medical Letter, Inc. in New York. This is a nonprofit publication for physicians and other allied health professionals. It issues two newsletters, *The Medical Letter on Drugs and Therapeutics* and *Treatment Guidelines from the Medical Letter*. They cover medications for the treatment of diseases, such as HIV, and cover new medications recently approved by the FDA. The information includes pharmacokinetics, clinical studies, dosage, adverse effects, and interactions. The website is https://secure.medicalletter.org/, and it is available as an online subscription.

Facts and Comparisons

Facts and Comparisons contains thousands of prescription and OTC medications and thousands of comparison charts and tables. It can be found online at www.factsandcomparisons.com. It is a reference for drug actions, indications, warnings and precautions, dosage and route of administration, adverse reactions, overdosage, interactions, contraindications, and patient (client) information. Medications are grouped by therapeutic category, and it also includes information on investigational medications. Facts and Comparisons is available as an annual subscription that includes monthly updates via a newsletter.

Hospital Pharmacist

Another valuable source of information on drugs is the clinical pharmacist. Consulting and educating have become an important part of pharmacy practice. The pharmacist is consulted when any question arises regarding medications, especially those that are newly approved.

Databases

A vast amount of information regarding medications, their proper use, possible drug side effects and interactions, and other important clinical considerations is available via the Internet. A site, such as https://medlineplus.gov/ can be accessed on smartphones and tablets. Databases, such as *Micromedex* and Facts and Comparisons' *CliniSphere*, are helpful tools that medical professionals use to access current pharmacologic information. Drug manufacturers also include drug information on their websites. Helpful Internet addresses include the following:

The American College of Clinical Pharmacy at www.accp.com

The American Heart Association at www.heart.org

The American Medical Association at www.ama-assn.org

The Centers for Disease Control and Prevention at www.cdc.gov

Drug Store News at www.drugstorenews.com

Facts and Comparisons at www.factsandcomparisons.com

Micromedex at www.micromedex.com

The National Cancer Institute at www.cancer.gov

The National Institutes of Health (NIH) at www.nih.gov

The National Library of Medicine at www.nlm.nih.gov

The Occupational Safety and Health Administration at wwwosha.gov

Prescribers' Digital Reference at www.pdr.net

PharmWeb at www.pharmweb.net

Pharmacy Times at www.pharmacytimes.com

US Pharmacist at www.uspharmacist.com

US Pharmacopeia at www.usp.org

The World Health Organization at www.who.int

> **! CAUTION**
>
> Keep in mind that medication information can be posted on the Internet by anyone, so the information may not always be accurate. It is a good idea to check reliable sources, such as governmental websites, and always verify information from two different sources. Other drug resource material is easily accessible by computer, including the USP-DI, PDR, current journal articles, and manufacturers' bulletins.

> **KEY CONCEPTS**
>
> - Federal regulations of medications protect consumers.
> - The federal Pure Food and Drug Act sets standards for quality and proper medication labeling.
> - The Food, Drug, and Cosmetic Act requires animal testing of medications.
> - The Controlled Substances Act established schedules for medications.
> - The US DEA enforces the Controlled Substances Act.
> - The US FDA developed a classification system related to medications' effects upon the unborn child.
> - State practice acts govern the ordering, dispersal, and administration of medications.
> - The role of the surgical technologist in medication handling may be specified by institutional policy.
> - The Joint Commission (formerly the Joint Commission on Accreditation of Healthcare Organizations [JCAHO]) evaluates and accredits healthcare facilities and sets policies, such as NPSGs.
> - Genetic factors are being used to predict a medication's action on patients, and thus are useful in medication development.
> - Medications must undergo testing that involves several phases (including animal testing) before being given FDA approval.
> - There are numerous medication references and databases, including the ones found on the Internet, that can be accessed for information.

■ LEARNING THE LANGUAGE (KEY TERMS)

Using your textbook and/or a medical dictionary, look up and write the definitions of each term.

AHFS drug information

controlled substances

DEA

Facts and Comparisons

FDA

generic

narcotics

OTC

PDR

pharmacogenetics/pharmacogenomics

prescription drugs

The Joint Commission

USP-NF

World Health Organization

■ REVIEW QUESTIONS

1. How does the federal government regulate medications?
2. What is the significance of the Pure Food and Drug Act of 1906?
3. What is the role of the FDA in drug regulation?
4. Why is the separation of some drugs into five schedules important?
5. What is the role of The Joint Commission in medication regulation? OSHA? CDC?
6. Use at least two medication references to research the indications and the side effects of the following medications:
   a. Heparin sodium
   b. Diazepam
   c. Ancef
7. Why is it important for surgical technologists to have an understanding of medications, even though they do not directly administer them to the patient?

CRITICAL THINKING

1. How does the DEA affect clinical practice?
2. Name three medications the surgeon uses during a procedure that are prepared on the back table.
3. How are medications for procedures obtained at your clinical site?

Scenario

The surgery is scheduled as an excision of a cyst from the right lower back. The surgeon requests Xylocaine 1% with epinephrine and Demerol for the local procedure.

1. What are the generic names for these medications?
2. Xylocaine is available in what strengths in addition to 1%?
3. Which of these medications is/are narcotics? What is/are the controlled substances schedules?
4. Which of the medications would have red on the label? What does this signify?

BIBLIOGRAPHY

Bardal S, Waechter J, Martin D: *Applied pharmacology*, St Louis, 2011, Saunders/Elsevier.

Fulcher EM, Fulcher RM, Soto CD: *Pharmacology: principles and applications*, ed 3, St Louis, 2012, Saunders/Elsevier.

Kee JL, Hayes ER, McCuistion LE: *Pharmacology: a patient-centered nursing process approach*, ed 8, St Louis, 2015, Saunders/Elsevier.

Skidmore-Roth L: *Mosby's drug guide for nursing students*, ed 11, St Louis, 2015, Mosby/Elsevier.

INTERNET RESOURCES

Acupuncture Today: http://acupuncturetoday.com.

American Association of Naturopathic Physicians: www.naturopathic.org.

Centers for Disease Control and Prevention: www.cdc.gov.

Facts and Comparisons: www.factsandcomparisons.com.

Healings ways: the teachings of Kenneth Cohen: http://qigonghealing.com.

Human Genome Project Information: www.genome.gov.

Kuhar D.T., Henderson D.K., Struble K.A., et al: Updated U.S. Public Health Service guidelines for the management of occupational exposures to HIV and recommendations for postexposure prophylaxis. Available at http://stacks.cdc.gov/view/cdc/20711. Accessed August 6, 2015.

Mayo Clinic, Mayo Clinic Healthy Lifestyle: www.mayoclinic.org/healthy-lifestyle.

MedicineNet.com: Definition of off-label use: www.medicinenet.com/script/main/art.asp?articlekey=4622.

National Center for Complementary and Integrative Health (NCCIH): www.nccih.nih.gov.

National Safety Compliance: http://osha-safety-training.net.

Occupational Safety & Health Administration: www.osha.gov.

Patents and Generics: www.news-medical.net/health/Drug-Patents-and-Generics.aspx.

Prescribers' Digital Reference: www.pdr.net.

Post-Exposure Prophylaxis (PEP): https://www.cdc.gov/hiv/risk/pep/index.html.

The Diane Rehm Show: *The Safety of Prescription Drugs Made Outside the US*: http://thedianerehmshow.org/shows/2014-02-20/safety-prescription-drugs-made-outside-us.

The New York Times: *Medicines Made in India Set Off Safety Worries*: www.nytimes.com/2014/02/15/world/asia/medicines-made-in-india-set-off-safety-worries.html?_r=0.

Springer Link, Medicine and Public Health: http://link.springer.com.

The Joint Commission: www.jointcommission.org.

The Joint Commission, Official "Do Not Use" List: www.jointcommission.org/facts_about_do_not_use_list.

The Journal of the American Medical Association: https://jamanetwork.com/journals/jama.

Thomson Reuters, Micromedex: www.micromedex.com.

Updated U.S. Public Health Service Guidelines for the Management of Occupational Exposures to Human Immunodeficiency Virus and Recommendations for Postexposure Prophylaxis: https://www.jstor.org/stable/10.1086/672271.

US Drug Enforcement Administration: www.dea.gov.

US Food and Drug Administration: www.fda.gov.

US National Library of Medicine: www.nlm.nih.gov.

US Pharmacopeial Convention, USP-NF: www.uspnf.com.

WebMD, Whole Medical Systems: An Overview: https://www.webmd.com/balance/guide/understanding-alternative-medicine.

World Health Organization: www.who.int/en.

World Health Organization, Patient Safety, Safe Surgery Saves Lives: https://www.who.int/publications/i/item/9789241598552.

Pharmacology Mathematics

OBJECTIVES

After completing this chapter, you should be able to do the following:

1. Define terminology, abbreviations, and symbols used in basic mathematics and measurement systems.
2. Convert civilian time to military time, and vice versa.
3. Use fractions in conversions and calculations.
4. Read and write decimals accurately.
5. Apply decimals in conversions and calculations.
6. Convert between fractions and decimals.
7. Define and discuss percentages.
8. Convert between percentages and decimals, and between percentages and fractions.
9. Define and compare ratios and proportions.
10. Apply ratios and proportions to solve problems.
11. Convert temperatures between the Fahrenheit and Celsius scales.
12. Discuss measurement systems, define the metric system of measurement, and explain how the metric system is used as the international standard.
13. Discuss other systems of measurement and their medical applications.
14. Identify symbols of measurement, and measurement equivalents.

OUTLINE

In this chapter, we look at basic mathematics, including military time, fractions, decimals, percentages, and ratios and proportions. We review how to solve simple problems, perform fundamental calculations, and make important conversions. Many surgical technology students are familiar with these principles; this chapter is designed as a refresher for students who need to practice their mathematical skills. Each rule is explained, and then examples are given to illustrate its principle. In addition, there are exercises, including specific surgical technology story problems, for students to practice the mathematical operations. This chapter also introduces students to measurement systems and how they are used in the medical setting. Students use basic mathematical skills to perform conversions in the systems of measurement. Knowledge of metric measurements and basic mathematical skills are necessary in pharmacology because they are used during surgical procedures, particularly when using implants and grafts and assisting the surgeon, as medications are administered from the sterile field.

 MAKE IT SIMPLE

Go to the end of this chapter and take the Mathematics Evaluation Pretest. This pretest has a variety of mathematical skills that are explained in the chapter. If you discover areas in which you believe you are weak, review those sections of this chapter to strengthen your skills.

MILITARY TIME

Hospitals and other medical institutions, along with law enforcement and the military, use a precise method of expressing time called *international* or military time. Military time uses a 24-hour scale without a.m. or p.m. designations (Fig. 3.1). It is similar to civilian time in the morning hours from midnight until noon. After noon it increases in 1-hour increments from 12, whereas civilian time starts over again with 1.

To convert military time to civilian time after noon, subtract 12. For example, 1900 hours becomes 7:00 p.m. (19 − 12 = 7).

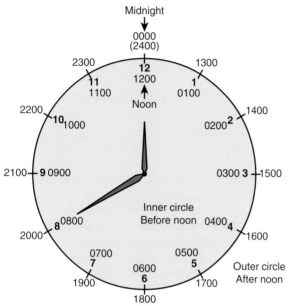

Fig. 3.1 Military/civilian clock. This 24-hour clock shows the time as 1140 (or 11:40 a.m.) and 2340 (or 11:40 p.m.).

TABLE 3.1	**Military and Civilian Times**			
Civilian Time	**Military Time**		**Civilian Time**	**Military Time**
Midnight[a]	0000		Noon	1200
1:00 a.m.	0100		1:00 p.m.	1300
2:00 a.m.	0200		2:00 p.m.	1400
3:00 a.m.	0300		3:00 p.m.	1500
4:00 a.m.	0400		4:00 p.m.	1600
5:00 a.m.	0500		5:00 p.m.	1700
6:00 a.m.	0600		6:00 p.m.	1800
7:00 a.m.	0700		7:00 p.m.	1900
8:00 a.m.	0800		8:00 p.m.	2000
9:00 a.m.	0900		9:00 p.m.	2100
10:00 a.m.	1000		10:00 p.m.	2200
11:00 a.m.	1100		11:00 p.m.	2300

[a]Midnight can be written two ways in military time: 2400, and read as "twenty-four hundred," or 0000 and read as "zero hundred."

To convert civilian time to military time after noon, add 12. For example, 1:00 p.m. becomes 1300 hours (1 + 12 = 13).

Military time is pronounced differently than civilian time. For example, 5:00 a.m. in civilian time, or 5 o'clock in the morning, is 0500 in military time and is pronounced as "oh-five-hundred" or "zero-five-hundred." In surgery, a procedure scheduled for 4 o'clock in the afternoon would be "sixteen-hundred hours" (1600) in military time. If the incision for this 4 o'clock case is made at 4:46 p.m., it would be written as 1646 and pronounced as "sixteen forty-six hours" in military time. Table 3.1 provides conversions between civilian and military times.

What if an event occurs at 9 minutes after midnight? In civilian time it would be written as 12:09 a.m. In military time it would be written as 0009 and pronounced as "zero-zero-zero-nine hours." If the event occurs at 9 minutes after noon, in civilian time it would be written as 12:09 p.m. In military time it would be written as 1209 and pronounced as "twelve-oh-nine hours."

MAKE IT SIMPLE

Notice that military time uses four digits to indicate the hours and minutes: the first two digits represent hours and the last two represent minutes.

NOTE: Midnight can be written two ways in military time: 2400 and read as "twenty-four hundred," or 0000 and read as "zero hundred."

QUICK QUESTION

You are assigned to a 2 p.m. case. How is this time written on the surgery schedule?
   Check your answer in Table 3.1.

FRACTIONS

A fraction is a number that represents one or more equal parts of a whole. The word comes from the Latin *fractio*, which means "to break into pieces." A fraction is a quotient—a number that can be written in an *a/b* or $\frac{a}{b}$ form, where *b* is never equal to 0. We say that *a* and *b* are the terms of the fraction, where *a* is the *numerator* and *b* is the *denominator*.

Example

One half = 1/2 = $\frac{1}{2}$ =

$\frac{1}{2}$ *a* = 1 is the numerator
      b = 2 is the denominator

Five sixths = 5/6 = $\frac{5}{6}$ =

$\frac{5}{6}$ *a* = 5 is the numerator
      b = 6 is the denominator

Five eighths = 5/8 = $\frac{5}{8}$ =

$\frac{5}{8}$ *a* = 5 is the numerator
      b = 8 is the denominator

We use fractions to express division of a whole into equal parts:

- The denominator tells how many equal parts into which the whole is divided.
- The numerator tells how many equal parts we are interested in.

Example

Imagine a pie divided into six equal parts, and five of those equal parts are eaten (Fig. 3.2).

$\frac{5}{6}$ Number of eaten parts
Number of equal parts into which the whole pie is divided

So

- $\frac{5}{6}$ of the pie is eaten

- $\frac{1}{6}$ of the pie remains

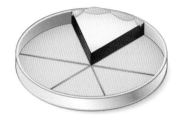

Fig. 3.2 A pie divided into six equal parts.

The larger the denominator, the smaller the pieces (fractions) in the whole.

Example

$\frac{1}{2}$ *is greater than* $\frac{1}{3}$

$\frac{1}{3}$ *is greater than* $\frac{1}{4}$

$\frac{1}{4}$ *is greater than* $\frac{1}{5}$

$\frac{1}{5}$ *is greater than* $\frac{1}{6}$

and so on.

❓ MAKE IT SIMPLE

If the denominators of two fractions are the same, the one with the higher numerator determines the higher fraction. If the numerators are the same, the one with the lower denominator determines the higher fraction.

Example

Imagine a circle divided into eight equal parts, and five of those equal parts are shaded (Fig. 3.3).

$\frac{5}{8}$ Number of shaded equal parts
Number of equal parts into which the whole circle is divided

So

- $\frac{5}{8}$ of the circle is shaded

- $\frac{3}{8}$ of the circle is not shaded

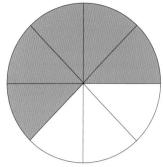

Fig. 3.3 A circle divided into eight equal parts.

If the numerator and the denominator are equal to each other, the fraction is equal to 1.

Examples

$$\frac{1}{1} = \frac{2}{2} = \frac{5}{5} = \frac{100}{100} = \frac{3569}{3569} = 1$$

If the numerator is less than the denominator, the value of the fraction is less than 1. Then the fraction is a proper fraction.

Examples

$$\frac{2}{3}\ \frac{3}{4}\ \frac{3}{5}\ \frac{99}{100}$$

If the numerator is greater than the denominator, the value of the fraction is more than 1. Then the fraction is an improper fraction.

Examples

$$\frac{3}{2}\ \frac{4}{3}\ \frac{12}{6}\ \frac{15}{10}$$

A mixed number is a combination of a whole number with a fraction.

Examples

$$1\frac{1}{2}\ \ 2\frac{1}{3}\ \ 5\frac{3}{7}\ \ 8\frac{49}{50}$$

NOTE: Any time the numerator of a fraction is zero, the value of the fraction is zero.

You can change a mixed number to an improper fraction in three steps.

Given the mixed number $2\frac{1}{2}$,

Step 1: Multiply the denominator of the fraction by the whole number:

Whole number $\times$ denominator $= 2 \times 2 = 4$

Step 2: Add the numerator to the result obtained in step 1:

Numerator $+ \left(\text{Step 1 result}\right) = 1 + 4 = 5$

Step 3: Use the result obtained in Step 2 as the numerator of the new fraction; use the original denominator as the new denominator:

$$\frac{\text{Step 2 result}}{\text{Original denominator}} = \frac{5}{2}$$

Thus, the mixed number of $2\frac{1}{2}$ is the same as the improper fraction $\frac{5}{2}$.

You can change an improper fraction to a mixed number in four steps.

Given an improper fraction $\frac{8}{5}$,

Step 1: Divide the numerator by the denominator:

$$\frac{\text{Numerator}}{\text{Denominator}} = \frac{8}{5} = 1 \text{ R3 (i.e., 1 with 3 left over)}$$

Step 2: Use the whole number obtained in Step 1 as the whole number of the mixed fraction:

$$\text{Whole number} = \text{Step 1 whole number} = 1$$

Step 3: Use the remainder (R) obtained in Step 1 as the numerator of the new fraction; use the original denominator as the new denominator:

$$\text{Fraction} = \frac{\text{Step 1 remainder}}{\text{Original denominator}} \frac{3}{5} = \frac{3}{5}$$

Step 4: Put the whole number and the fraction together to get the mixed number:

$$1 \text{ and } \frac{3}{5} = 1\frac{3}{5}$$

Thus, the improper fraction $\frac{8}{5}$ is the same as the mixed number $1\frac{3}{5}$.

If you multiply or divide the numerator and the denominator of a fraction by the same nonzero number, you get an equivalent fraction.

Example

$$\frac{3}{4} = \frac{3 \times 2}{4 \times 2} = \frac{6}{8}$$

$$\frac{6}{8} = \frac{6 \div 2}{8 \div 2} = \frac{3}{4}$$

Thus, $\frac{3}{4}$ and $\frac{6}{8}$ are equivalent fractions.

A fraction is in its *lowest terms* when no nonzero number except 1 can be evenly divided into both the numerator and the denominator. Reducing fractions to their lowest terms is *always* the last step in mathematical problem solving.

Example

In the fraction $\frac{10}{12}$ both the numerator and the denominator can be evenly divided by 2. When this is accomplished, the resulting fraction, $\frac{5}{6}$, is an equivalent fraction to the original and also its lowest terms.

Addition and Subtraction of Fractions

To add (or subtract) fractions whose denominators are the same, just add (or subtract) the numerators and keep the denominators the same.

Examples

$$\frac{2}{5} + \frac{1}{5} = \frac{2+1}{5} = \frac{3}{5} \quad \frac{2}{5} - \frac{1}{5} = \frac{2-1}{5} = \frac{1}{5}$$

To add (or subtract) fractions whose denominators are not the same, first convert the fractions to equivalent fractions with the lowest common denominators, then add (or subtract) the numerators. This can be done in three steps. Given the problem $\frac{1}{2} + \frac{1}{3} = ?$,

Step 1: Find the lowest common denominator of $\frac{1}{2}$ and $\frac{1}{3}$. The lowest number divisible by both 2 and 3 is 6, so 6 is the lowest common denominator.

Step 2: Change the fractions to equivalent fractions using 6 as the new denominator:

$$\frac{1}{2} = \frac{1 \times 3}{2 \times 3} = \frac{3}{6}$$

and

$$\frac{1}{3} = \frac{1 \times 2}{3 \times 2} = \frac{2}{6}$$

Step 3: Now perform your operation, and add the two new fractions because they have the same denominators (remember to always reduce to lowest terms):

$$\frac{3}{6} + \frac{2}{6} = \frac{5}{6}$$

In this example, $\frac{5}{6}$ is in lowest terms.

Example

$$\frac{1}{2} - \frac{1}{3} = \frac{3}{6} - \frac{2}{6} = \frac{1}{6}$$

$$\frac{3}{4} + \frac{1}{8} = \frac{6}{8} + \frac{1}{8} = \frac{7}{8}$$

To add (or subtract) mixed numbers, convert the mixed numbers to improper fractions, find the lowest common denominator, and add (or subtract) as usual. Then convert the answer, if it is an improper fraction, to a mixed number. This can be done in four steps.

Given the problem $4\frac{2}{3} + 1\frac{1}{6} = ?$,

Step 1: Convert the mixed numbers to improper fractions.

$$4\frac{2}{3} = \frac{14}{3} \text{ and } 1\frac{1}{6} = \frac{7}{6}$$

Step 2: Find the lowest common denominator of $\frac{14}{3}$ and $\frac{7}{6}$. The lowest number divisible by both 3 and 6 is 6, so 6 is the lowest common denominator.

Step 3: Change the fractions to equivalent fractions using 6 as the new denominator.

$$\frac{14}{3} = \frac{14 \times 2}{3 \times 2} = \frac{28}{6} \text{ and } 7/6 \text{ already has 6 as its denominator.}$$

Step 4: Now perform your operation, and add the two new fractions because they have the same denominators (and convert back to a mixed number because that is the lowest term for this fraction):

$$\frac{28}{6} + \frac{7}{6} = \frac{28 + 7}{6} = \frac{35}{6} = 5\frac{5}{6}$$

Examples

$$6\frac{3}{4} - 2\frac{1}{3} = \frac{27}{4} - \frac{7}{3} = \frac{81}{12} - \frac{28}{12} = \frac{53}{12} = 4\frac{5}{12}$$

$$2\frac{1}{5} + 2\frac{1}{10} = \frac{11}{5} + \frac{21}{10} = \frac{22}{10} + \frac{21}{10} = \frac{43}{10} = 4\frac{3}{10}$$

Multiplication and Division of Fractions

To multiply two fractions, multiply the numerators by the numerators and the denominators by the denominators. The results are the new fraction/answer. Remember to always reduce to lowest terms.

Examples

$$\frac{2}{3} \times \frac{1}{4} = \frac{2 \times 1}{3 \times 4} = \frac{2}{12} = \frac{1}{6}$$

$$\frac{1}{7} \times \frac{1}{8} = \frac{1 \times 1}{7 \times 8} = \frac{1}{56}$$

To divide two fractions, invert the divisor, then multiply.

Examples

$$\frac{1}{5} \div \frac{3}{8} = \frac{1}{5} \times \frac{8}{3} = \frac{8}{15}$$

$$\frac{5}{12} \div \frac{1}{3} = \frac{5}{12} \times \frac{3}{1} = \frac{15}{12} = 1\frac{3}{12} = 1\frac{1}{4}$$

NOTE: To remember the rule for division of fractions:
The number you are dividing by
Turn upside down and multiply.

To multiply or divide mixed numbers, first convert them to improper fractions, then multiply or divide.

Examples

$$1\frac{1}{4} \times 2\frac{1}{8} = \frac{5}{4} \times \frac{17}{8}$$
$$= \frac{85}{32}$$
$$= 2\frac{21}{32}$$

$$3\frac{1}{3} \div \frac{2}{12} = \frac{10}{3} \div \frac{2}{12}$$
$$= \frac{10}{3} \times \frac{12}{2}$$
$$= \frac{120}{6}$$
$$= 20$$

DECIMALS

Decimal numbers are written by placing digits (0, 1, 2, 3, 4, 5, 6, 7, 8, 9) into place value columns that are separated by a decimal point, as shown in Table 3.2. The place value columns are read in sequence from left to right as multiples of decreasing powers of 10:

- Numbers to the left of the decimal point represent values greater than 1.
- Numbers to the right of the decimal point represent values less than 1.
- The number sequence is added.
  The number 652.345 is represented as:

			decimal point
hundreds	tens	ones	↓
(6×100) +	(5×10) +	(2×1)	●
600 +	50 +	2	●
tenths	hundredths	thousandths	
$(3 \times 1/10)$ +	$(4 \times 1/100)$ +	$(5 \times 1/1000)$	
3/10 +	4/100 +	5/1000	

NOTE: Notice that each place value is a power of 10. This can also be written using **exponents**. These are shortcuts to show multiplication of a number times itself. For example, 10×10 can be written as 10^2. Any number with an exponent of 0 is equal to one. So, $10^0 = 1$. The above-mentioned multiples of 10 can be written as:

$$(6 \times 10^2) + (5 \times 10^1) + (2 \times 10^0) + (3 \times 10^{-1}) +$$
$$(4 \times 10^{-2}) + (5 \times 10^{-3})$$

TABLE 3.2   Decimal Place Values

Ten thousands			10^4
Thousands			10^3
Hundreds			10^2
Tens			10^1
Ones			10^0
Decimal point			
Tenths			10^{-1}
Hundredths			10^{-2}
Thousandths			10^{-3}
Ten thousandths			10^{-4}
Hundred thousandths			10^{-5}
Millionths			10^{-6}
or			
Ten thousands	10,000.	=	10^4
Thousands	1000.	=	10^3
Hundreds	100.	=	10^2
Tens	10.	=	10^1
Ones	1.	=	10^0
Decimal point	.	=	
Tenths	0.1	=	10^{-1}
Hundredths	0.01	=	10^{-2}
Thousandths	0.001	=	10^{-3}
Ten thousandths	0.000 1	=	10^{-4}
Hundred thousandths	0.000 01	=	10^{-5}
Millionths	0.000 001	=	10^{-6}

Remember:

$$10^2 = 10 \times 10 \text{ or } 100$$
$$10^1 = 10$$
$$10^0 = 1$$
$$10^{-1} = 1/10$$
$$10^{-2} = 1/100$$

The decimal 652.345 can be read as "six-hundred fifty-two point three four five." It can also be read as "six-hundred fifty-two and three-hundred forty-five thousandths." Notice that:
- The word "and" is used for the decimal point.
- The decimal fraction is named for the rightmost place in the place column sequence.
- The suffix "-th" is used to signify fractions.

Examples

5.45 is read as five "and" forty-five hundredths

7.0 is read as seven or seven "and" 0 tenths

The **relative value** of a decimal number is determined by looking at the spaces to the left of the decimal point. The more spaces, the higher the value. When comparing two decimal numbers with the same spaces to the left of the decimal point, the first place where they differ determines the relative value of each number. To compare decimal numbers, write the numbers with each decimal point aligned. For example, compare 45.67 and 46.78.

Examples

Write   4**5**.67
           4**6**.78

Begin with the numbers to the left of the decimal and compare. In these numbers, 6 is larger than 5. As the larger number determines the higher value, 4**6**.78 is larger than 4**5**.67.

Compare 45.67 and 45.78. Now both numbers to the left of the decimal point are the same. So, we must look at the numbers to the right of the decimal point.

Write: 45.**6**7
          45.**7**8

Begin with the numbers to the right of the decimal point and compare. In these numbers, 7 is larger than 6. As the larger number again determines the higher value, 45.**7**8 is larger than 45.**6**7.

❓ QUICK QUESTION

Which decimal has the higher value: 0.6, 0.66, or 0.62?
Refer to the relative value explanation on the previous page.

Addition and Subtraction of Decimals

To add or subtract decimal numbers, line up the decimal points and carry out the calculations.

Examples

24.531 + 2.798 =

     ↙ — align the decimal points

    24.531
     2.798
   ‾‾‾‾‾‾‾
    27.329

5.04 − 1.213 =

     5.040 ← add a zero as a place holder
   − 1.213
   ‾‾‾‾‾‾‾
     3.827

NOTE: Adding zeros to the right of a number on the right side of the decimal point does not change its value. Adding zeros to the left of a number on the left side of the decimal point does not change its value. This practice is used when adding, subtracting, multiplying, and dividing decimals. However, The Joint Commission has stated in the "Do Not Use" abbreviation list that a trailing zero may be used only when required to demonstrate the level of precision of the value being reported, such as for laboratory results, imaging studies that report size of legions, or catheter/tube sizes. It may not be used in medication orders or other medication-related documentation.

Multiplication and Division of Decimals

To multiply two decimals, carry out the multiplication, then add the number of decimal places from the right of the decimal point in the original two numbers. This total is the number of decimal places from the right of the decimal point in the product (answer).

Examples

```
   0.07        2 decimal places
 × 2.1        +1 decimal places
  007
  014
 0.147         3 decimal places
```

```
  0.00051       5 decimal places
 ×   0.04      +2 decimal places
 0.0000204      7 decimal places
                add zeros
```

To divide decimals by whole numbers, carry out the long division. Align the decimal point of the quotient directly above that of the dividend.

Examples

```
    3.09
 5) 15.45
    15
    45
    45
     0
```

```
    3.3
 3) 9.9
    9
    9
    9
    0
```

If the divisor is a decimal, convert it to a whole number before dividing. To do this, move the decimal point of the divisor and that of the dividend the same number of places to the right.

Examples

```
            2.5
2.5) 6.25  =  25.) 62.5
              50
              125
              125
                0
```
Divisor ——▼ ┌─┐ ▼—— Whole number
One place value
(1) 2.5 × 10 = 25
(2) 6.25 × 10 = 62.5
Dividend ——↑

```
            20.
.25) 5  =  25.) 500.
            50
            00
```
Divisor ——▼ ┌─┐ ▼—— Whole number
Two place values
(1) .25 × 100 = 25
(2) 5 × 100 = 500
Dividend ——↑

When more than one operation (addition, subtraction, multiplication, division, exponents) must be carried out, use the order of operations:

Parentheses

Exponents

Multiplication

Division

Addition

Subtraction

? MAKE IT SIMPLE

To remember the order of operations, use the phrase, "Please excuse my dear Aunt Sally," or the initials PEMDAS.

To convert fractions to decimals, divide the numerator by the denominator.

Examples

```
        0.25
1/4 = 4) 1.00
        8
        20
        20
         0
```

```
        0.666...
2/3 = 3) 2.0000    = 0.6̄6̄
        1 8
        20
        18
        20
```

NOTE: When the answer is a nonterminating repeating number, you may signify this with a line over the repeating numerals.

To convert decimals to fractions, the decimal numeral expressed becomes the numerator and the decimal place (tenth, hundredths) becomes the denominator.

Examples

0.95   95 is the decimal expressed and becomes the numerator. 1/100 or hundredths is the decimal place expressed and becomes the denominator

thus $0.95 = \dfrac{95}{100}$

0.05   05 is the decimal expressed and becomes the numerator. 1/100 or hundredths is the decimal place expressed and becomes the denominator

thus $0.05 = \dfrac{5}{100} = \dfrac{1}{20}$ (always reduce to lowest terms)

NOTE: To round to the nearest tenth, carry the division out to the next decimal value after tenths, which is hundredths. If this number is 5 or greater, round the number in tenths up. If this number is less than 5, the number in tenths place remains the same.

To compare the values of two or more decimals to determine which is larger (or smaller), place the decimals in a column and align the decimal points. Fill in with zeros to the *right* of the decimal point so all decimals have the same number of digits. The larger decimal will have the largest digit in the greatest column (the decimal place farthest left).

Examples

Compare 0.000350 and 0.000082.

0.000350

0.000082

Align them with equal numbers of digits. Because the 3 is in the ten-thousandths place and the 8 is in the hundredth-thousandths place, the 3 is larger. Thus 0.000350 is the larger decimal.

Compare 0.012 and 0.0045.

0.0120

0.0045

Align them with equal numbers of digits. Because the 1 is in the hundredths place and the 4 is in the thousandths place, the 1 is larger. Thus 0.012 is the larger decimal.

PERCENTAGES

Percentages are special types of fractions that mean "per every hundred." Thus the denominator of a percentage is always understood to be 100 and is shown by the symbol % rather than being written.

A percentage can be written as a fraction by putting the number expressed as the numerator and the denominator as 100. It can be written as a decimal by putting down the number expressed and moving the decimal point two places to the left, thus signifying hundredths.

 MAKE IT SIMPLE

It is easier to calculate percentages if they are first converted to fractions or decimals.

Examples

$25\% = \dfrac{25}{100}$ or $\dfrac{1}{4}$

$25\% = 0.25$

$56\% = \dfrac{56}{100} = \dfrac{14}{25}$

$56\% = 0.56$

In other words, when you drop the % sign, either replace it with a denominator of 100 or a decimal place of hundredths. When you add the % sign, either drop the denominator of 100 or move the decimal point two places to the right.

Examples

$0.33 = 33\%$

$0.33 = 33/100$

$0.17 = 17\%$

$0.17 = 17/100$

To find the percent of a number, change the percent to a decimal or fraction, replace the "of" with the times (×) sign, and multiply.

Examples

10% of 100

$= 0.10 \times 100 = 10$

or 0.10 can be expressed as 10/100, which is reduced to 1/10 × 100 = 10

50% of 10

$= 0.50 \times 10 = 5$

or 0.50 can be expressed as 50/100, which is reduced to 1/2 × 10 = 5

Try these:

9 is what percent of 27?

$\dfrac{9}{27} = \dfrac{1}{3} = 0.333$ or 33.3%

5 is what percent of 25?

$\dfrac{5}{25} = \dfrac{1}{5} = 0.20 = 20\%$

Table 3.3 lists common fractions, decimals, and percentages.

RATIO AND PROPORTION

A ratio is a comparison of two numbers, *a* and *b*, expressed as:

$$\text{a:b or a/b or } \dfrac{a}{b}$$

Examples

A two-to-one ratio is expressed as:

$$2\!:\!1 \text{ or } 2/1 \text{ or } \dfrac{2}{1}$$

A one-to-one thousand ratio is expressed as:

$$1\!:\!1000 \text{ or } 1/1000 \text{ or } \dfrac{1}{1000}$$

A **proportion** is a statement of equality between ratios: *a/b = c/d or a:b = c:d*. See Insight 3.1 for more on ratios. In any proportion, the product of the means must equal the product of the extremes:

$$a \times d = b \times c$$

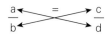 where a and d are the extremes and b and c are the means

or

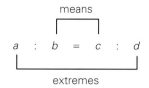

INSIGHT 3.1 Ratios Used in Surgery

You will see a ratio expressed on a split-thickness skin graft procedure with the skin graft mesher. The mesher uses plates or special rollers to cut "slits" into the donor skin graft. This meshing allows the graft to be enlarged when it is stretched. The graft can then cover a greater area of the recipient site, and epithelial tissue will grow in between the slits. Mesher plates are available in a variety of expansion ratios, such as 1:2, 1:3, and even 1:9.

TABLE 3.3 Common Fractions, Decimals, and Percentages

Fraction	Decimal	Percentage (%)
$\frac{1}{2}$	0.5	50
$\frac{1}{4}$	0.25	25
$\frac{3}{4}$	0.75	75
$\frac{1}{3}$	0.333[a]	$33\frac{1}{3}$
$\frac{2}{3}$	0.666[a]	$66\frac{2}{3}$
$\frac{1}{5}$	0.2	20
$\frac{2}{5}$	0.4	40
$\frac{3}{5}$	0.6	60
$\frac{4}{5}$	0.8	80
$\frac{1}{10}$	0.1	10
$\frac{1}{1}$	1.0	100

[a]0.333 and 0.666 are nonterminating decimals. This means the number patterns 0.333 and 0.666 go on forever.

Examples

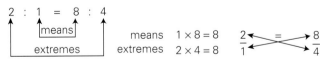

$$2 : 1 = 8 : 4$$

means: $1 \times 8 = 8$
extremes: $2 \times 4 = 8$

$$\frac{2}{1} \times\!\!\!\!\!\times \frac{8}{4}$$

Proportions can be used to solve for an unknown term when the other three terms are known. This can be done in four steps:

Step 1: Let x be the unknown.

Step 2: Set up the proportion with the terms that are given (known).

Step 3: Multiply the means and the extremes.

Step 4: Solve for x.

Examples

Given $2:3 = x:9$, what is x?

$\dfrac{2}{3} = \dfrac{x}{9}$ Let x be the unknown, set up the proportion

$3x = 2 \times 9$ Multiply the means and the extremes

$3x = 18$

$x = 18/3$ Divide both sides of the proportion by the same number (3) in order to have x alone on one side

$x = 6$ Answer

Given $4:16 = 1:x$

$\dfrac{4}{16} = \dfrac{1}{x}$ Let x be the unknown, set up the proportion

$1 \times 16 = 4x$ Multiply the means and the extremes

$16 = 4x$ Divide both sides of the proportion by the same number (4) in order to have x alone on one side

$4 = x$ Answer

You can use ratios and proportions to calculate the quantities of medications. To do this, you must know that strength is a ratio—it is always expressed as units of substance per unit or units of volume—for example, the strength of meperidine (Demerol) may be 100 mg of meperidine per 1 mL of solution. And sometimes we express strength per hundred units of another substance. For example, a 5% saline solution is 5 g of sodium chloride (NaCl) per 100 g of water.

> **NOTE:** One cubic centimeter of water weighs 1 g, so a 5% solution of saline is also 5 g/cc.

Example

The physician prescribed 50 mg of Demerol. The Demerol solution that the anesthesia provider has is a strength of 100 mg/mL. How many milliliters of that solution are needed?

This relationship can be expressed in the proportion $100:1 = 50:x$, or

$\dfrac{100 \text{ milligrams}}{1 \text{ milliliter}} = \dfrac{50 \text{ milligrams}}{x \text{ milliliter}}$ x is the unknown amount of solution needed, set up the proportion

$100 \times x = 50 \times 1$ Multiply the means and the extremes

$100x = 50$ Solve for x by dividing both sides of the proportion by 100 so x stands alone on one side

$x = 50/100$ or $\dfrac{1}{2}$ milliliter   Answer

You can also use proportions to solve other calculation problems. For example, the physician will be giving the patient medications that are prescribed according to weight in kilograms (kg). You know the patient weighs 150 pounds (lb), but how many kilograms is this?

First, you must know three parts of the proportion, so you research and find that 1 kg is equal to 2.2 lbs.

This relationship can be expressed in the proportion 1:2.2 = x:150

$$\frac{1 \text{ kg}}{2.2 \text{ lbs}} = \frac{x \text{ kg}}{150 \text{ lbs}}$$ x is the unknown, and set up the proportion

$1 \times 150 = x \times 2.2$ Multiply the means and the extremes

$150 = 2.2x$ Divide both sides of the proportion by 2.2 to leave x alone on one side

$x = 68.18$ kg   Answer

Sometimes we can think of ratios in terms of parts of a whole. In this case, it is easy to think about percentages.

Example

You want to make up a 3:3:4 solution of saline, Lincocin, and Gentamicin. (1) What percentage of the solution does each ingredient represent? (2) If you wanted to make up 200 mL of this solution, how many milliliters of saline would you use? Of Lincocin? Of Gentamicin?

(a) A 3:3:4 solution means that there are three parts to three parts to four parts (i.e., you need a total of 3 + 3 + 4 = 10 parts of whole solution).

By convention, the parts are listed in the same order as the ingredients, so you have:

3 parts of saline in 10 parts of solution = 3/10 = 30/100 = 30%

3 parts of Lincocin in 10 parts of solution = 3/10 = 30/100 = 30%

4 parts of Gentamicin in 10 parts of solution = 4/10 = 40/100 = 40%

Total parts of solution = 100%

(b) You want 200 mL of solution, so you multiply each ingredient's percentage by 200:

Saline (30%) 0.30 × 200 mL = 60 mL

Lincocin (30%) 0.30 × 200 mL = 60 mL

Gentamicin (40%) 0.40 × 200 mL = 80 mL

Total = 200 mL

You want to make up a 1:1:3 solution of saline, antibiotic A, and antibiotic B, respectively. What percentage of the solution does each ingredient represent?

1:1:3 solution means one part to two parts to three parts. That is:

1 + 1 + 3 = 5 total parts in the solution

The parts are listed in the same order as the ingredients, so you have:

1 part of saline in 5 parts of solution = 1/5 = 20/100 = 20%

1 part of antibiotic A in 5 parts of solution = 1/5 = 20/100 = 20%

3 parts of antibiotic B in 5 parts of solution = 3/5 = 60/100 = 60%

Total parts of solution = 100%

Another way to use proportions for calculations is to use the standard dilution equation. This is expressed as

$$\frac{C_1}{C_2} = \frac{V_2}{V_1} \text{ or } C_1 \times V_1 = C_2 \times V_2$$

where C stands for concentration in percent and V stands for volume. Thus

C_1 = concentration 1

C_2 = concentration 2

V_1 = volume 1

V_2 = volume 2

Example

The procedure calls for 60 cc of 1/2% contrast media. How much saline and how much contrast media do you need to make the required amount of solution when you have 1%?

In this problem, you are being asked for a dilution, so you start by sorting out what you know from what you do not know:

$C_1 = \dfrac{1}{2}$ or .5% asked for contrast media

$C_2 = 1\%$ have on hand contrast media

$V_1 = 60$ asked for volume

$V_2 = x$ unknown volume of saline (solve this unknown first)

Now you can write the standard dilution equation as:

$$C_1 \times V_1 = C_2 \times V_2$$
$$\frac{1}{2} \times 60 = 1 \times x$$
$$30 = x$$
$$x = 30 \text{ cc of saline is needed}$$

But we are not finished with the problem. It also asks how much of the 1% contrast media we need. If you add 30 cc of saline and the total amount you want is 60 cc, that means that 60 − 30 cc = 30 cc of the 1% contrast media is needed.

TEMPERATURE CONVERSIONS

In medicine, we use two scales to measure temperature (Fig. 3.4): the Fahrenheit scale and Celsius (centigrade) scale. In the Fahrenheit scale, the boiling point of water is 212 °F and its freezing point is 32 °F. In the Celsius scale the boiling point of water is 100°C and its freezing point is 0°C. Nine degrees on the Fahrenheit scale corresponds to 5° on the Celsius scale. Using these ratios, the following formulas (Table 3.4) were developed to convert temperatures from one scale to the other.

$$C = 5 / 9 \left(F - 32 \right)$$

$$F = \left(9 / 5C \right) + 32$$

where C is the Celsius temperature and F is the Fahrenheit temperature.

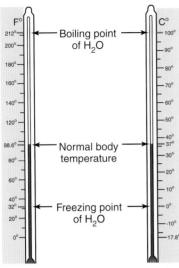

Fig. 3.4 Fahrenheit and Celsius scales.

TABLE 3.4 Temperature Conversions

To Convert From	Use the Formula	Operation Means
Fahrenheit to Celsius	$C = \dfrac{5}{9}(F - 32)$	1. Subtract 32 from the Fahrenheit temperature 2. Multiply this number by 5/9
Celsius to Fahrenheit	$F = \dfrac{9}{5}C + 32$	1. Multiply the Celsius temperature by 9/5 2. Add 32 to the result

QUICK QUESTION

Your temperature is 40°C. Use this value in the correct formula to see if you have a fever, as $F = (9/5 \times 40/1) + 32$. What is your temperature in degrees Fahrenheit?

Temperature is important in many aspects of the surgical setting, and readings may be given in Fahrenheit or Celsius degrees. The surgical patient's body temperature is of vital importance and is constantly monitored. Normal body temperature is 98.6 °F or 37°C. Preoperatively, an elevated temperature could signify an infection or other health problem. This could result in the postponement of the surgical procedure. Intraoperatively, the body temperature is monitored by anesthesia personnel. An abnormal body temperature—whether below normal (*hypothermia*) or elevated (*hyperthermia*)—alters the basal metabolic rate, interfering with blood pressure, heart rate, circulation, and so on. Hyperthermia can also indicate life-threatening situations, such as malignant hyperthermia (see Chapter 15). Postoperatively, temperature is monitored for the same reasons, and an elevated temperature at this time may indicate a wound infection. Another surgical aspect of temperature is the sterilization of instruments and equipment. Here, temperature along with pressure and time is monitored for proper sterilization. Temperature is also important for the surgical environment. Each surgical room is kept at 68 °F to 75 °F

(20°C–24°C) to discourage the growth of bacteria that can cause surgical site infections. It is also important to keep the room at this temperature range for the comfort of surgical personnel who are working under surgical lights attired in full scrub apparel. A cool environment decreases the chance that perspiration will drip from a surgical team member onto the sterile field.

? MAKE IT SIMPLE

To assist your understanding of temperature in the Celsius scale, remember this: 30 is warm, 20 is nice, 10 is cold, and 0 is ice.

NOTE: Temperature of	F	C
Boiling water	212°	100°
Normal body temperature	98.6°	37°
Freezing point of water	32°	0°

MEASUREMENT SYSTEMS

Although the surgical technologist does not administer medications directly to the patient, the technologist is responsible for obtaining medicines and mixing them for use in the sterile field. For example, you may have to mix antibiotics in an irrigation solution. This may require you to calculate measurements and perform some conversions. Therefore, you will need to know conversion equivalents and be able to perform the calculations involved in such conversions.

The metric system of measurement is the most commonly used in medicine. However, the surgical technologist should be familiar with other systems. They include the apothecary and household systems and measurements of some medications that are based on their strengths.

The Metric System

The metric system (also called the *International System*) is the international standard of weights and measures used by more than 90% of developed countries. Introduced by the French in the 18th century, today it is the preferred system for prescribing and administering medications. It is also used extensively in the healthcare field. For example, the *United States Pharmacopeia* uses it exclusively, and all specimens sent to pathology are weighed and measured in metric terms. The metric system allows a way to calculate small drug dosages, and most manufacturers use this system for calibration in the development of new drugs. Most medications used in surgery are dispensed using the metric system of measurement.

In the metric system, length, volume, and weight (mass) are measured against certain defined units called *base units*:

Length—the *meter* (m)
Volume—the *liter* (L)
Weight—the *gram* (g)

Each of these base units is divided into smaller and larger units based on multiples of 10, and these multiples are indicated by prefixes (Table 3.5).

Any prefix can be used with any base unit to indicate a measurement. For example, 1 **mm** = 0.001 m, 1 **mL** = 0.001 L, and 1 **mg** = 0.001 g; similarly, 1 **km** = 1000 m, 1 **kL** = 1000 L, and 1 **kg** = 1000 g. However, you will be most concerned with only a few of them—particularly "micro-," "milli-," and "centi-."

Because metric is based on the decimal system, conversions are very easy. You just have to recognize the correct multiple of 10. Then you can use the appropriate unit conversion (Table 3.6). To convert within the metric system, you can move the decimal point to the right or left, depending on converting from smaller to larger (or larger to smaller) units (Fig. 3.5).

Metric Comparisons

The meter is approximately 39.37 inches, just over a yard (36 inches). It is a linear measure used for lengths, including heights and widths. For example, patient height is measured in meters, whereas tumors, flaps, and defects are measured as lengths and widths—usually in centimeters or millimeters (hundredths or thousandths of meters). Note that when a length measure is multiplied by another length measure, the result is an area, which is a *square measure*. For example, a defect that is 10 cm by 5 cm has an area of 5 × 10 = 50 cm².

The meter is related to volume by *cubic measure*. When 1 cm is multiplied by itself 3 times—1 cm × 1 cm × 1 cm—it becomes the volume 1 cc (1 cm³), which is approximately the same size as a sugar cube. When length, width, and height (or depth) are multiplied together, the result is measured in cubic terms. Thus, a block of tissue that is 5 cm long, 3 cm wide, and 1 cm deep is 5 × 3 × 1 = 15 cm³.

The liter is a fluid (or liquid) measure approximately equal to a quart (1 L = 1.06 qt). Most medicines in surgery are in liquid form, including intravenous and irrigation solutions (often measured in liters), and many antibiotic solutions (usually measured in milliliters or thousandths of liters). However, in medicine we call a cm³ a "cc" (short for cubic centimeter, of course). This liquid measure of volume is related to the solid measure by one simple definition: 1 cc = 1 cm³ = 1 mL. In surgery, the liquid measure used comes from the metric system as liters (L) and milliliters (mL). These measurements are seen on intravenous bags and medication labels. The abbreviation "mL" is safer to use than "cc" because "cc" can be confused with other abbreviations such as "u" or "00."

TABLE 3.5 Metric Prefixes

Prefix (Abbreviation)	Multiply Base Unit by
micro (μ)	0.000001 (or 1/1,000,000)
milli (m)	0.001 (or 1/1000)
centi (c)	0.01 (or 1/100)
deci (d)	0.1 (or 1/10)
Unit	Meter, liter, gram
deka (da)	10
hecto (h)	100
kilo (k)	1000

TECH TIP

The term *cc* is often used verbally in surgery when referring to amounts of irrigation solution, such as "We used 400 ccs of irrigation," or when asking for equipment, such as a "10-cc syringe."

The gram is a small unit of mass (or weight), which is much less than an ounce (30 g is approximately 1 oz). For a mental picture, consider a paper clip; it weighs approximately a gram. In this case, it is easier to think in terms of kilograms. One kilogram is 2.2 lb (picture a 2-lb can of coffee). It is worth knowing that 1 cc (1 mL) of water weighs 1g, which means that aqueous solutions measured in weight percentage (g/100 g) can also be reckoned in grams per milliliter of solution. You will encounter gram or milligram measures when working with drugs in

TABLE 3.6 Unit Conversions

Unit Conversion

Length
1 meter = 1000 millimeters	1 m/1000 mm = 1	or	1000 mm/1 m = 1
1 meter = 100 centimeters	1 m/100 cm = 1	or	100 cm/1 m = 1
1 meter = 1,000,000 micrometers (microns)	1 m/1,000,000 μm = 1	or	1,000,000 μg/1 m = 1
1 millimeter = 1000 micrometers (microns)	1 mm/1000 μm = 1	or	1000 μg/1 mm = 1

Volume
1 liter = 1000 milliliters	1 L/1000 mL = 1	or	1000 mL/1 L = 1
1 kiloliter = 1000 liters	1 kL/1000 L = 1	or	1000 L/1 kL = 1

Weight (Mass)
1 gram = 1000 milligrams	1 g/1000 mg = 1	or	1000 mg/1 g = 1
1 gram = 1,000,000 micrograms	1 g/1,000,000 μg = 1	or	1,000,000 μg/1 g = 1
1 milligram = 1000 micrograms	1 mg/1000 μg = 1	or	1000 μg/1 mg = 1
1 kilogram = 1000 grams	1 kg/1000 g = 1	or	1000 g/1 kg = 1

Additional options for converting within the metric system

kilo	hecto	deka	unit	deci	centi	milli	X	X	micro
1000.	100.	10.	1	.1	.01	.001	.0001	.00001	.00001

→

When converting from larger units to smaller units (such as L to mL) – move to the right

←

When converting from smaller units to larger units (such as mL to L) – move to the left

Or just memorize the most often used conversions in surgery

Volume	mL to L	Move decimal 3 to the left as: 5000.0 mL = 5.0 L
	L to mL	Move decimal 3 to the right as: 3.0 L = 3000.0 mL
Length	cm to mm	Move decimal 1 to the right as: 6.0 cm = 60.0 mm
	mm to cm	Move decimal 1 to the left as: 200.0 mm = 20.0 cm
Weight	kg to g	Move decimal 3 to the right as: 11.0 kg = 11,000.0 g
	kg to mg	Move decimal 6 to the right as: 0.1234 kg = 12,3400.0 mg
	g to kg	Move decimal 3 to the left as: 1973.0 g = 1.973 kg
	g to mg	Move decimal 3 to the right as: 7.0 g = 7000.0 mg
	mg to kg	Move decimal 6 to the left as: 54,321.0 mg = 0.054321 kg
	mg to g	Move decimal 3 to the left as:17,010.0 mg = 17.010 g

Fig. 3.5 Metric system conversions.

powder form, such as antibiotics, that must be reconstituted (dissolved) in water.

NOTE: You will use kilogram measures when calculating dosages determined by body weight. It is important to be able to convert a patient's weight from pounds to kilograms. There are 2.2 lbs in 1 kg, so to convert pounds to kilograms, divide the weight by 2.2.

TECH TIP

One way to remember your pounds to kilograms conversion is to note you will weigh a lot less in the metric system. For example, a patient who weighs 143 lbs weighs only 65 kg. So, if your conversion comes out with the kilogram weight more than the pound weight, you know it is incorrect and you might have your conversion reversed.

QUICK QUESTION

Can you convert your weight from pounds to kilograms? Refer to the *Note* feature mentioned earlier.

The metric system is by far the most important measuring system in the world—and the most important to you. It lets you measure—and calculate with—small and large quantities of any kind without having to multiply by such ill-behaved conversion factors as 12 in/ft, 2 pints in a quart (and 4 quarts in a gallon), and 16 oz/lb. All you have to do is multiply and divide by 10, which is mostly a matter of moving the decimal point the correct number of places in the proper direction. Eventually, you will find yourself thinking in it. But if you are not already used to it, you will find it helpful to compare metric measures with common measures. For example, if you already know how long an inch is, you can easily picture that length as about 2.5 cm. Box 3.1 lists some of the more common equivalents, giving approximate conversions.

MAKE IT SIMPLE

One cubic centimeter is the amount of space occupied by 1 mL of liquid. Thus 1 cc = 1 mL (Fig. 3.6).

BOX 3.1 Approximate Measurement Equivalents

Weight
1 kilogram = 2.2 pounds
1 gram = 15 grains
1 ounce = 30 grams
1 grain = 60 milligrams

Volume
1 kiloliter = exactly 1000 liters
1 liter = approximately 1 quart
1 milliliter = 1 gram = 1 cubic centimeter
1 fluid ounce = 8 fluid drams = 30 milliliters
1 gallon = approximately 4 liters
1 pint = approximately 500 milliliters
1 quart = 2 pints = approximately 1000 milliliters
1 gallon = 4 quarts = approximately 4000 milliliters
1 teaspoon = 60 drops
1 minim = 1 drop

Length
1 meter = 39.37 inches = approximately 1 yard
1 yard = 3 feet = 36 inches
1 inch = 2.54 centimeters

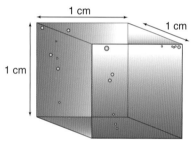

Fig. 3.6 A cubic centimeter filled with water (1 cc = 1 mL here).

INSIGHT 3.2 Apothecary and Household Systems of Weights and Measures

The apothecary system was the system of weights and measures used for writing medication orders in ancient Greece and Rome and in Europe during the Middle Ages. It is rarely used today. The apothecary system is based on everyday items (such as the weight of a grain of wheat) and uses lowercase Roman numerals. For example, 4 grains would be written as gr. Some medications continue to use this system, so the basic units of measure of the apothecary system are given:
Volume—the *minim* (fluid)
Weight—the *grain*
   A minim is approximately equal to one drop. (Because drops vary according to the dropper used, this measurement is not always accurate. For accuracy, a calibrated dropper should be used.) Larger quantities are multiples of the minim:
60 minims = 1 fluid dram
8 fluid drams = 1 fluid ounce
1 pint = 16 fluid ounces
2 pints = 1 quart
4 quarts = 1 gallon
   The grain was based on the average weight of a grain of wheat. Larger quantities are multiples of the grain:
20 grains (xx) = 1 scruple
3 scruples = 1 dram
60 grains = 1 dram
12 ounces = 1 pound
8 drams = 1 ounce
   Note that in the apothecary system 12 ounces equals 1 pound rather than 16 ounces (as in avoirdupois weight).
   Although household measurements are used primarily for administering over-the-counter medications—and never in surgery—it is useful to see how they compare with more accurate standard measures:
1 teaspoon = 5 milliliters = 5 cubic centimeters = 1 fluid dram
1 tablespoon = 1/2 fluid ounce = 4 fluid drams = 15 milliliters = 15 cubic centimeters
2 tablespoons = 1 fluid ounce = 30 milliliters = 30 cubic centimeters

The apothecary and household systems were used more in the past. It is not necessary to learn conversions from these measurement systems because medications are prepared and administered primarily from the metric system. These systems can be used for comparisons because they are more familiar until you are proficient with the metric system (Insight 3.2).

Fig. 3.7 shows measuring equipment used in surgery.

Other Standardized Measurements (Doses)

Some medications are measured directly by their strengths (i.e., they are measured in *units* based on their potency). A common medication measured in units is insulin. There are special insulin syringes calibrated to these units. In surgery, several antibiotics, including penicillin and bacitracin, are also measured in units. These medications are used in antibiotic irrigation solutions during surgical procedures (see Chapter 5). Other medications measured in units are those that affect coagulation. One is heparin, an anticoagulant administered intravenously to the patient by anesthesia personnel during vascular cases. Heparin is also used diluted in saline on the back table. Another is topical thrombin, a hemostatic agent, which comes

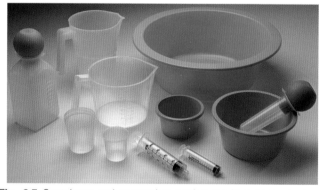

Fig. 3.7 Containers and measuring equipment in surgery, such as basins in various sizes, medicine cup, specimen cup, pitchers, and syringes. Courtesy Frank Pronesti T/A heirloomstudio.com.

in different strengths and preparations and is used to stop bleeding (see Chapter 9).

Other measurements used to indicate quantity of medicine prescribed are the international unit (IU) and the milliunit (mU). The international unit is used to measure vitamins and chemicals. The milliunit, which is one thousandth (.001 or

TABLE 3.7 Symbols of Measurement

Metric System

Meter	m
Liter	L
Centimeter	cm
Cubic centimeter	cc
Millimeter	mm
Gram	g
Kilogram	kg
Milligram	mg
Milliliter	mL
Kiloliter	kL
Microgram	µg
Micron (micrometer)	µm
Milliequivalent	mEq

Apothecary System

Minim	m, min, ℳ
Grain	gr
Dram	dr, ℨ
Fluid dram	fl dr, ℥
Drop	gtt
Ounce	oz
Pint	pt
Quart	qt
Gallon	gal
Pound	lb
Scruple	scr, ℈

Household System

Teaspoon	tsp
Tablespoon	tbsp
Ounce	oz
Pint	pt
Quart	qt
Gallon	gal
Inch	in
Yard	yd

As discussed in Chapter 2, some symbols are not being used with medication orders in an effort to decrease medication errors. However, the surgical technologist should be familiar with symbols because hospital policies vary on their use.

1/1000) of a unit, is used for dosages of oxytocin (Pitocin). Pitocin is used in childbirth to stimulate the uterus to contract (see Chapter 8). Another measurement of medications according to their strength is the *milliequivalent* (mEq). A milliequivalent is equal to 1/1000 (0.001) of a chemical equivalent, a measurement associated with electrolytes. Concentrations of electrolytes are often expressed as milliequivalents per liter. Electrolytes are essential for metabolic activities in the body and for normal function of body cells. A common electrolyte administered to the surgical patient is potassium chloride (KCl), which is necessary for the transmission of nerve impulses, control of heart rhythm, and fluid balance. Low potassium levels can pose a risk to the surgical patient undergoing general anesthesia. KCl is administered in milliequivalents preoperatively or by anesthesia personnel. See Table 3.7 for symbols of measurement.

KEY CONCEPTS

- Military time is used by hospitals and other medical institutions, and it uses a 24-hour scale without a.m. or p.m. designations.
- Surgical technologists may use fractions, decimals, and percentages, together with ratios and proportions, to solve problems and perform calculations and conversions.
- A fraction is a number that represents one or more equal parts of a whole and can be written as a quotient a/b.
- Fractions may be proper, improper, or expressed as mixed numbers.
- Decimals are numbers written by placing digits into value columns that are separated by a decimal point.
- Exponents are shortcuts to showing multiplication of a number times itself.
- Percentages are special types of fractions that mean "per every hundred" and are shown by the symbol %.
- A ratio is a comparison of two numbers expressed as $a{:}b$, a/b, or $\frac{a}{b}$.
- A proportion is a statement of equality between ratios expressed as $a{:}b = c{:}d$ or $a/b = c/d$.
- Two temperature scales are used in medicine, the Fahrenheit and Celsius.
- Conversion from one temperature scale to the other can be accomplished by using one of the following formulas: $C = 5/9(F - 32)$ or $F = 9/5\,C + 32$.
- The metric system is the international standard of weights and measures.
- In the metric system the base units are represented by length—meter, volume—liter, and weight—gram.
- Other measurements include medications measured by strength, such as units, international unit, milliunit, and milliequivalent.

▌ LEARNING THE LANGUAGE (KEY TERMS)

Using your textbook and/or a medical dictionary, look up and write the definitions of each term.

Celsius scale	metric system
civilian time	military time
decimal point	percentage
exponent	proportion
Fahrenheit scale	ratio
fraction	relative value

MATHEMATICAL EVALUATION PRETEST

The following test includes the various mathematical skills explained in this chapter. Take the test and compare your answers with those given at the end. If you have difficulty with some of the questions, review that section in the chapter to improve your skills.

1. Write 5:10 a.m. in military time. _____
2. Write 0010 in civilian time. _____
3. Write 1/10,000 as a decimal. _____
4. Write 3 5/8 as an improper fraction. _____
5. Write 50% as a fraction in lowest terms. _____
6. Write 35% as a decimal number. _____
7. Which decimal number is smaller, 0.151 or 0.251? _____
8. Write 7/10 ÷ 3/10 as a mixed number. _____
9. Write 5 3/4 ÷ 23 as a fraction and as a decimal. _____
10. Round 7.2235 to the nearest hundredth. _____
11. Write 3/8 as a decimal number. _____
12. Write an equivalent fraction for 5/9. _____
13. 2 3/4 + 3 1/8 = _____
14. 32 ÷ 0.5 = _____
15. 8.25 × 0.022 = _____
16. 0.655 − 0.011 = _____
17. Write 0.77 as a percentage. _____
18. 2:3 = 10:x, x = _____

19. Write 96 °F in Celsius. _____
20. Write 41°C in Fahrenheit. _____

Answers to Mathematical Evaluation Pretest:
1. 0510
2. 12:10 a.m.
3. 0.0001
4. 29/8
5. 1/2
6. 0.35
7. 0.151
8. 21/3
9. 1/4, 0.25
10. 7.22
11. 0.375
12. 10/18
13. 47/8
14. 64
15. 0.1815
16. 0.644
17. 77%
18. 15
19. 35.56
20. 107.6

REVIEW QUESTIONS

1. Explain the difference in calculating military and civilian times.
2. In the fraction 7/8:
   A. Which number represents the numerator?
   B. Which number represents the denominator?
   C. What type of fraction is this?
3. In the fractions 7/8 and 1/6, what is the least common denominator?
4. What is meant by "the order of operations"?
5. In the number 22.0453:
   A. What is the place value of 3?
   B. What is the place value of 5?
6. Complete the following sentences:
   A. The rule for division of fractions states "the number you are dividing by _____".
   B. Percentages are fractions that mean "per every _____".
   C. In a proportion, "the product of the means equals _____".
7. Explain why the metric system is the preferred measurement system.

CRITICAL THINKING

1. Why is military time "safer" to use in the medical setting?
2. Dr. Kim is giving his patient propofol (Diprivan). The dosage is 2 mg/kg of patient's weight. The patient weighs 176 lbs. How much of the medication is given?
3. The procedure calls for 50 cc of 1% contrast media. You have 25 cc of 2% contrast media. How much saline and how much of the 2% solution are mixed for the proper amount and strength of the required contrast media?
4. The patient's body temperature is 39°C. What is this in Fahrenheit degrees? Will the patient's elective surgical procedure be performed? Why or why not?

BIBLIOGRAPHY

Fulcher EM, Fulcher RM, Soto CD: *Pharmacology: principles and applications*, ed 3, St Louis, 2012, Saunders/Elsevier.
Johnston M: *Pharmacy Calculations: the pharmacy technician series*, Upper Saddle River, Pearson.
Key JL, Hayes ER, McCuistion LE: *Pharmacology: a patient-centered nursing process approach*, ed 4, St Louis, 2015, Saunders/Elsevier.
Olsen JL, Giangrasso AP, Shrimpton D, et al: *Medical dosage calculations*, ed 9, Upper Saddle River, 2007, Pearson/Prentice Hall.
Pickar GD, Abernethy AP, editors: *Dosage calculations*, ed 8, New York, 2008, Thompson Delmar.

INTERNET RESOURCES

AAA Math: www.aaamath.com.

Calculate Hours, Military time converter—Army time converter—24 hour clock converter: www.calculatehours.com/Military_Time_Converter.html.

Metric System, How to learn the metric system: https://themetricsystem.info/how-to-learn.

Space Archive, Military time: www.spacearchive.info/military.htm.

wikiHow: www.wikihow.com.

4

Medication Administration

OBJECTIVES

After completing this chapter, you should be able to do the following:

1. Define terms and abbreviations related to medication administration.
2. Identify the role of the surgical technologist in medication administration.
3. Explain the six "rights" of medication administration.
4. List and discuss the steps of medication identification used in surgery.
5. Explain aseptic techniques for delivery of medications to the sterile field.
6. Describe the procedure for labeling drugs on the sterile back table.
7. Discuss how to properly handle medications.
8. Identify supplies used in medication administration in surgery.
9. Discuss standard precautions and sharps safety in relation to medication administration.

OUTLINE

The role of the surgical technologist in medication administration varies from state to state and differs from facility to facility. As a surgical technologist, you should have firsthand knowledge of medication administration legislation in your state.

 TECH TIP

Do not depend on hearsay or someone else's understanding or opinion regarding the limits of your practice. Use your computer competence and the easy availability of the Internet to read the pertinent legislative statutes for yourself. Ask for assistance at your facility's medical library or from the reference librarian at any public library. Remember, professional surgical technologists should be highly knowledgeable regarding their own practice.

Institutional policies and procedures regarding medication handling and administration should be clearly understood as well. All staff members have a duty to know and adhere to established medication policies and procedures. Handling medications is a critical function in the surgical technologist's job description. Several different types of medications are obtained and passed to the surgeon routinely during a procedure, and the surgical technologist must be knowledgeable regarding such drugs.

NOTE: The limits of legal authority for the surgical technologist to perform the indicated roles described in this text are controlled by each state through its statutes, case law, regulatory law, attorney general opinions, and medical licensing boards. Discussion of these sources of law is beyond the scope of this text. Except as otherwise noted, this book describes the general practice of surgical technology in the United States, not the legal authority for such practice. It is the surgical technologists' responsibility to consult the limitations in their area on acts described in this book.

SURGICAL TECHNOLOGIST'S ROLES IN MEDICATION ADMINISTRATION

Administration of drugs from the sterile field is a team effort. Each team member has a particular role in the process (Box 4.1). Most commonly, medications used from the sterile field are obtained by the *circulator* (a nonsterile team member) and delivered to the *scrub person* (a sterile team member). The scrub person is responsible for passing the medication to the surgeon for administration during the surgical procedure. Each team member is responsible for accurately identifying all medications used from the sterile field during a surgical procedure.

Circulating Role

The surgical technologist in the circulating role obtains medications as specified on the surgeon's preference card, delivers those medications to the sterile field as needed, and documents the medications used from the sterile field during an operation. The circulator must be sure that the medication obtained is the exact drug and strength specified on the preference card. The circulator must also inspect the container for integrity and expiration date. The circulator must maintain strict sterile technique when transferring medications to the scrub person. All medications must be properly identified, both by the scrub and by the circulator. The circulator is responsible for documenting all medications used from the sterile field according to institutional policy.

Scrub Role

The surgical technologist in the scrub role correctly identifies and accepts medications from the circulator, immediately labels (Fig. 4.1) those medications, and passes medications to the surgeon, as requested. Accurate identification and immediate labeling of all drugs accepted onto the sterile field are crucial. If medications are not clearly identified, they should be discarded immediately, and a new dose should be obtained. This practice is essential to avoid possible drug administration error. The surgical technologist must clearly state the name and strength of a medication when passing it to the surgeon.

THE SIX "RIGHTS" OF MEDICATION ADMINISTRATION

The six "rights" of medication administration have been established to help avoid medication errors (Box 4.2). Team members must work together to ensure that the right drug is given in the right dose, by the right route, to the right patient, and at the right time. It is also important to ensure that all medications given are accurately documented.

Right Drug

Drugs that are routinely needed on the sterile field during a procedure should be clearly specified on the surgeon's preference card. The information is initially obtained directly from the surgeon and entered into the electronic preference card by a qualified member of the surgery department staff. Electronic preference cards are one component of computer software programs used in surgery, and the format may vary by institution. The information stated on the preference card must be accurate, including correct spelling and strength. If handwritten preference cards are used, information must be written legibly to avoid confusion. Preference cards should be updated, as needed, to reflect any changes in routine medications. Additional drugs are obtained in response to verbal orders by the surgeon, during the procedure.

In addition, some medications used in surgery, such as Depo-Medrol and Solu-Medrol (two brand names for methylprednisolone, see Chapter 8), are easily confused because they may sound similar. Other drugs may have similar spellings, such as Tobrex and TobraDex (see Chapter 10). The Institute

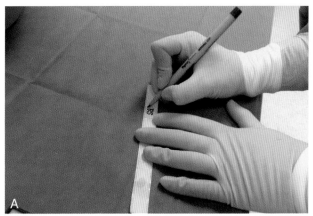 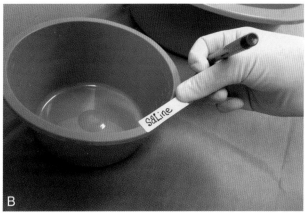

Fig. 4.1 (A) and (B) The scrubbed surgical technologist labels medications immediately.

for Safe Medication Practices maintains a list of confused drug names, which includes look-alike and sound-alike name pairs and serves as a resource for clinical practice. The surgical technologist must always clarify the name of the requested medication if there is any doubt.

When any medication is delivered to the sterile back table, it must be carefully identified by both the circulator and scrub and labeled immediately and accurately by the scrubbed surgical technologist. All medication containers must be labeled, including delivery container (such as a syringe) and intermediate containers (often a medicine cup or basin). Careful, mindful attention must be consistently practiced in the identification and labeling of drugs to prevent medication errors.

> **! CAUTION**
>
> When accepting a medication, especially an antibiotic or an iodine-based contrast medium, the scrubbed surgical technologist should ask the circulator if the patient has any medication allergies. This team effort helps to ensure that patients do not get a medication to which they are allergic.

Surgical technologists must always state the name and strength of the drug aloud as they hand it to the surgeon; this practice serves as confirmation that the medication is correct. The name of the drug should be spoken aloud even though the syringe (or other delivery container) is labeled. Using two processes, audible and visual, provides an additional level of patient safety. If there is ever *any* question as to the identity of a medication on the back table, it must be discarded and a new dose of the intended medication must be obtained, identified, and labeled.

Right Dose

The actual dose of a medication is a factor of both its amount (volume) and its strength (concentration), which is explained in more detail in Chapter 1 (see Insight 1.2). For example, you might see an order for 30 mL (amount) of 0.5% (strength) lidocaine with epinephrine 1 mg/mL (1:1000) on a surgeon's preference card. This information must be clearly specified and clearly understood. It is especially important when the drug must be mixed or diluted on the sterile back table. For example, suppose a surgeon requests 0.5 mL of 1% phenylephrine diluted in 20 mL of saline for vasoconstriction. Further suppose that 1% phenylephrine is available in 1-mL vials only. If the entire 1-mL vial (instead of the 0.5 mL specified) is mixed with the correct amount (20 mL) of saline and dispensed to the sterile field, the dosage of phenylephrine administered will be *twice* the desired dose.

> **! CAUTION**
>
> Always use a leading zero to accurately label medications in concentrations of less than 1%. For example, write "0.5% lidocaine" *not* ".5% lidocaine."

Written protocols may be instituted and posted to eliminate common confusions about some medications. Heparin (a systemic anticoagulant) is an excellent example of a medication

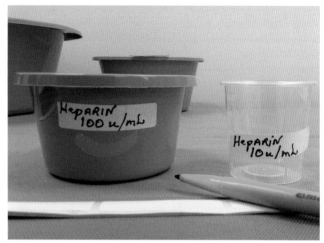

Fig. 4.2 When different strengths of heparin are needed from the sterile back table, immediate and clear labeling is crucial.

that is available in a number of different strengths in the same volume (see Chapter 9). During insertion of a venous access port, different strengths of heparin may be needed from the sterile back table: 100 units/mL and 10 units/mL may be used, each concentration with a specific purpose. Given the 10-fold difference in heparin concentration, immediate, accurate, and complete labeling is crucial (Fig. 4.2). In addition, the scrubbed surgical technologist must understand the reasons or purposes for the various strengths of heparin required to know which concentration to hand at the appropriate time. In this case, a department routine or protocol for heparin dosages in venous access procedures may be established and posted to minimize the potential for error.

The surgical technologist serves a key role in the prevention of administration of the wrong dosage of a medication from the sterile field. In addition to ensuring correct identification and labeling, the scrubbed surgical technologist provides the final safety check for intended dosage by stating out loud and clearly the name and strength of the medication, as it is handed to the surgeon.

Right Route

Most medications administered in surgery are given intravenously, usually by the anesthesia care provider. However, many other medications may be injected or applied topically by the surgeon at the surgical site. Different administration routes may require different preparations and concentrations of a medication. The preference card should clearly state administration route or form, so that the proper form of the drug for a particular route may be obtained. For example, the preference card for cystoscopy may state that 2% lidocaine jelly is needed for local anesthesia (see Chapter 13). Although the preference card should clearly state "for topical application," it may also be safely assumed that properly educated surgical team members know that jelly, a semisolid form of the drug, is intended for topical application, not injection (Fig. 4.3). In a situation of a novice practitioner or a person with a knowledge deficit, careful reading of the medication label will reveal that this form of lidocaine

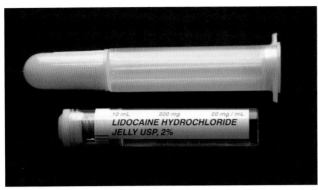

Fig. 4.3 Syringe prefilled with 2% lidocaine hydrochloride jelly. (Courtesy Sheryl Olson. From Auerbach PS, editor: *Wilderness medicine*, ed 6, St Louis, 2012, Elsevier.)

is intended for topical use only. This situation also provides an excellent example of the importance of always reading the medication label carefully. When in doubt, the surgical technologist *must* clarify the information stated on the preference card.

Another common example demonstrating the use of the right form of a drug for the right route is 1% lidocaine with epinephrine 1 mg/mL (1:1000) for local anesthesia for procedures such as breast biopsy. Again, the administration route may not be stated clearly on the preference card because the drug specified is formulated for injection. If for some unusual reason a team member does not know that a local anesthetic agent is injected for breast biopsy, careful reading of the medication label will provide the necessary information.

Another common medication, Cortisporin (see Chapter 5), is specifically formulated for administration by two different routes used in surgery. Neomycin/polymyxin B/hydrocortisone ophthalmic suspension is formulated for administration into the eye and neomycin/polymyxin B/hydrocortisone otic suspension is intended for use in the external ear canal. (Fig. 4.4). The surgical technologist must read the drug label carefully to ensure that the correct form of this drug is available for the intended administration route.

A crucial example of the importance of the right dose for the right route in surgery occurs during procedures on the middle ear. The surgical technologist must exercise particular caution when identifying, labeling, and handling medications for middle ear surgery because two significantly different strengths of epinephrine (a hormone that is a powerful vasoconstrictor, see Chapter 8) are present on the sterile back table. For example, in tympanoplasty, epinephrine 1 mg/mL (1:1000) is administered on tiny pieces of Gelfoam (see Chapter 9) for topical hemostasis in the middle ear, whereas a local anesthetic with dilute epinephrine (1% lidocaine with epinephrine 0.001% or 0.0005%) is injected for hemostasis over a larger area. Both solutions are used for hemostasis, but in significantly different strengths, intended for significantly different routes. In addition, both solutions are clear. For the correct medication to be passed at the correct time, both solutions must be accurately identified and labeled, and the surgical technologist *must* know the route of administration for both strengths of epinephrine. If epinephrine 1 mg/mL (1:1000) is mistakenly injected, deadly tachycardia and hypertension may result (Insight 4.1).

The scrubbed surgical technologist must observe the delivery of these medications to the sterile field and immediately label each drug—its identity and strength—as it is accepted into the sterile field to avoid errors. In addition, topical-strength epinephrine 1 mg/mL (1:1000) must never be kept in a syringe on the back table. Rather, a shallow container (such as a sterile Petri dish) should be used for topical epinephrine to prevent the drug from being mistakenly drawn up into a syringe for injection.

Right Patient

All surgical patients must be accurately identified before being transported into the operating room. Tools, such as The Joint Commission's Universal Protocol and the World Health Organization's Surgical Safety Checklist (Fig. 4.5), are used in the operating room to ensure that the correct surgical procedure will be performed on the correct patient. This process also includes relevant information about the patient, such as a history of drug allergies or hypersensitivity to a particular drug. The surgical procedure and operating surgeon are verified, and the preference card, containing medication orders for that specific procedure, is kept available in the operating room for reference. In addition, a surgical safety "time out" is conducted just before the incision to further verify that the intended surgical procedure is being performed on the correct patient. Diligence and care taken to properly identify the patient will help to ensure that the correct patient receives the medications intended for administration during a surgical procedure.

Right Time

In surgery, the surgeon (or as delegated to the surgical first assistant) administers all medications at the surgical site. This practice prevents the vast majority of medication *timing* errors

Form: otic suspension sterile drops

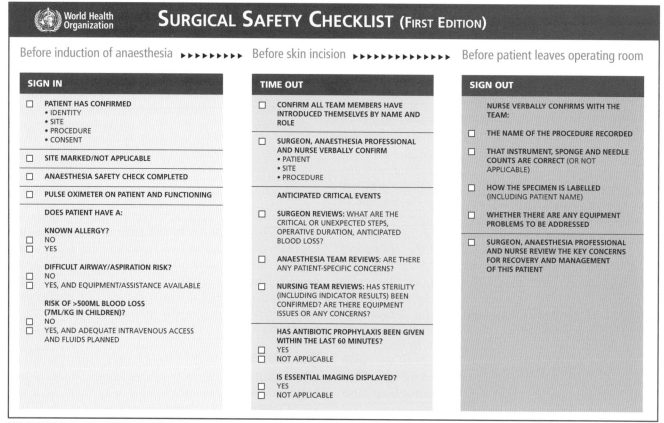

Fig. 4.4 Cortisporin Otic label. Cortisporin Otic suspension is now called neomycin/polymyxin B/hydrocortisone otic suspension. (From Morris DG: *Calculate with confidence*, ed 5, St Louis, 2010, Elsevier.)

Fig. 4.5 The World Health Organization's Surgical Safety Checklist. (WHO, 2015, available from https://www.who.int/teams/integrated-health-services/patient-safety/research/safe-surgery/tool-and-resources.)

during surgery (for drugs administered from the sterile back table). The purpose of the drug, when stated on the preference card, often indicates the timing of administration. For example, if 1% lidocaine with epinephrine 0.001% is listed on the preference card for a local anesthetic, it will be administered before incision. In addition, it may be administered periodically throughout the procedure as needed (pro re nata [PRN]) for patient comfort. If 0.5% bupivacaine with epinephrine 0.001% is listed on the preference card for postoperative pain control, it may be administered at the beginning of the procedure or at the time of wound closure. Some routine medications (e.g., contrast media for cholangiography, antibiotics for irrigation, heparinized saline) are obtained and labeled during case setup and passed to the surgeon at the appropriate time. The surgeon may request a drug by verbal order during any procedure. In

such a case the medication is obtained, labeled, and passed to the surgeon from the sterile back table for administration, as soon as requested.

Right Documentation

It is also crucial that medications given from the sterile table are accurately documented on the operative record. The circulator will document all medications delivered to the field, and the surgical technologist in the scrub role will verbally provide a final total of the amount of each medication administered for the circulator to note in the record. When a medication is repeatedly administered during a procedure, such as a local anesthetic, the scrubbed surgical technologist must also maintain an accurate ongoing total of the amount of medication being used throughout the procedure.

TECH TIP

Use a sterile marking pen on the field to keep a written tally of the amount of medications used during the procedure.

MEDICATION IDENTIFICATION

Both the scrub and the circulator are responsible for correctly identifying medications delivered to and used from the sterile field. This dual responsibility minimizes the potential for errors in medication administration, as does following a logical series of steps (Box 4.3) to properly identify drugs. The first step in medication identification is to carefully read the label on the medicine container (see Chapter 2 for examples of medication labels). The team member obtaining the drug reads the label initially and checks the container for cracks or discolored contents. If there is any doubt as to the integrity of the container, the medication should not be used. Rather, it should be returned to the pharmacy with a note indicating the specific concern. The medication label contains important information about the drug, as Table 4.1 shows. The most crucial information is the drug name (both generic and trade), strength, amount, and expiration date. Special handling instructions (such as refrigeration or keeping medication from direct light), the drug form, and intended administration route are also key pieces of

drug information contained on the label (for more detail see Chapter 2 and Fig. 4.6). The circulator reads vital label information aloud just before delivery to the sterile field and shows the label to the surgical technologist in the scrub role. Finally, the scrub repeats the label information aloud to confirm the correct drug. The drug should be delivered to the sterile field only after the steps described have been completed. Alternatively, both scrub and circulator may read the information aloud together before delivery of the medication to the sterile field.

! CAUTION

All medications delivered to the sterile field must be labeled immediately to avoid errors and to help ensure patient safety.

DELIVERY TO THE STERILE FIELD

Principles of asepsis (sterile technique) must be followed when delivering and receiving medications into the sterile field. Medications frequently used from the sterile back table are packaged in different types of containers, including vials and ampules (Fig. 4.7), and aseptic delivery methods vary by type of container. One of the most common containers is a glass or plastic vial, with a rubber stopper encased in a metal cap, and covered by an outer plastic cap. The plastic cap is popped off without touching the rubber stopper underneath. The circulator can draw up the drug (if in liquid form) with a syringe and hypodermic needle and then empty the contents of the syringe into a sterile medicine cup held by the scrub. The circulator should handle only the outside of the vial and should not touch the rubber stopper unless it is being removed. Alternatively, the circulator may hold the vial in an inverted position, while the scrub withdraws the drug from the vial, with a syringe and needle, using the two-handed technique (Fig. 4.8). The scrubbed surgical technologist should first draw some air into the syringe, then puncture the rubber stopper with the needle and inject air into the vial, which will allow the contents of the vial to enter the syringe rapidly. In addition, the hypodermic needle used to puncture the vial should be a larger needle, such as 18 gauge, to permit rapid filling of the syringe. After the medication is in the syringe, the 18-gauge needle is removed and replaced with the correct gauge needle for injection (such as a 25-gauge needle).

If a drug is in powder form in a vial, the circulator must reconstitute it, and the resulting liquid is withdrawn from the vial with a syringe and delivered to the sterile field, as described earlier.

BOX 4.3 Steps for Medication Identification

Circulator reads label
Circulator reads label aloud to scrub
Circulator shows label to scrub
Scrub states medication information aloud
Scrub accepts medication
Scrub labels medication containers immediately

? QUICK QUESTION

What does it mean to reconstitute a powdered medication? See the section on drug forms or preparations in Chapter 1.

TABLE 4.1 Sample Information Contained on a Medication Label

Type of Information	Example
Name (brand and generic)	bupivacaine HCl (Sensorcaine)
Strength	0.5%
Amount	50 mL
Expiration date	01/2022
Administration route	Injection
Manufacturer	AstraZeneca
Storage directions	Store at room temperature
Warnings or precautions	Federal law prohibits dispensing without prescription
Lot number	1234567
Schedule (only if drug is a controlled substance)	(C-I to C-V, see Chapter 2)

If a syringe is used to draw up and inject the reconstituting agent and to withdraw the mixture, extra care must be taken not to touch the sides of the plunger (Fig. 4.9). If unsterile hands

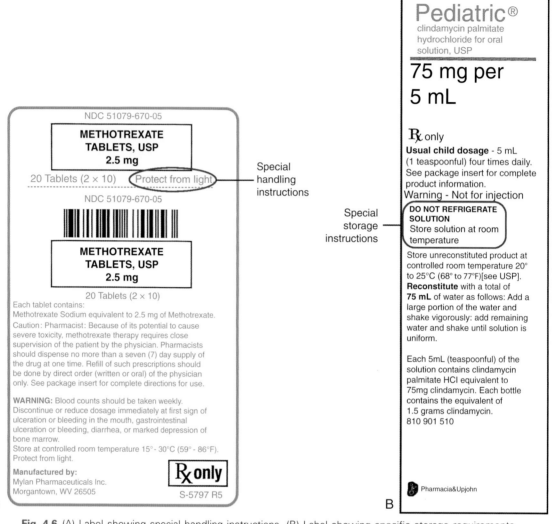

Fig. 4.6 (A) Label showing special handling instructions. (B) Label showing specific storage requirements. (From Macklin D, Chernecky CC, Infortuna MH: *Math for clinical practice*, ed 2, St Louis, 2011, Elsevier.)

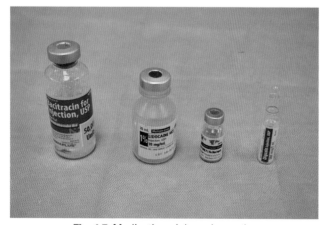

Fig. 4.7 Medication vials and ampule.

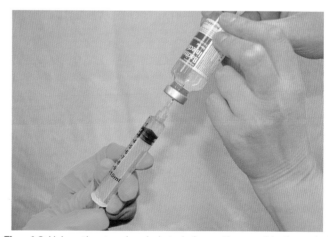

Fig. 4.8 Using the two-handed technique, the scrubbed surgical technologist may draw up medication from a vial held by the circulator.

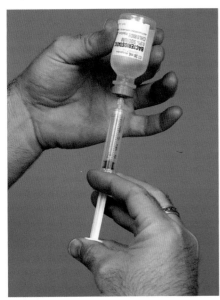

Fig. 4.9 Unsterile hands must not touch the syringe plunger. (From Fulcher EM, Fulcher RM, Soto CD: *Pharmacology: principles and applications*, ed 3, St Louis, 2012, Saunders.)

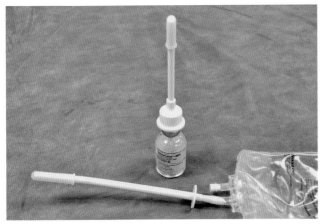

Fig. 4.10 A sterile, disposable pour spout (decanter) is used to deliver medication contained in a bag of intravenous fluid or a medication vial. The decanter is grasped by the hub, and the prong is inserted into the injection port.

touch the plunger, the plunger contaminates the inside of the barrel as it moves down the barrel when injecting. If the drug mixture is then drawn into the syringe barrel, it too becomes contaminated.

Sterile disposable pour spouts (decanters) are commercially available to facilitate sterile delivery of medications contained in vials and in bags of intravenous solution (Fig. 4.10). Medications may be added to a bag of intravenous solution, such as 1 g of an antibiotic into 1000 mL of normal saline, and disposable spouts called bag decanters are used to deliver the solution to the sterile field aseptically. Vial decanters are used to deliver medications contained in vials. Decanters provide a greater margin of safety by increasing the distance between the circulator (nonsterile person) and the scrubbed surgical technologist during medication delivery. If decanters are not available, the circulator should draw up the medication from the vial as described previously.

Pouring directly from a vial into a sterile medication cup is discouraged, because it is extremely difficult to verify that the rubber stopper was removed in a manner that did not contaminate any area of the vial lip.

Some medication vials and ampules are available in sterile packages, which can be opened directly onto the sterile field. The scrub is responsible for showing the medication label and expiration date to the circulator, before opening the vial and drawing up the contents. Alternatively, the scrub may pour a medication directly from a sterile vial into a sterile medication cup, within the sterile field.

Some medications are available in an ampule, a sealed glass container with a narrowed neck. The top of an ampule is broken off at the neck, and a sterile filter needle attached to a syringe is inserted to aspirate and withdraw the medication. The filter needle has a one-way filtering device at the base of the needle to prevent any broken glass pieces being drawn into the syringe. The filter needle is then replaced with a regular hypodermic needle before the medication is distributed to the sterile field. Special care should also be used when breaking the glass ampule because glass may cut unprotected hands. Gauze or plastic protective caps are recommended to prevent injury during opening. A glass ampule should be broken away from the body to help to prevent injury from the broken edge (Fig. 4.11). Some glass ampules also come packaged sterile for use on the back table, such as the liquid component used to make polymethylmethacrylate (bone cement). Once again, care must be taken to protect the gloved hands. After the ampule is broken, the item used to protect the hands should be discarded from the sterile field to avoid accidental transfer of glass particles into the surgical wound.

Although not technically considered a medication, saline irrigation is often delivered to the sterile field from a pour bottle. The bottle cap should be lifted straight up and off, and the entire

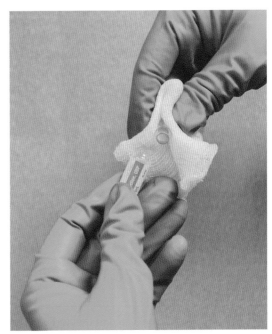

Fig. 4.11 Breaking a medication ampule. Carefully break the neck of the ampule in a direction away from you.

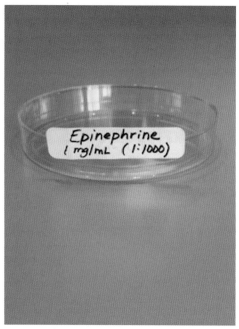

Fig. 4.12 A medication intended for topical application, such as epinephrine 1 mg/mL (1:1000) should be kept in a shallow container, such as a Petri dish, rather than a syringe. For example, Gelfoam pledgets are dipped into topical epinephrine 1 mg/mL (1:1000) for hemostasis in the middle ear.

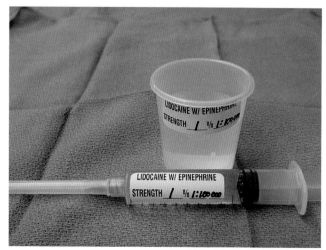

Fig. 4.13 Preprinted medication labels used in the sterile field.

contents poured immediately. Unused portions should not be saved for later use because sterility cannot be ensured. If the bottle is recapped, its contents are considered unsterile because of potential contamination of the bottle lip during replacement of the cap.

To avoid potential contamination, the circulator must take care not to lean over the sterile field when delivering medications or solutions. The scrub should hold containers away from the sterile table when accepting medications to assist the circulator in maintaining a safe distance from the field.

Several different types of containers are available to store medications and solutions on the sterile back table (see Fig. 3.7). Medicine cups, pitchers, basins, or syringes may be used, depending on the volume of medication needed.

Medications intended for topical administration (such as thrombin or epinephrine 1 mg/mL [1:1000]) should *never* be kept in a syringe on the back table. Syringes are used to inject medications. Some topical medications are fatal if injected. Use a labeled shallow container, such as a plastic Petri dish, to store topical medications. The use of a shallow container will make it more difficult to accidentally draw up a topical medication into a syringe. In addition, a shallow container provides easy access to the medication when needed (e.g., when dipping pieces of Gelfoam into the medication for topical application) (Fig. 4.12).

MEDICATION LABELING ON THE STERILE BACK TABLE

Once a medication has been delivered to the sterile back table, it is no longer in its original container, so it must be labeled immediately. Most drugs used from the sterile field are clear in color;

thus, they are easily confused if not clearly marked. There are different methods of labeling medications on the sterile back table, but the most important point is that each medication must be labeled—in the intermediate storage container (such as pitcher or medicine cup) and in any delivery vehicle (such as a syringe). The Joint Commission National Patient Safety Goal 3, NPSG.03.04.01, requires that all medication containers in the sterile field be labeled. The most accurate medication labeling method is the use of preprinted medication labels available from sterile supply manufacturers (Fig. 4.13). If preprinted labels are not available, a sterile skin marking pen may be used to write on blank labels. If blank labels are not available, sterile skin adhesive strips may be used. Regardless of the labeling method used, proper identification of all medications in the sterile field is an absolutely crucial step in preventing medication administration errors.

📌 TECH TIP

When placing the adhesive medication label on a syringe, be sure to place it on the syringe barrel opposite the volume markings so that you can always read the amount of medication used during the procedure.

Occasionally, the scrubbed surgical technologist may be replaced during a procedure (e.g., for shift change or lunch relief). All medications must be plainly labeled and reported to the new scrub. If there is any doubt as to the identity of a solution, it must be discarded, and new medication must be obtained.

There is no acceptable excuse for the presence of unlabeled (unidentified) medications on the sterile back table. Improper or inadequate labeling of drugs may be considered negligent. Negligence is defined in the Miller-Keane *Encyclopedia and Dictionary of Medicine, Nursing and Allied Health* as "failure to do something that a reasonable person of ordinary prudence would do in a situation or the doing of something that such a person would not do." By this definition, it is "reasonable" to expect that the correct medication will be obtained, identified, and passed to the surgeon and that a "prudent" person will perform these duties. This means that reason and prudence are everyone's responsibility, whatever the situation. This is not always easy. The rapid pace of events in surgery often pressures team members to accomplish difficult tasks in a hurry. However, the process of medication identification should never be compromised, nor should staff become complacent about routine medications. If a question or doubt arises regarding a medication, it must be clarified and resolved immediately. If the medication seems wrong or the dose appears to be incorrect, verify it with the physician before using it. It is better to be certain about the drug—even if it means provoking the surgeon—than to make an error and thus cause harm to the patient.

> ### 📌 TECH TIP
>
> Do not be embarrassed to admit ignorance or confusion, and always admit an outright error. Honesty and integrity are vital characteristics in healthcare professionals. If you make a medication error, acknowledge it at once so that corrective measures may be taken. Notify the surgeon immediately. Then follow institutional policy. Usually when a medication error occurs, the unit supervisor is notified, and an incident or occurrence report is completed. Above all, immediate action is taken to correct the error. The surgical technologist's primary focus in medication administration is patient safety.

HANDLING MEDICATIONS

When medications have been delivered to the sterile field and labeled, some additional handling may be necessary. Occasionally, the surgeon may order that two medications be mixed for concurrent administration. For example, an anti-inflammatory agent and a long-acting local anesthetic agent may be mixed for injection into a joint at the conclusion of an arthroscopy. Some medications may be diluted before use, such as Hypaque (a radiopaque contrast medium, see Chapter 6), which may be diluted with equal parts of injectable saline, as ordered on the preference card. It is vital that the surgical technologist read the preference card carefully and use basic math skills (see Chapter 3) to ensure the correct mixture or dilution of medications at the sterile back table. All containers (such as medicine cups) must be labeled for the original medications, and a separate container must be clearly labeled indicating the mixture or diluted medication. The administration container, usually a syringe, must be labeled with complete information on the mixture or dilution. The final check for accuracy is performed when the scrubbed surgical technologist states the complete mixing or dilution information, when handing the medication to the surgeon.

Other medications may require reconstitution before use (see Chapter 9). An example is topical thrombin, which is available in a sterile kit with a spray nozzle (Fig. 4.14). The kit contains a vial of thrombin, a vial of diluent (an inert diluting agent; saline), and a syringe with spray nozzle. The scrub draws the diluent into a syringe and injects it into the thrombin vial. The mixture is shaken until the thrombin is dissolved and drawn into the syringe. The nozzle is attached to enable administration to large oozing surfaces, such as the liver.

Special caution is required when handling controlled substances in surgery. Institutional policies regarding handling and disposal of controlled substances (see Table 2.1) must be in compliance with federal law; thus, policies must be understood and followed by all staff members.

SUPPLIES

Syringes and hypodermic needles are used frequently in surgery to draw up, measure, and administer medications. A syringe has

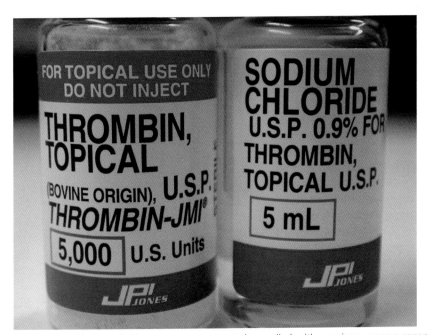

Fig. 4.14 Topical thrombin is available as a spray pump, to be applied with a syringe, or as a reconstituted powder to saturate absorbable Gelfoam. (From Dockery GD, Crawford ME: *Lower extremity soft tissue & cutaneous plastic surgery*, ed 2, Edinburgh, 2012, Elsevier.)

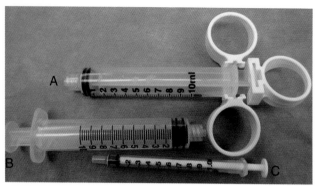

Fig. 4.15 Types of syringes. (A) A 10-mL finger-control Luer-lock syringe. (B) A 10-mL Luer-lock syringe. (C) A 1-mL plain-tip tuberculin syringe.

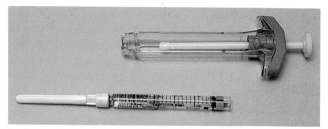

Fig. 4.16 A Tubex syringe, glass carpule, and needle. (From Potter P, Perry A: *Basic nursing: essentials for practice*, ed 5, St Louis, 2003, Mosby.)

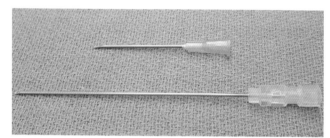

Fig. 4.17 Hypodermic needles, 1½-inch and 3-inch.

three basic parts: the barrel (or outer portion), plunger (inside portion), and tip. The barrel of the syringe is marked or calibrated to indicate the amount of medication contained in the syringe. The amount of medication in the syringe is measured from the innermost edge of the rubber tip on the end of the plunger. The most common sizes of syringes routinely used in surgery range from 1 to 60 mL. Some syringes have a finger-control attachment on the barrel and plunger to provide ease of motion and more precise control when injecting (Fig. 4.15). The most common type of syringe *tip* used in surgery is the Luer-lock tip, which has a screw-type locking mechanism used to securely attach a hypodermic needle. Plain-tip or "slip-tip" syringes are also available, but these are used for specific purposes. For example, a plain-tip syringe may be attached to a spinal needle for subclavian venipuncture during a venous access procedure. Various sizes of syringes are used for various purposes, so consult the surgeon's preference card for specific information. In general, 1-mL (called a TB or tuberculin syringe) and 3-mL syringes are used to inflate the tiny balloon on the end of an embolectomy catheter. By far the most common syringe size used in the operating room is a 10-mL syringe. That size syringe is used for a number of purposes, including inflating the cuff on a tracheostomy tube and injection of a local anesthetic agent throughout a surgical procedure. Thirty-milliliter syringes are most frequently used to inject saline irrigation and contrast media into the common bile duct, inflate a 30-mL balloon on a Foley catheter, or administer heparinized saline through an arterial irrigation catheter.

Special syringes are available for particular purposes. For example, a Tubex syringe has a metal or plastic device used to accommodate a carpule of medication for injection (such as lidocaine or heparin). A carpule is a glass tube with a rubber cap that is penetrated by a special needle attached to the Tubex syringe (Fig. 4.16). Another type of special syringe is a dual-syringe device used to deliver two medications simultaneously, such as those used to form a fibrin sealant (see Chapter 9).

Hypodermic needles are used to draw up and administer drugs. A hypodermic needle has three basic parts: the hub (which fits onto a syringe), shaft, and tip (the beveled end of the shaft). Needles vary in diameter (gauge) and length (measured in inches). The larger the gauge of a needle, the smaller

the diameter of the lumen (inside channel). Thus an 18-gauge needle has a much larger lumen than a 25-gauge needle. Most hypodermic needles used in surgery are disposable and are color-coded by size at the plastic hub for ease in identification. Sizes of hypodermic needles routinely used in surgery range from 27-gauge needles (used in ophthalmology) to larger 18-gauge needles (used to draw up medications). Color-coding for size may vary by manufacturer, but several companies use the same colors to indicate size. The three needle sizes most frequently used at the sterile field are 18 gauge (pink), 22 gauge (gray), and 25 gauge (blue). The most common hypodermic needle length used in surgery is 1.5 inches (Fig. 4.17). Shorter, ⅝-inch needles may be used for superficial injections, whereas longer needles (3-inch), called spinal needles, may be used from the sterile field for specific purposes, such as aspiration of cysts or to inject fluid to distend the shoulder joint for a shoulder arthroscopy.

SHARPS SAFETY

Standard precautions state that used needles must never be recapped because most needle-puncture injuries are the result of attempting to recap a used needle. It is also dangerous, though, to leave an unsheathed hypodermic needle exposed on the sterile table during a surgical procedure. Use of syringes and needles within the sterile field differs from other situations, in that the same syringe and needle combination may be used repeatedly during a surgical procedure. An example is the use of local anesthesia during a breast biopsy, when the agent is administered into progressively deeper tissue layers to enable deeper dissection. For prevention of injury from the needle while not in use, it must be recapped between injections. In addition, more than 10 mL of local anesthetic may be required, which necessitates refilling of the syringe. For the refilling of

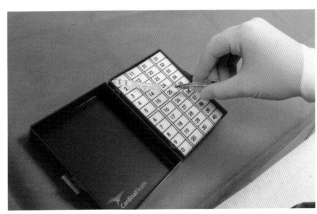

Fig. 4.18 If a needle must be recapped for protection for reuse during an operation, such as the periodic injection of local anesthetic for patient comfort, use a one-handed recapping technique.

a syringe at the sterile field, the smaller hypodermic needle used for injection is recapped, removed from the syringe, and replaced with a larger needle to draw up additional amounts of the agent. The larger needle is then recapped, removed from the syringe, and replaced with the smaller needle for injection. Both situations require recapping of hypodermic needles at the sterile field. To prevent injury, the surgical technologist must use a one-handed recapping technique (Fig. 4.18) or a recapping device intended for that purpose. Specialized self-shielding needles are also available for use from the sterile field (see *AST Guidelines for Best Practices for Sharps Safety and Use of the Neutral Zone*, 2017).

KEY CONCEPTS

- The role of the scrubbed surgical technologist in medication administration is to identify, accept, label, and clearly state the medication when passing it to the surgeon.
- Each facility's established policies and procedures must always be understood and followed.
- In addition, the surgical technologist must be aware of state regulations regarding specific practices.
- Consistent application of the six "rights" of medication administration will reduce the potential for drug errors.
- The surgical technologist in the scrub role must never accept a medication without properly identifying it.
- Aseptic technique must be used when delivering or accepting drugs into the sterile field.
- Accurate and immediate labeling of drugs on the sterile back table is required to minimize potential for errors.

LEARNING THE LANGUAGE (KEY TERMS)

Using your textbook or a standard medical dictionary, look up and write the definitions of each term.

carpule   diluent

REVIEW QUESTIONS

1. What is the role of the surgical technologist in medication administration when serving in the scrub role? As the circulator?
2. Give examples of applications of the six "rights" of medication administration in surgery.
3. Which steps would you use to correctly identify medications that are going to be used from the sterile back table during a surgical procedure?
4. How do the principles of sterile technique apply to medication delivery to the sterile field?
5. How would you label drugs on your sterile back table?
6. What items are used to facilitate medication administration from the sterile back table?

CRITICAL THINKING

Scenario 1

It is 0725, and the patient has just been brought into the operating room. The circulator is in a hurry because the patient has come into the room late and the surgeon is in the department. The circulator asks you to put the medication containers at the edge of the sterile back table, so she can pour the solutions, as soon as she has time, and you can continue setting up for the procedure.

Is this safe practice? Justify your answer.

List a better alternative to her request.

Scenario 2

Marilu Lin is a 10-year-old girl undergoing a type II tympanoplasty procedure. The back table and Mayo stand are set up, but the procedure has not yet begun. You are asked to relieve the surgical technologist in the scrub role and start the case. She has several medications on the back table, but none of them are labeled.

1. What should you do?
2. Which medications do you expect to be on the back table?
3. What is the purpose for each medication?
4. What route is used for each?
5. What could happen if these two medications are switched and the epinephrine 1 mg/mL (1:1000) is injected?

BIBLIOGRAPHY

Association of Surgical Technologists: *AST Guidelines for best practices for sharps safety and use of the Neutral Zone*, 2017, Guideline VI, Littleton, CO. AST

Fulcher EM, Fulcher RM, Soto CD: *Pharmacology: principles and applications*, ed 3, St Louis, 2012, Saunders/Elsevier.

Hatlie MJ, Sheridan SE: The medical liability crisis of 2003: must we squander the chance to put patients first? *Health Aff* 22(4): 37–40, 2003.

INTERNET RESOURCES

BD, United States, Syringes and Needles, Products, Safety Needles: www.bd.com/hypodermic/products/safety_needles.asp.

Drugs.com, Neomycin, Polymyxin B, Hydrocortisone Ophthalmic Suspension Prescribing Information: www.drugs.com/cdi/cortisporin-ophthalmic-suspension-drops-suspension.html.

Drugs.com, Professionals, Cortisporin Otic Suspension Prescribing Information: www.drugs.com/pro/cortisporin-otic-suspension.html.

Institute for Safe Medication Practices: ISMP's List of Confused Drug Names: www.ismp.org/Tools/confuseddrugnames.pdf.

Medline Plus, Drugs, Herbs and Supplements, Methylprednisolone Sodium Succinate Injection: www.nlm.nih.gov/medlineplus/druginfo/meds/a601157.html.

Single Entity Injectable Drug Products: https://www.fda.gov/drugs/information-drug-class/single-entity-injectable-drug-products.

efficacy
half-life

potency

FIVE MORE "RIGHTS" OF MEDICATION ADMINISTRATION

The six rights to medication administration are described previously in this chapter. Their importance for patient safety is reflected by frightening statistics. A medical error is defined by the National Coordinating Council for Medication Error Reporting and Prevention as "any preventable event that may cause or lead to inappropriate medication use or patient harm, while the medication is in the control of the healthcare professional, patient, or consumer." The reality is that serious preventable medication errors are estimated to occur in more than 3.2 million inpatient admissions and 3.3 million outpatient visits in the United States each year. Inpatient costs are approximately $16.4 billion and outpatient costs are estimated at $4.2 billion annually. The Institute of Medicine estimates 7000 deaths occur annually because of preventable medication errors. These statistics verify that five additional "rights" of medication administration are important for providing patient safety. Surgical first assistants may not be the primary professional involved in the actual medication administration; however, they can assist with clarifying and verifying information before, during, and after a medication is given. These five additional "rights" are the right patient assessment before administration, right documentation of the medication given, patient's right to education about the medication before it is administered, right evaluation of the medication's effect, and patient's right to refuse the medication.

> **WEBSITES TO HELP TO AVOID MEDICATION ERRORS:**
> Electronic drug resource: www.epocrates.com
> FDA MedWatch: www.fda.gov/safety/MedWatch/default.htm
> Institute for Safe Medication Practice: www.ismp.org
> Medline Plus: Drugs, Supplements, and Herbal Information: www.nlm.nih.gov/medlineplus/druginformation.html
> National Coordinating Council for Medication Error Reporting and Prevention: www.nccmerp.org

MEDICATION ADMINISTRATION FROM THE STERILE FIELD

Intraoperative administration of medications to the surgical patient presents a unique situation unlike any other medical environment, especially for the advanced practitioner functioning as a surgical first assistant. Different personnel administer medications to the patient through several routes, often at the same time. Although surgical first assistants might not perform the actual administration of medications, it is important that they are aware of the effects any medication can have on the patient.

Personnel who fulfill the role of the surgical first assistant will have different educational and clinical backgrounds ranging from medical school to physician's assisting, nursing, and surgical technology. These different backgrounds and employment disciplines dictate different regulatory agencies, under which each professional practices, in regard to administration of medications. State statutes will supersede any other regulatory agency regarding limitations of practice; however, when there is no statute regulating specific personnel, it is usually the individual facility that regulates the practice. All personnel practicing as surgical first assistants should be aware of the policies or bylaws regulating their practice. For example, the surgical first assistant functioning as an independent practitioner may be regulated by the medical staff bylaws of the facility. However, the surgical first assistant employed by the facility may be regulated by that facility's policies and procedures.

The process of administering medications at the sterile field requires a team effort. Medications will pass through at least two other people, the circulator and scrub person, before being delivered to the surgeon. The medication will almost always be in a container different from its original—usually a syringe, medicine cup, basin, or pitcher on the field. For the prevention of medication errors, strict policies and procedures have been developed for delivery of medications onto the sterile field (as described in this chapter). The surgeon and the surgical first assistant may be the last line of defense to avoid medication errors, therefore each should be aware of and follow all of these procedures. The person who administers the medication *always* has the right to question the procedure and decide whether the medication will be given or a new medication obtained. It is always in the best interest of the patient to discard any questionable medication (see Box 4.A).

NOTE: When medications are administered from the sterile field, it is important to communicate to the anesthesia care provider, the name of the agent and amount given. For example, when a local anesthetic agent that contains epinephrine is administered, the anesthesia care provider should be notified immediately and verbally advised as to the amount of the medication ultimately injected (which is also noted on the operative record). This is important because epinephrine acts as a vasoconstrictor and can affect the patient's blood pressure.

DRUG-RESPONSE RELATIONSHIPS

As discussed in Chapter 1, all medications have systemic effects on the patient. It is important for the surgical first assistant to be aware of these effects, as well as the duration and safe dosages of medications. This pharmacologic principle is known as the *dose-time-effect relationship*. Drug effects are a result of the dose administered and the time from absorption to elimination. Medication dosage, time the medication is absorbed by the body, and the duration of action are all interrelated and interdependent. The duration of a medication's effect is based on the half-life of the medicine. Elimination half-life (T), also called *biologic half-life*, is the time it takes for 50% of a drug to be cleared from the bloodstream. Each drug has a unique half-life dependent on its characteristics. Certain conditions, such as decreased liver or renal function, will alter the half-life of medications. It is important to note that a medication may go through many of its half-lives before it no longer has a therapeutic effect on the body. This must be recognized when calculating subsequent doses of the same medication to maintain a therapeutic level of its desired effects. Some half-lives are of short duration, such as those used in general anesthesia (a few minutes). Others may have a half-life of several days, such as those used to treat hypothyroidism. Therefore, drugs with long half-lives are dosed less frequently than those with short half-lives. Essentially, drugs with short half-lives are said to leave the body quickly—in 4 to 8 hours. Drugs with long half-lives are said to leave the body more slowly—in more than 24 hours, and there is a greater risk for accumulation of these medications in the bloodstream and toxicity. A common example in the surgical setting is the administration of heparin sodium to achieve

---

BOX 4.A **Guidelines for Administering Medications From the Sterile Field**

Always be aware of the process of delivering medications to the sterile field
Always read the label on the device you receive, which contains the medication
Always confirm name and strength of the medication with the scrub person
Always inform anesthesia personnel when administering medications
Always be aware of any patient allergies
Always be aware of the amount of the medication administered
Never administer medications that are discolored or contain sediment
Never administer medications that are contaminated with other materials from the sterile field
Never administer a medication from any unlabeled container
Never administer a medication when there is any doubt about its identification or strength

---

TABLE 4.A **Heparin Sodium Route of Administration Comparison**

	Subcutaneous	Intravenous
Onset	0.5–1 hours	5 min
Peak	2 hours	10 min
Duration	8–12 hours	2–6 hours

---

anticoagulation during vascular surgery. It has a relatively short half-life of approximately 60 to 90 minutes and so would have to be administered frequently to maintain its initial effect.

Other terms related to drug effects are efficacy and potency. Drug efficacy is the degree to which a drug is able to produce its desired effects. Potency is the relative concentration required to produce that effect, as in how much of the drug is needed.

Bioavailability is the extent to which an administered amount of a drug reaches the site of action and is available to produce the drug effects (as described in Chapter 1). This is influenced by drug absorption and distribution to the site of action. Bioavailability is important in pharmacokinetics because it must be taken into consideration when calculating medication doses, especially those administered via nonintravenous routes. For intravenous administration, the bioavailability of the drug is considered to be 100% because it reaches systemic circulation immediately. Factors that affect bioavailability are form of the medication given (tablet, liquid, inhalation, etc.); route of administration (enteral, parenteral, etc.); gastrointestinal motility; food, herbals, and other drugs given; and liver function. Using heparin sodium as an example, see Table 4.A for a comparison of onset, peak, and duration when given subcutaneously and intravenously.

ADVANCED PRACTICES: REVIEW QUESTIONS

1. All of the following statements are true concerning patient effects from medication administration except:
   a. All medications have a systemic effect.
   b. Topical medications affect only the localized area.
   c. Liver function influences medication effects.
   d. The time a medication is given influences its effect.
2. When there is no state statute or federal law regulating an individual profession, what organization regulates healthcare workers in regard to medication administration?
   a. OSHA (Occupational Safety and Health Administration)
   b. The Joint Commission
   c. Healthcare facilities
   d. Health department
3. The duration of a medication's effect is based on the medication's:
   a. Dosage
   b. Strength
   c. Half-life
   d. Administration route

4. The bioavailability of an intravenous medication is considered to be what percent?
   a. 15
   b. 25
   c. 50
   d. 100
5. Explain why it is important to notify the anesthesia provider when a medication is administered at the sterile field.
6. Explain the pharmacologic principle known as the dose-time-effect relationship.
7. Which medication has the greater opportunity to become toxic in the body, drugs to treat hypothyroidism or heparin? Why?
8. List the guidelines for administering medications from the sterile field.

ADVANCED PRACTICES: BIBLIOGRAPHY

Fulcher EM, Fulcher RM, Soto CD: *Pharmacology: principles and applications*, ed 3, St Louis, 2012, Saunders/Elsevier.

Kee JL, Hayes ER, McCuistion LE: *Pharmacology: a patient-centered nursing process approach*, ed 8, St Louis, 2015, Saunders/Elsevier.

Skidmore-Roth L: *Mosby's drug guide for nursing students*, ed 11, St Louis, 2015, Mosby/Elsevier.

ADVANCED PRACTICES: INTERNET RESOURCES

Drugs.com, Professional, Medfacts, Heparin: www.drugs.com/ppa/heparin.html.

Food and Drug Administration: Drugs, Drug Safety and Availability, Medication Errors Related to CDER-Regulated Drug Products: www.fda.gov/drugs/drugsafety/medicationerrors/.

MerriamWebster.com, Bioavailability: www.merriamwebster.com/dictionary/bioavailability.

National Coordinating Council for Medication Error Reporting and Prevention: www.nccmerp.org.

National Quality Forum: Preventing Medication Errors: www.qualityforum.org/Publications/2010/12/Preventing_Medication_Errors_CAB.aspx.

The Joint Commission: www.jointcommission.org.

US Drug Enforcement Administration: www.dea.gov.

UNIT II

Applied Surgical Pharmacology

Many medications are used in surgery each day. This unit provides an introduction to the medications you will frequently encounter as a surgical technologist. We look at antibiotic, diagnostic agents, diuretics, hormones, and fluid and irrigation solutions. We also examine medications that affect blood coagulation, medications used as ophthalmic agents, and those used in labor and delivery. To understand these agents, you will need to be familiar with basic anatomy and physiology, so we review some of these principles as well. Once you know the generic and brand names of common surgical medications and their categories, it will be easier for you to recognize their purposes, action, administration routes, and proper handling to provide safe patient care. Note the generic name of the medication is given first with a brand name in parentheses after it. It is important for you to recognize generic names because medications may have more than one brand name.

5

Antibiotics

OBJECTIVES

After completing this chapter, you should be able to do the following:

1. Define terms and abbreviations related to antibiotics and antimicrobial therapy.
2. Discuss the broad term *antimicrobial* and its several categories of agents.
3. Define and explain healthcare-associated infections (HAIs) and surgical site infections (SSIs).
4. State the purposes of antibiotic therapy in surgery.
5. Identify and discuss various ways in which antimicrobials work.
6. Explain antibiotic resistance.
7. Discuss common categories of antibiotics used in surgery and give examples of each.

OUTLINE

Before the discovery of antimicrobial agents, surgical patients often died from postoperative wound infections. It was not known that bacteria were the cause of surgical wound infections, so there was no concept of aseptic surgical practice. Discovery of the existence of bacteria and their role in surgical wound infections eventually led to the development of modern aseptic practices (also known as *sterile techniques*). The incorporation of sterile techniques into surgical practice helped to reduce, but not completely eliminate, postoperative wound infections. The discovery of antimicrobial agents and their ability to treat surgical wound infections has saved countless lives. Although many antimicrobial agents have been developed, there has also been a dramatic increase in the number of bacterial species that are now resistant to many of these agents, causing a disturbing resurgence of deadly infections.

The broad term *antimicrobial* applies to several categories of agents. These include antibacterials, antiprotozoals, antifungals, antiparasitics, and drugs, such as sulfa and mercury (Insight 5.1). Because bacteria are the cause of surgical wound infections, the only category of antimicrobial agents routinely used in surgery are antibacterials, commonly referred to as *antibiotics*.

 MAKE IT SIMPLE

The word "antibiotic" takes its name from the Greek words *anti*, which means "against," and *bios*, which means "life." Using medical terminology word-building techniques can help you learn the meaning of many new words. When the prefix *anti-* is combined with other root words, the meaning of these terms for medication categories becomes clearer. For example, the word anti/bacteri/al indicates pertaining to; against; bacteria, which is more precise than the more commonly used term antibiotic.

Healthcare-associated infections (HAIs) are a major public health concern, and the Centers for Disease Control and Prevention (CDC) provides up-to-date information on this issue. It is estimated that 30% of all HAIs in hospitalized patients in the United States are *surgical site infections (SSIs)*. An SSI is defined as an infection that occurs at or near a surgical incision within 30 days of the procedure (or within 1 year if an implant was placed). Most SSIs are caused by six types or species of bacteria (Table 5.1). The most common causative agent of SSI is *Staphylococcus aureus*, which is present in the nose and on the skin of approximately 25% of healthy persons. An SSI is a potential complication of nearly every surgical intervention,

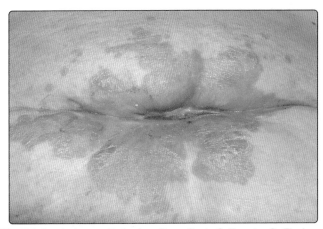

Fig. 5.1 Surgical wound infection. (From Currie G, Douglas G: *Flesh and bones of medicine*, St Louis, 2012, Elsevier.)

TABLE 5.1   Pathogens Associated With Surgical Site Infection

Pathogen	Percentage of SSIs (%)
Staphylococcus aureus	30
Coagulase-negative Staphylococcus	13.7
Enterococcus species	11.2
Escherichia coli	9.6
Pseudomonas aeruginosa	5.6
Enterobacter species	4.2

SSI, Surgical site infection.

particularly because most surgical procedures penetrate the body's first line of defense: the skin. SSIs may range from minor to serious; they may even be deadly, depending on several factors. Each day in the operating room, surgical technologists vigilantly apply their knowledge of sterile techniques as part of the team effort to prevent SSIs.

Antibiotics are effective tools used to supplement the conscientious practice of sterile techniques. As such, antibiotics are used in surgery: (1) to help prevent SSIs, and (2) to treat infections caused by bacterial pathogens (disease-causing microbes) (Fig. 5.1). It is important to remember that antibiotics are *adjuncts* that assist the patient's own defenses to prevent—or diminish the severity of—an SSI. When used to help prevent SSIs, antibiotics may be prescribed for the surgical patient preoperatively, intraoperatively, or postoperatively.

These agents may be administered during surgery from the sterile back table in the form of topical irrigation or application of an antibiotic ointment for surgical dressings. The use of topical antibiotic irrigation at the surgical site has been almost routine in some cases. However, the increase in antibiotic resistance has caused some discussion about the careful use of antibiotics. Further study is ongoing to determine whether this practice is effective at reducing SSIs.

! CAUTION

The availability of antibiotic therapy is *never* considered a substitute for the consistent, mindful, and meticulous practice of sterile techniques. Prevention of all SSIs is the goal in this vital aspect of safe surgical patient care.

The Surgical Care Improvement Project (SCIP) is a quality partnership developed by the Centers for Medicare and Medicaid Services and the CDC in collaboration with representatives of several national organizations. One aspect of this project focuses on reducing SSIs, and one of its goals is to increase compliance for proven effective measures related to use of antibiotics, such as:

- Selection of the proper antibiotic
- Timing antibiotic administration before the incision
- Timing discontinuation of the antibiotic after surgery
- Identification of the person responsible for these actions
- Verification of antibiotic names, times of administration, and documentation

The Surgical Patient Checklist (see Chapter 4, Fig. 4.5) developed by the World Health Organization is a tool that can be used to help to ensure compliance with established standards for antibiotic administration. The checklist has three sections: before the induction of anesthesia, before the skin incision, and before the patient leaves the operating room. Under each section is a list of tasks to be accomplished and verified. The second section of the checklist contains a task to confirm that antibiotic administration has been accomplished within the optimal time frame.

So what are these crucial agents known as *antibiotics*, and where do they come from? Antibiotics are derived from natural chemicals (or *metabolites*) produced by microorganisms that inhibit the growth of other microorganisms. In nature, these chemicals are thought to provide the microbe with a competitive advantage for survival (Fig. 5.2). Microorganisms that produce antimicrobial substances include fungi (and molds, a type of fungi) and bacteria. These natural chemicals are identified, cultured, extracted, and purified for medicinal use in a pharmaceutic laboratory. Penicillin is a natural chemical produced by *Penicillium chrysogenum*, a fungus. Bacitracin and the polymyxins are examples of natural agents produced by bacteria of the genus *Bacillus*. A natural substance may be altered in the laboratory to produce semisynthetic (see Chapter 1) antibiotics, such as some penicillins and the aminoglycosides. Cephalosporins are derived from a substance produced by the mold *Cephalosporium acremonium*, found in the ocean near a sewage outflow. Alterations of existing agents result in families and generations of antibiotics. Each antibiotic in a family is

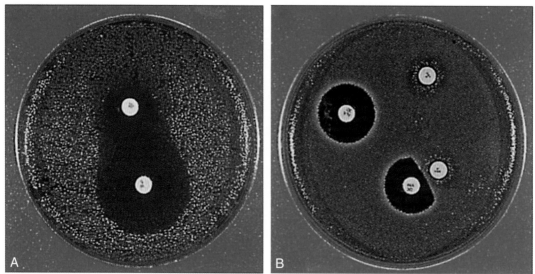

Fig. 5.2 Testing for culture and sensitivity. This is a common method of determining which antibiotics are effective against a specific bacterium or fungus. Various types of antibiotic agents impregnated on paper are positioned in the culture medium, which has been inoculated with the microorganism (A). Note the areas of no colonization around some of the paper discs (B). (From Goering R, Dockrell H, Zuckerman M, et al: *Mim's medical microbiology*, ed 5, London, 2013, Saunders Elsevier Ltd.)

similar to the original chemical but can be used to treat different types of infections because it has different properties. Other antimicrobial chemicals, such as sulfonamides and fluoroquinolones, are developed in the laboratory by chemical synthesis; these are classified as synthetic antibacterial agents.

MICROBIOLOGY REVIEW

SSIs are caused by the introduction of pathogenic microorganisms into a susceptible host (Fig. 5.3) via a route of transmission. The pathogen must have a source, means of transmission, and susceptible host to cause an infection. The source of pathogenic microorganisms may be *endogenous* or *exogenous*—the infectious microbe may come from the patient's own bacteria (endogenous) or from outside the patient (exogenous). For example, among the most common causative agents of SSIs are bacteria known as *S. aureus*, which are frequently present on the patient's skin (endogenous source) and may be carried into the surgical site during the course of the operation. Exogenous sources of pathogenic microbes include surgical personnel and the environment.

> **! CAUTION**
>
> A rare but documented example of an exogenous source of infectious microbes is various bacteria carried under artificial fingernails. Such microbes are thought to be introduced into the surgical site by glove tears commonly associated with long fingernails. Long and/or artificial nails are prohibited in surgery, and team members who choose to wear them are failing to follow policies established to prevent SSIs.

Surgical instruments that are not properly cleaned before sterilization may carry viable microbes into a surgical wound, and thus are another example of an exogenous source of pathogens. Regardless of the source, many other factors influence the

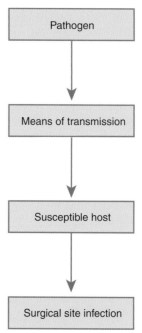

Fig. 5.3 Infection cycle. Source of pathogenic microbe plus transmission route plus susceptible host equals infection.

surgical patient's susceptibility to an infection, including general health, nutritional status, operative site, and duration of the surgical procedure.

If an SSI occurs, treatment requires prompt identification of the causative microorganism and selection of an appropriate antimicrobial agent. Pathogenic microorganisms causing SSIs are identified by several methods. Common methods used to identify pathogens include Gram staining and culture and sensitivity (C&S). A broad-spectrum antibiotic is prescribed to begin treatment, while awaiting the results of identification testing. Occasionally, during a surgical procedure, such as an incision and drainage, a sample of abscess fluid may be subjected to an immediate Gram stain process (Insight 5.2). A Gram stain is a rapid identification test that assists the physician in prescribing an initial course of antibiotic therapy based on the probable pathogen causing the infection. Gram staining is a way of distinguishing types of bacteria. In combination with *morphology* (the study of shapes), it can be used to identify many common bacteria. Bacteria occur in many shapes, most of which may be placed in three major groups: bacilli (also known as *rods* [oblong shaped]), cocci (round or spherical), and spirals (Fig. 5.4). Table 5.2 lists some common microorganisms classified by Gram stain and morphology. Medically relevant gram-positive microbes are usually cocci (but sometimes rods) and gram-negative microbes are usually rods (but sometimes cocci).

C&S is the process of growing microbes in culture to determine the infecting pathogen and exposing the pathogen to various antibiotics to determine which agent will best inhibit the pathogen's growth. For C&S to be performed, a fluid or tissue specimen is obtained with a swab from the infection site and placed in one or more culture tubes for transport to the microbiology

TABLE 5.2 Pathogenic Microorganisms by Gram Staining and Morphology

Gram-Positive (Stain Purple)	Gram-Negative (Stain Pink)
Cocci (Round)	
Staphylococcus aureus	Neisseria meningitidis
Staphylococcus epidermidis	
Streptococcus pneumoniae	
Streptococcus pyogenes	
Enterococcus faecium	
Enterococcus faecalis	
Bacilli (Rods)	
Clostridium	Klebsiella
Listeria	Bacteroides
Actinomyces	Escherichia coli
	Pseudomonas
	Proteus
	Salmonella
	Serratia
	Haemophilus influenzae

INSIGHT 5.2 Gram Staining

Gram staining is a differential staining procedure, which means it is used to distinguish between two types of bacteria. The Gram stain procedure was developed in 1884 and is still widely used today. A specimen containing the pathogenic microorganism to be identified is swabbed onto a slide and fixed. Crystal violet is applied first, staining all cells a bluish purple. Gram iodine is then applied to the slide as a mordant—an agent that increases the cell's affinity for the primary stain. The slide is then rinsed with acetone or alcohol, decolorizing the cells. Next, safranin, a red counterstain, is applied. Only cells that were decolorized pick up the red counterstain. The cell walls of gram-positive bacteria do not decolorize, remaining purple. Gram-negative bacteria lose the purple stain during decolorization, so they appear red or reddish-pink after application of safranin.

laboratory (Fig. 5.5). Note that separate culture tubes are available for aerobic (in oxygen) and anaerobic (lacking oxygen) testing. In the laboratory, the culture swab is used to spread the fluid sample onto nutrient agar and differential (distinguishing) media in Petri dishes called *plates*. This process is called *inoculation*. The inoculated plates are incubated for 24 to 48 hours, after which they can be examined for microbial growth. Miniaturized reaction containers allow laboratory personnel to identify causative microbes faster and more easily. Once the microbe has been isolated, it is grown in a pure culture and exposed to different antibiotics. This process of successive exposure to antibiotics to determine which agent is most effective against it is called *sensitivity testing*. The conventional method of sensitivity testing is the Kirby-Bauer disk diffusion test. Because of the emergence of multidrug-resistant (MDR) pathogens and the resulting need to start definitive treatment quickly, various methods of more

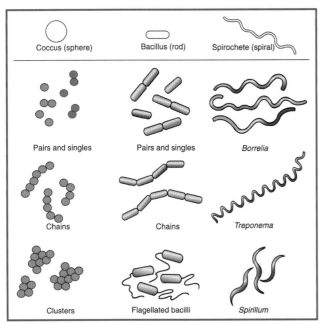

Fig. 5.4 Three basic shapes of bacteria. (From Robinson, Bird DL: *Essentials of dental assisting*, ed 5, St. Louis, 2013, Saunders.)

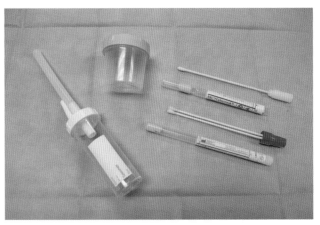

Fig. 5.5 Lukens trap, specimen container, culture swabs, and tubes.

rapid identification are now available. Rapid identification kits currently on the market include Enterotube II, VITEK system, and the BBL Crystal system.

> TECH TIP

Tissue and fluid may also be sent in the appropriate sterile container to the laboratory for C&S processing (see Fig. 5.5).

When the causative microorganism is identified and tested for antibiotic sensitivity, more definitive therapy can be initiated. To be effective, an antimicrobial agent must have *selective toxicity* (i.e., it must act against pathogenic microorganisms without harming host cells). Antibiotics must target structures and functions in pathogenic microorganisms that differ from those of host cells. We can better understand selective toxicity by reviewing the structural differences between host cells and bacterial pathogens. Bacteria are one-celled organisms that do not have a fully developed nucleus. This means they are classified as *prokaryotes*. (A karyote is a nucleus. A *prokaryote* is an early, or "pre" nucleus.) Multicellular organisms, including fungi, plants, and animals, are classified as *eukaryotes* ("true" karyotes). Both prokaryotic and eukaryotic cells have a plasma membrane that encloses the cell and preserves its integrity. Thus, it both protects the cell and regulates the movement of materials in and out of the cell.

Prokaryotes differ from eukaryotes because they have a cell wall in addition to the plasma membrane. This cell wall provides a potential location for antibiotic therapy (Fig. 5.6).

Prokaryotic cells also differ from eukaryotic cells in the structures responsible for protein synthesis—the *ribosomes*. These tiny structures assemble or synthesize proteins from amino acids. Both prokaryotes and eukaryotes have ribosomes, but prokaryotic ribosomes are smaller than eukaryotic ribosomes. This size difference offers another avenue of action for antibiotics; antibiotics that bind to the smaller bacterial ribosomes do not bind to the larger ribosomes of the eukaryotic host cells.

ANTIMICROBIAL ACTION

Mechanisms and Types

The goal of antibiotic administration is to assist the patient's immune system to subdue the infection, so antibiotic therapy does not have to kill all of the infecting microorganisms. Antimicrobial agents may work against pathogenic microorganisms by five different mechanisms, as summarized in Box 5.1. Some agents, such as cephalosporins, penicillins, vancomycin, and bacitracin, keep bacteria from synthesizing adequate cell walls. They can stop cell walls from forming or inhibit the synthesis process, so the walls are too weak to maintain vital functions. Some antibiotics, such as aminoglycosides, macrolides, and tetracyclines, interfere with protein synthesis. This means they bind to prokaryotic ribosomes, thus preventing the assembly of critical proteins. Polymyxins and some antifungal agents work by disrupting the bacterial cell membrane, causing leakage

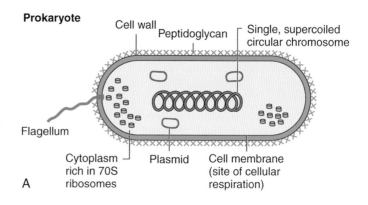

Prokaryote

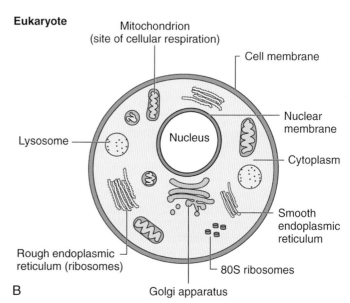

Eukaryote

Fig. 5.6 Eukaryotic cells are encased in a plasma membrane, whereas prokaryotic cells have a cell wall in addition to a plasma membrane: (A) prokaryotic cell; (B) eukaryotic cell. (From Murray PR, Rosenthal KS, Pfaller MA: *Medical microbiology*, ed 7, Philadelphia, 2013, Elsevier.)

BOX 5.1   Methods of Antimicrobial Action
Inhibit cell wall synthesis
Interfere with protein synthesis
Alter cell membrane function
Inhibit production of nucleic acids (ribonucleic acid or deoxyribonucleic acid)
Interfere with cell metabolism

of materials necessary for cell function. A few agents, such as fluoroquinolones and some antivirals, inhibit production of the nucleic acids (ribonucleic acid [RNA] or deoxyribonucleic acid [DNA]) that are necessary for bacterial replication. Still other agents interfere with bacterial cell metabolism. For example, sulfonamides take the place of a vital substance needed to produce folic acid.

We classify antimicrobial agents as *bactericidal* or *bacteriostatic*. Bactericidal agents kill bacteria. These include agents such as the aminoglycosides, cephalosporins, and penicillins. Bacteriostatic agents inhibit bacterial growth, relying on the host's own immune system to take over once the pathogenic microorganism is suppressed. Bacteriostatic agents include the macrolides and tetracyclines. Antimicrobial agents are also classified by their *spectrum* of activity. A *broad-spectrum* antibiotic has a wide range of activity—usually effective against both gram-negative and gram-positive bacteria. *Narrow-spectrum* antibiotics have a smaller range of activity—often effective against only one category of microorganisms, gram-negative or gram-positive. *Limited-spectrum* antibiotics are effective against just one species of microorganism.

Antibiotic Resistance

Microorganisms multiply rapidly, can mutate, and can adapt to new environments and hosts. Unfortunately, certain pathogenic microorganisms have also developed an alarming capacity to survive despite treatment (Insight 5.3). Approximately 70% of bacteria that cause HAIs are resistant to at least one of the agents used to treat these infections. *Antibiotic resistance* is the ability of some strains of pathogenic microbes to prevent or withstand the activity of antimicrobial agents. Antibiotic resistance mechanisms generally fit into four major categories:

- The microorganism may manufacture microbial enzymes that inactivate the antibiotic.
- The cell membrane may be altered to prevent the antibiotic from entering the cell.
- The target area, such as ribosome, may be altered so that the agent is no longer effective.

- The microorganism may add a substance to the antibiotic, which inhibits its ability to reach its desired binding site.

For example, some bacteria produce an enzyme known as *penicillinase*. This enzyme breaks down part of the chemical structure of penicillin, making the drug ineffective (Fig. 5.7). Penicillinase is produced by a number of microbes, including two common strains of staphylococci. Thus, these microorganisms have become resistant to treatment with penicillin. When antibiotic resistance appears as a bacterial trait, pharmaceutic manufacturers attempt to develop new forms of the antibiotic capable of withstanding the bacterial resistance mechanism. For example, methicillin (which is not broken down by penicillinase) was developed to treat some of the gram-positive pathogenic microbes. However, a strain of *S. aureus* developed a resistance to it. This strain is known as *methicillin-resistant S. aureus (MRSA)*. Methicillin is no longer in clinical use, having been replaced by other penicillins (such as flucloxacillin, dicloxacillin, and oxacillin). However, the term continues to be used to represent *S. aureus* strains resistant to all penicillins. This resistant strain of bacteria is difficult to treat with the traditional first-line agents. Similarly, one group of enteric (digestive tract) bacteria developed resistance to vancomycin. These bacteria are known as *vancomycin-resistant enterococci (VRE)*.

New "superbugs" (see the section on advanced practices) are emerging that have developed resistance, usually to two or more current antibiotics. Scientists have identified a plasmid (a segment of bacterial DNA) that confers resistance to six antibiotics. Multiple antibiotic resistance is found in a number of pathogens, including a strain of the tubercle bacillus (TB), the pathogen that causes tuberculosis. This strain of TB resists several powerful antibiotics used to treat it, including isoniazid and rifampicin. An alarming new strain of bacteria normally found in the intestinal tract has been identified, carbapenem-resistant *Enterobacteriaceae* (CRE) (Fig. 5.8). Of particular concern is that transmission of this microbe has been documented

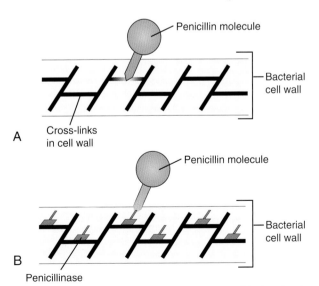

Fig. 5.7 Penicillinase inactivates penicillin. (A) Penicillin breaks down cross-links in bacterial cell wall. (B) Penicillinase breaks down a portion of penicillin structure, inactivating it.

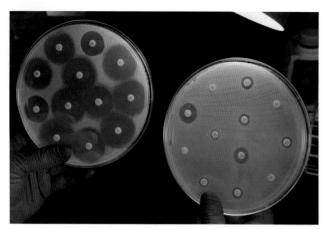

Fig. 5.8 Centers for Disease Control and Prevention staff show two plates growing bacteria in the presence of discs containing various antibiotics. The isolate on the left plate is susceptible to the antibiotics on the discs and is therefore unable to grow around the discs. The one on the right has a carbapenem-resistant Enterobacteriaceae that is resistant to all of the antibiotics tested and is able to grow near the disks. (Fig. courtesy James Gathany and Public Health Image Library at phil.cdc.gov.)

INSIGHT 5.4 NDM-1

NDM-1 stands for New Delhi metallo-beta-lactamase 1, an enzyme first identified in a strain of *Klebsiella* and now found in three other groups of common gram-negative bacteria (*Escherichia*, *Enterobacter*, and *Acinetobacter*). The NDM-1 enzyme inactivates agents in the broad class of antibiotics categorized as beta-lactams, which includes penicillins, cephalosporins, and carbapenems. In addition, pathogens containing NDM-1 also frequently contain resistance mechanisms to other major antibiotics as well—truly earning the title of "superbugs" for pathogens that have obtained this enzyme.

---

through properly reprocessed duodenoscopes. See the section on advanced practices for more information on CRE.

Pathogenic microorganisms with unique resistance mechanisms are being continually identified (Insight 5.4). The major cause of concern in antibiotic resistance is that microbes are capable of developing resistance mechanisms to prevent or inactivate agents much faster than scientists can develop new agents. This is no longer a "drug for every bug." It is generally accepted that there will be increasing morbidity and mortality because of infections with resistant microbes for a significant time to come.

The rapid development of resistant pathogens is linked to the misuse of antimicrobial agents. Misuse includes the widespread practice of inappropriate prescribing, such as prescribing antibiotics for colds, which are viral infections (not treatable with antibiotics). When normal host bacteria are frequently exposed to antibiotics, they have many opportunities to develop resistance; this means an antibiotic may be ineffective against a subsequent bacterial infection because the resistant trait has pervaded the host's bacterial population. Similarly, when patients do not take necessary antibiotics as prescribed—regularly and in the right dose—they give pathogens a chance to develop resistance. Weaker pathogens may be destroyed, but stronger, mutated strains may survive and reproduce (Fig. 5.9).

ANTIBIOTIC AGENTS

Many antibiotics are available to treat a wide variety of infectious processes. However, in this text we focus on the main categories of antibiotics (Box 5.2). Antibiotics are usually administered intravenously both before and during a surgical procedure to help prevent SSIs. Antibiotics may also be administered topically from the sterile field, often in the form of irrigating solutions or as ointments. Antibiotics are also prescribed for postoperative use, to be administered intravenously or orally, to prevent or treat infection. Here, we look at some common categories of antibiotics, together with their origins, mechanisms of action, surgical uses, and bacterial resistance mechanisms against the agent.

! CAUTION

Always label your medications on the sterile field with the name and strength. Antibiotics are generally clear liquids and can be easily confused when multiples are used during a procedure.

BOX 5.2 Major Groups of Antibiotics

Aminoglycosides
Beta-lactams
Penicillins
Cephalosporins
Carbapenems
Monobactams
Fluoroquinolones
Macrolides
Tetracyclines

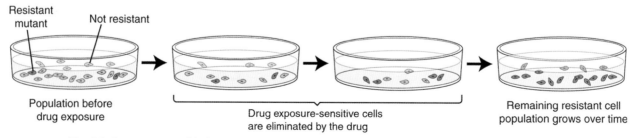

Fig. 5.9 Exposure to antibiotics can produce resistant microorganisms. (From VanMeter KC, Hubert RJ: *Microbiology for the healthcare professional*, ed 2, St Louis, 2016, Elsevier.)

Beta-Lactams

Beta-lactams are a large class of antibiotics that are similar in chemical structure, all containing a structure known as a *beta-lactam ring*. All drugs in this class act on bacteria by inhibiting a penicillin-binding protein (called *transpeptidase*) that makes cross-links during the formation of bacterial cell walls. Inhibition of that protein leads to the formation of weak cell walls, making bacteria vulnerable to rupture (referred to as *lysis*) and subsequent cell death. Because of their mechanism of action, beta-lactams are considered bactericidal. Unfortunately, most agents in this class are not effective against MRSA.

The primary resistance mechanism that some bacteria have acquired is the ability to make the enzyme beta-lactamase, which breaks the beta-lactam ring of these antibiotics' chemical structure (Fig. 5.10). To overcome this resistance mechanism, synthetic compounds known as *beta-lactamase inhibitors* are added to some of these drugs. For example, clavulanic acid is added to amoxicillin, sulbactam is added to ampicillin, and tazobactam is added to piperacillin. These beta-lactam compounds (clavulanic acid, tazobactam, and sulbactam) have little antibacterial action themselves, but they are able to irreversibly bind to many beta-lactamases, thus providing effective treatment. This series of events illustrates the complexity of the fight to treat infections caused by antibiotic-resistant bacteria. Bacteria adapt all too quickly to the changes made in agents used to treat them.

The beta-lactam class includes three major groups of antibiotics: penicillins, cephalosporins, and carbapenems. In addition, the small category known as *monobactams*, which contains only one agent, is also included in this large class of antibiotics.

Penicillins

Penicillin was the first of the true antibiotics (Insight 5.5). Originally extracted from the mold *Penicillium*, this antibiotic is available in several natural and semisynthetic forms effective against a wide variety of gram-positive and gram-negative microbes. Four basic categories of penicillins are available: natural penicillins, penicillinase-resistant penicillins, aminopenicillins, and broad-spectrum penicillins. Penicillins may be given orally or by intramuscular or intravenous injection, depending on the agent. Penicillins may be prescribed before dental or other medical procedures to prevent bacterial infection to the heart

(endocarditis) in patients with prosthetic heart valves. Allergic reactions to penicillin are common, with cross-reactivity among penicillins and some of the cephalosporins. Some species of bacteria have become resistant to penicillin by producing penicillinase, an enzyme that breaks down the drug molecule, inactivating it. Table 5.3 lists some of the penicillins by category.

Natural penicillins include penicillin G, penicillin V, and penicillin G benzathine. Advantages of natural penicillins are low cost and low toxicity. Natural penicillins display a relatively narrow spectrum of action, primarily against gram-positive microbes.

Penicillinase-resistant penicillins are semisynthetics that include nafcillin and oxacillin. This class of penicillins was developed to be effective against strains of bacteria that produce penicillinase. However, some bacteria have developed a means of resistance against penicillinase-resistant penicillins. MRSA is resistant to all penicillinase-resistant penicillins.

Aminopenicillins have been chemically altered by adding an amino group, which makes them effective against gram-negative species, but they are not penicillinase resistant. These semisynthetics include ampicillin and amoxicillin.

Broad-spectrum penicillins include piperacillin and ticarcillin, both of which are effective against *Pseudomonas*. The action of both these agents is enhanced with the addition of a beta-lactamase inhibitor, as previously discussed. Broad-spectrum penicillins are semisynthetics that have been chemically altered to be effective against strains of gram-negative microbes.

Cephalosporins

Cephalosporins are broad-spectrum antibiotics derived from the fungus *C. acremonium*. Cephalosporins are classified into five generations based on different ranges of activity. Each newer generation has greater gram-negative antimicrobial properties and has a longer half-life. This means doses are needed less frequently. The generations are the following:

- *First-generation cephalosporins* are active against many gram-positive and some gram-negative microbes.
- *Second-generation cephalosporins* are effective on a wider variety of gram-negative, but fewer gram-positive, organisms.
- *Third-generation cephalosporins* have a wider range of activity against gram-negative microbes than second-generation agents, but are less effective on gram-positive organisms. They may be used in treating some HAIs.

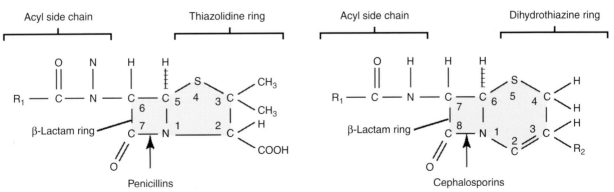

Fig. 5.10 General structures of penicillins and cephalosporins, the most important classes of beta-lactam antibiotics. The presence of a hydrophilic R1 group, as in ampicillin, increases activity against Gram-negative bacteria. The *arrow* indicates the bond that is broken during hydrolysis by beta-lactamase. (From Rosenthal KS: *Rapid review microbiology and immunology*, ed 3, St Louis, 2011, Elsevier.)

INSIGHT 5.5 Yesterday and Today: The Discovery of Penicillin

Penicillin, discovered by Alexander Fleming in 1928, was the first of the "wonder drugs" known as *antibiotics*. It revolutionized medicine by fighting bacterial infections, which could be deadly complications to any type of wound. A chain of events led to the development of this wonder drug. Prominent in these events were men who would lay the foundations for modern-day bacteriology.

In the 1850s a French chemist named Louis Pasteur began work with microscopic organisms called bacteria (or germs). By 1870 he proved that disease in silkworms was caused by germs. He then reasoned that germs could also cause disease in animals, including humans. Because Pasteur was not a physician, though, he kept his research centered on animals. Another event took place when a highly respected Scottish surgeon named Joseph Lister became interested in Pasteur's work. He reasoned that germs could get into surgical wounds and cause postoperative problems: pus, swelling of tissue, fevers, and (all too often) death. Lister added a surgical link to the chain by using chemicals to kill germs in the operating room. His methods, which included spraying the room with carbolic acid, yielded impressive results. Lister's germ-killing chemicals were the first antiseptics. In the meantime, the chain of events strengthened as a German physician, Robert Koch, worked on the role played by bacteria in disease. It was he who proved that specific germs causing diseases in animals caused them in humans as well. In 1876 Koch identified the germ that causes anthrax, showing that it affects cattle, sheep, and people. Then in 1882 he isolated the tuberculosis germ, a common killer of that time.

In 1893 an influential British Army Medical School physician named Almroth Wright forged another link in the chain when he began the search for a typhoid vaccine. He was concerned that this disease was a serious threat to soldiers in the field. Spread by unsanitary conditions that contaminated water, milk, or food, typhoid killed 10% to 30% of its victims at that time. Wright took 6 years to produce a successful vaccine. Then the army authorities refused to use it on a large scale. As a result, thousands of British troops contracted typhoid during the Boer War (1899–1902), and more troops died of this disease than from battle wounds. Shocked and bitterly chagrined, Wright resigned from the Medical School and joined the faculty at St. Mary's Hospital in London. There he created a department to study germs, immunity, and vaccines. In 1910 Wright hired a new research worker—Alexander Fleming.

To develop vaccines, Fleming and the staff of Wright's "Inoculation Department" took blood and pus samples from patients with ulcers, boils, and sores. They kept their samples in Petri dishes filled with agar (a gelatin made from seaweed). Fleming was particularly interested in a pus-producing bacterium called *Staphylococcus*, which is commonly found on the skin. He prepared many microscopic slides from these germ samples. One day Fleming noticed a mold growing on one of his samples. Molds are simple, nonflowering organisms from the fungi family; they can float freely in the air, and this one had blown onto his Petri dish by accident. This "spoiled" sample was special, though: *around the area of the mold was a wide, clean area—no staphylococci.* Even beyond this clean area, the staphylococci were dissolving. Clearly, something from the mold was killing the disease-causing germs. Fleming found out the killer mold was a common one, often found on ripened cheese, stale bread, and rotting fruit. It was from the group of molds called *penicillia*, so Fleming named his discovery "penicillin." However, when he announced his discovery to the rest of the department, no one was impressed. Even Wright showed little enthusiasm. Fortunately, Fleming continued his research, growing more of the mold and testing it on a variety of bacteria. Some were not affected, but a number of them were destroyed. Among those affected were the germs that cause pneumonia, scarlet fever, meningitis, diphtheria, and gonorrhea. Then Fleming took the next step. He went on to test the mold on human blood and found it did not kill white blood cells. He successfully used it topically on a lab assistant to cure an eye infection. Fleming was no chemist, though, so he had problems extracting and purifying the mold. This left him thinking that the new medicine was good for topical use only. When he presented a paper on penicillin to a medical audience in 1929, he was met with indifference. Fleming's interest waned, and his work was directed along other paths.

Ten years later a team of Oxford medical researchers picked up where Fleming left off. The Oxford team took samples of penicillin to the United States, sought backing, and found manufacturers for the new antibiotic. The mass production of this wonder drug in the United States was to save millions of Allied soldiers' lives during World War II. After the war, penicillin and its "wonder-full" derivatives were to change the history of medicine forever.

TABLE 5.3 Penicillins	
Generic Name	**Trade Name**
Natural Penicillins	
penicillin G	Pfizerpen
penicillin G benzathine	Bicillin L-A
Penicillinase-Resistant Penicillins	
nafcillin	Nallpen, Unipen
oxacillin	Bactocill
Aminopenicillins (Not Penicillinase-Resistant)	
ampicillin	N/A
ampicillin-sulbactam	Unasyn
amoxicillin	Amoxil, Trimox
amoxicillin-clavulanate	Augmentin
Broad-Spectrum Penicillins	
piperacillin-tazobactam	Zosyn

- *Fourth-generation cephalosporins* have an expanded spectrum on both gram-positive and gram-negative microorganisms. Many can cross the blood-brain barrier and are effective against meningitis. They are also used against *Pseudomonas aeruginosa.*
- *Fifth-generation cephalosporins* are a new "generation," although the term is not universally used at this time. The US Food and Drug Administration (FDA) has approved one agent, ceftaroline (Teflaro), in this category. It is effective against MRSA and vancomycin-resistant *S. aureus*, and it is used to treat acute skin infections and community-acquired bacterial pneumonia. It is not effective against gram-negative bacteria that produce some of the more advanced resistance factors. Ceftaroline is administered as a prodrug.

QUICK QUESTION

What does the term *prodrug* mean? See the sections on pharmacokinetics and biotransformation in Chapter 1 to check your answer.

Cephalosporins are used as prophylaxis in a variety of surgical procedures, and several of these agents are specifically recommended as part of the SCIP measures. Administration is oral, intramuscular, or intravenous, depending on the particular cephalosporin. Some cephalosporins may be used as topical irrigation solutions in surgery. Bacterial resistance to cephalosporins is conferred by the production of an enzyme (cephalosporinase) that changes the chemical structure of the agent, inactivating it. Table 5.4 lists some of the cephalosporins by generation.

Carbapenems

These beta-lactam antibiotics have a wide spectrum of activity against many gram-positive, gram-negative, and anaerobic bacteria. There is some variation of activity among these agents, but most carbapenems are not effective against *Enterococcus faecium* and MRSA. These antibiotics are considered as the last line of defense against a number of MDR bacteria. Carbapenems are indicated only for serious gram-negative infections, especially *polymicrobic infections* (caused by several different microbes) and infections caused by bacteria resistant to other antibiotics. Unfortunately, the bacterial species most responsible for SSIs (see Table 5.1) have developed multiple resistance factors, including the enzyme beta-lactamase, that interfere with the action of carbapenems. The first approved agent in this class is imipenem (Primaxin). Other carbapenems include meropenem (Merrem) and ertapenem (Invanz).

Monobactams

Aztreonam (Azactam) is the only drug in this small class of beta-lactams called *monobactams*. Aztreonam is the totally synthetic form of an antibiotic originally isolated from *Chromobacterium violaceum*. It is used for infections caused by gram-negative bacteria, including *Pseudomonas*. Because of its slightly different chemical structure, it is considered safe to use in patients who have an allergy to the other beta-lactams. It is available for intramuscular or intravenous injection.

Aminoglycosides

Aminoglycosides are derived from various strains of *Actinomyces* bacteria. The bactericidal action of agents in this category is attributed to two mechanisms: (1) interfere with protein synthesis by binding to bacterial (prokaryotic) ribosomes, and (2) create small holes in bacterial cell membranes causing leakage. Generally, aminoglycosides are active only against aerobic, gram-negative bacteria, but they can also provide some activity against some gram-positive bacteria, such as Staphylococcus species, including some methicillin-resistant strains. Otherwise, they are not very active against gram-positive organisms. All aminoglycosides are contraindicated if the patient has a history of hypersensitivity or toxic reactions to any aminoglycoside. Major adverse effects include nephrotoxicity and ototoxicity.

> ### ❓ QUICK QUESTION
>
> What is meant by the terms *nephrotoxicity* and *ototoxicity*? See the section in Chapter 1 on pharmacodynamics to check your answers.

Approximately 10% of patients receiving aminoglycosides may experience ototoxicity in the form of damage to the sensory cells of the inner ear, which may be permanent. An estimated 10% of patients may experience nephrotoxicity because of damage of the cell membrane of renal tubules. This adverse effect is usually mild and may be reversible if the agent is discontinued. Aminoglycosides are poorly absorbed orally, but are almost completely absorbed when applied topically during surgical procedures. Intramuscular and intravenous injections are the most common administration routes for aminoglycosides. Aminoglycosides are indicated for short-term treatment of serious infections caused by susceptible organisms. Such infections include bacterial septicemia, as well as infections of the respiratory tract, bones and joints, central nervous system (meningitis), skin, and soft tissue. Aminoglycosides may also be prescribed for intraabdominal infections.

Among the drugs in the aminoglycoside category are amikacin, gentamicin, neomycin, and tobramycin, as listed in Table 5.5. Amikacin is often effective even when strains of susceptible organisms are resistant to other aminoglycosides. Gentamicin is available in cream and ointment, ophthalmic solution and ointment, and solution for injection. Neomycin is used topically *only* in the form of drops (ophthalmic) or ointment because of significant adverse effects associated with systemic absorption. Often neomycin is used in combination with other agents, such as polymyxin B and dexamethasone in Maxitrol, an ophthalmic suspension. Tobramycin is also

TABLE 5.4 Cephalosporins

Generic Name	Trade Name
First Generation	
cefazolin	Ancef, Kefzol
cephalexin	Keflex
Second Generation	
cefoxitin	N/A
cefonicid	N/A
cefotetan	N/A
cefuroxime	N/A
Third Generation	
cefotaxime	N/A
ceftazidime	Fortaz, Tazicef
ceftriaxone	N/A
Fourth Generation	
cefepime	N/A
Fifth Generation	
ceftaroline	Teflaro

TABLE 5.5	**Aminoglycosides**
Generic Name	**Trade Name**
amikacin	N/A
gentamicin	Garamycin
tobramycin	Tobrex Ophthalmic

TABLE 5.6	**Fluoroquinolones**
Generic Name	**Trade Name**
ciprofloxacin	Cipro
ofloxacin	N/A
levofloxacin	N/A
besifloxacin	Besivance
moxifloxacin	N/A

available in an ophthalmic preparation under the trade name Tobrex (see Chapter 10).

Bacterial resistance to aminoglycosides is conferred by the production of enzymes that modify the chemical structure of the agent, inactivating it.

> **! CAUTION**
>
> Suffixes can help you understand some antibiotic names by class, but not always! Antibiotic names that end in the suffix "-mycin" (such as tobramycin, an aminoglycoside) usually indicate chemicals derived from *Streptomyces*, a genus of bacteria present in soil. However, not all antibiotics that end in "-mycin" are aminoglycosides. Macrolide antibiotics (see Table 5.7) end in "-mycin" too, as do other antibiotics, such as vancomycin, daptomycin, and clindamycin. In addition, the similar suffix "-micin" is used to indicate antibiotics derived from *Micromonospora*, a genus of bacterial also found in soil. Gentamicin (an aminoglycoside) is derived from *Micromonospora*, so not all aminoglycosides are derived from *Streptomyces*.
>
> The class of various antibiotics is vitally important when dealing with patients who have known hypersensitivity to a particular class of antibiotic agents. If a surgeon's preference card indicates a routine order for an antibiotic, always check the patient's allergies and the most current available information regarding cross-reactivity between antibiotic classes!

Fluoroquinolones

Fluoroquinolones are a category of synthetic antibiotics that inhibit DNA gyrase, a protein necessary for bacterial replication. They are classified as first, second, third, and fourth generation. Fluoroquinolone antibiotics have a relatively low toxicity and a broad spectrum of activity against both gram-positive and gram-negative aerobes. However, both MRSA and VRE are resistant to fluoroquinolones. They are given orally or intravenously for systemic infections, urinary tract infections (UTIs), and osteomyelitis. Many of the fluoroquinolones are also formulated for ophthalmic use (see Chapter 10).

Agents include ciprofloxacin (Cipro, second generation), ofloxacin, enoxacin, levofloxacin, moxifloxacin, and besifloxacin (Besivance) (Table 5.6).

Macrolides

Macrolides, which include the erythromycins, are a group of broad-spectrum agents that inhibit bacterial protein synthesis by binding to the prokaryotic ribosomal subunit. Bacteriostatic for most bacteria, macrolides are bactericidal for several gram-positive bacteria, such as *Legionella*. Bactericidal activity is explained by the fact that these antibiotics can penetrate the cell walls of gram-positive organisms. Macrolides may be obtained from isolates of *Streptococcus erythreus* or may be synthesized in the laboratory.

TABLE 5.7	**Macrolides**
Generic Name	**Trade Name**
erythromycin	Erythrocin
azithromycin	Zithromax
clarithromycin	N/A

> **🔖 TECH TIP**
>
> Macrolide antibiotics are derived from strains of *Streptomyces*, so they end in the suffix "-mycin." However, you can tell a macrolide antibiotic name because it has the word part "thro" in front of the "-mycin" suffix.

Macrolides are only partially metabolized and are excreted almost unchanged in bile. Most macrolides are administered orally; however, erythromycin is available in topical ointment and solution, as well as in an ophthalmic ointment for local infections and for newborns to prevent gonococcal infections. Bacterial resistance is primarily caused by changes in bacterial cell wall permeability, such as some strains of *Pseudomonas*, which have developed resistance to erythromycin. When a strain of bacteria becomes resistant to one macrolide antibiotic, they are resistant to all agents in this category. Macrolide antibiotics include the natural erythromycin (Erythrocin) and the semisynthetic azithromycin (Zithromax) and clarithromycin, as listed in Table 5.7.

Tetracyclines

Tetracyclines were the first broad-spectrum antibiotics, originally obtained from cultures of *Streptomyces*. Bacteriostatic in action, tetracyclines bind to the bacterial ribosomal subunit, interfering with protein synthesis. Originally effective against many gram-positive and gram-negative bacteria, some common bacteria have developed resistance to tetracyclines. Resistance factors are carried in plasmids (pieces of bacterial DNA), which are widely distributed among many bacteria. The mechanism of resistance is somewhat novel in that these bacteria have developed the ability to actively pump these antibiotics out of the cell unchanged (called *tetracycline-specific efflux pumps*) (Fig. 5.11). Tetracycline-resistant bacteria include MRSA, VRE, and *Pseudomonas*, so use is significantly limited; they are primarily used to treat acne and rickettsial infections. Tetracycline hydrochloride is administered orally because no parenteral form is available.

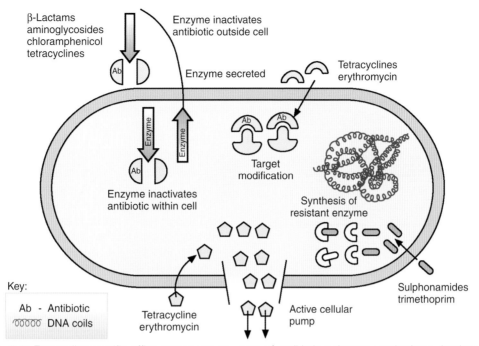

Fig. 5.11 Tetracycline-specific efflux pumps are one type of antibiotic-resistance mechanisms developed in bacteria. (From Eley B, Soory M, Manson JD: *Periodontics*, ed 6, St Louis, 2010, Churchill Livingstone, Elsevier.)

Minocycline may be administered intravenously if the oral route is not feasible. Doxycycline may be administered orally or intravenously.

A new subclass of tetracyclines has been developed, called *glycylcyclines*. Designed to overcome known bacterial resistance mechanisms, the first agent in this category is tigecycline (Tygacil). It is available for intravenous administration and is reserved for use in complicated infections, such as intraabdominal infections caused by *Escherichia coli*, VRE, and MRSA. Tetracycline antibiotics are listed in Table 5.8.

Miscellaneous Antibiotics

Many other antibiotics are available for prophylaxis and treatment of infections caused by susceptible microorganisms. Miscellaneous agents presented in this chapter include sulfonamides, several individual agents, and combination agents.

Sulfonamides

Sulfonamides, more commonly known as *sulfa drugs*, are not strictly considered to be antibiotics because these chemicals did not originate in a microorganism. Sulfonamides are laboratory-synthesized chemicals that interfere with cell metabolism by inhibiting bacterial synthesis of folic acid. Introduced in 1935 by Gerhard Domagk, sulfonamides are the oldest of the chemotherapeutic agents. They are in limited use today (owing to increasing microbial resistance) but are still prescribed for community-acquired pneumonia, nonobstructive UTIs, severe burns, and superficial eye infections. Sulfonamides are administered orally, topically, and, occasionally, intravenously. Resistance is conferred

TABLE 5.8   Tetracyclines

Generic Name	Trade Name
tetracycline	N/A
minocycline	Minocin
doxycycline	Vibramycin
tigecycline	Tygacil

by altering bacterial cell wall permeability, thus preventing the agent from entering the bacterium. Examples of sulfonamides include silver sulfadiazine, sulfamethoxazole, sulfasalazine, and sulfacetamide sodium. Sulfamethoxazole is also combined with trimethoprim (another antibacterial) and is available under the trade names Bactrim and Septra. Silver sulfadiazine (Silvadene cream) is a topical antimicrobial agent containing sulfa and silver salts that is used in dressings for burn patients.

> **? QUICK QUESTION**
>
> Because silver sulfadiazine (Silvadene cream) is a combination of sulfa and silver salts, it can be considered as derived from which drug source(s)? See the section on drug sources in Chapter 1 to check your answer.

Individual Agents

A number of individual agents are unique or are in a class of only a few agents (Table 5.9).

TABLE 5.9 Individual Agents	
Generic Name	**Trade Name**
bacitracin	N/A
clindamycin	Cleocin
daptomycin	Cubicin
linezolid	Zyvox
metronidazole	Flagyl
mupirocin	N/A
polymyxin B sulfate	N/A
quinupristin and dalfopristin	Synercid
vancomycin	Vanocin

Bacitracin is an antibacterial polypeptide derived from the strain of bacterium *Bacillus subtilis* that interferes with bacterial cell wall synthesis. It is effective against a wide range of gram-positive and a few gram-negative microorganisms. It has similar properties to penicillin and is effective against staphylococci and streptococci. Intramuscular injection is associated with nephrotoxicity, a serious adverse effect, so its use is strictly limited. Bacitracin is used as a topical ointment to prevent or treat minor skin infections and it is available in combination with other medications (such as polymyxin B) in a topical ophthalmic ointment form to treat eye infections.

Clindamycin (Cleocin) is the synthetic analogue of the natural antibiotic lincomycin, so it is classified as a lincosamide antibiotic. It is active against gram-positive aerobic and anaerobic bacteria. It is bacteriostatic and inhibits protein synthesis by binding to the bacterial ribosomes. Used to treat infections in patients who are allergic to penicillin, clindamycin may be administered orally or intravenously. It is often used in combination with a bactericidal agent to treat severe infections caused by gram-positive microbes. Its high affinity for bone makes it an option for treatment of osteomyelitis caused by susceptible bacteria. Because clindamycin is very effective at reducing normal intestinal bacteria, as well as pathogens, a serious adverse effect has emerged, which has resulted in an FDA "Black Box" warning regarding use of this agent. The FDA warns that *Clostridium difficile*-associated diarrhea (CDAD), ranging from mild to severe, is a potential adverse effect from use of almost all antibiotics. However, the warning indicates that treatment with clindamycin has been associated with a higher incidence of severe colitis, which may be fatal. Microbial resistance is obtained by changes in bacterial ribosomal structure, which prevents the agent from binding.

Daptomycin (Cubicin) is a newer antibiotic derived from *Streptomyces roseosporus* and is classified as a cyclic glycopeptide. Its mechanism of action allows it to bind irreversibly to the cell membranes of susceptible gram-positive bacteria. Daptomycin is indicated for complicated skin infections and for bacteremia (bloodstream infection), particularly those caused by MRSA.

Linezolid (Zyvox) is the only agent in a unique class called *oxazolidinones*. A synthetic chemical, Zyvox inhibits bacterial protein synthesis by an entirely different mechanism of action from other agents, targeting a specific ribosomal subunit. It is administered intravenously or orally and is used to treat infections caused by MRSA, VRE, and some streptococci. It is bacteriostatic against enterococci and staphylococci and bactericidal against most streptococci. Resistance to linezolid is conferred by altering the site of action (ribosomal subunit).

Metronidazole (Flagyl) is a synthetic antibiotic classified as a nitroimidazole. It is administered as a prodrug that becomes activated in the presence of anaerobic microbes, producing toxins that damage bacterial DNA. It is bactericidal against anaerobic gram-positive and gram-negative bacilli. It may be administered intravenously for prophylaxis in colorectal procedures when contamination from enteric anaerobic bacteria is possible. Metronidazole is also administered intravenously to treat postoperative SSIs caused by susceptible anaerobic bacteria, but conversion to oral administration as soon as possible is recommended. It is effective in treating CDAD. Bacterial resistance is accomplished by the production of enzymes and by changes in cell membrane permeability.

Mupirocin ointment 2% is a naturally occurring antibiotic produced by fermentation using the organism *Pseudomonas fluorescens*. It inhibits protein synthesis by binding to a bacterial enzyme. It is active against a wide range of gram-positive bacteria, including *S. aureus*, *Streptococcus pyogenes*, and MRSA. It may be used to treat nasal colonization of MRSA. In surgery, it may be used for intranasal packing placed after septoplasty.

Polymyxin B sulfate (generic name only) and colistin (polymyxin E) are related lipopeptide antibiotics derived from *Bacillus polymyxa*. These agents are bactericidal and effective against nearly all species of gram-negative bacilli except *Proteus*. They work against bacteria by increasing the permeability of the cell membrane. Polymyxin B had been in limited use for a very long time but has been identified as a drug of "last resort" to treat infections caused by some strains of MDR gram-negative bacteria. It is used to treat infections of the bloodstream (bacteremia), meninges, and urinary tract caused by susceptible strains of *P. aeruginosa*. Polymyxin B sulfate is available in powder form, which is reconstituted for topical ophthalmic, intravenous, intramuscular, or intrathecal (spinal; see Chapter 13) administration. It is measured in units rather than milligrams. Microbial resistance is rare.

Quinupristin/dalfopristin (Synercid) is a combination of two semisynthetic agents derived from pristinamycin. Synercid is bactericidal, inhibiting protein synthesis by binding to bacterial ribosomes. It is used to treat complicated skin and skin structure infections caused by methicillin-susceptible *S. aureus* or *S. pyogenes*. Synercid is administered intravenously in a solution of 5% dextrose in water over a period of 60 minutes.

Vancomycin (Vancocin) is a glycopeptide antibiotic derived from *Amycolatopsis orientalis* and used to treat severe infections caused by MRSA. It is bactericidal, but only against gram-positive bacteria. Vancomycin inhibits cell wall synthesis by binding to a molecule that is needed to form cross-links in the cell wall. Vancomycin also alters cell membrane permeability and interferes with RNA synthesis. It is administered intravenously and is active against staphylococci, streptococci, and enterococci. Bacterial resistance occurs by altering the bacterial binding site, as seen in VRE. A new synthetic agent, telavancin (Vibativ), is derived from vancomycin. Telavancin is used to treat serious skin infections and hospital-acquired or ventilator-associated pneumonia caused by susceptible gram-positive bacteria.

KEY CONCEPTS

- Antibiotics are antimicrobial agents used in surgery for prophylaxis against wound infections. They are also given to treat postoperative SSIs. Despite meticulous aseptic technique, SSIs may arise when pathogenic microorganisms are transmitted to a susceptible host. When that happens, the causative microbe will be identified and tested for antibiotic sensitivity before a definitive course of antibiotic therapy is selected.

- Antibiotics work against microbes in five major ways. The agent may inhibit bacterial cell wall synthesis, impede protein synthesis, interfere with nucleic acid (RNA or DNA) synthesis, alter bacterial cell wall function, or disrupt bacterial cell metabolism. Antibiotics may be bacteriostatic or bactericidal and may have a broad, narrow, or limited spectrum of activity. Some bacteria have developed resistance to some leading antibiotics, making treatment protocols difficult. Antibiotics may be administered orally, intramuscularly, intravenously, or topically, depending on the agent.

- Major categories of antibiotics include aminoglycosides, cephalosporins, fluoroquinolones, macrolides (erythromycins), oxazolidinones, penicillins, and tetracyclines. Several other categories of antibacterials are in use today, as well as several unique agents. Surgical technologists should become familiar with antibiotics used routinely during surgery.

LEARNING THE LANGUAGE (KEY TERMS)

Using your textbook or a standard medical dictionary, look up and write the definitions of each term.

antibiotic resistance
bactericidal
bacteriostatic
culture and sensitivity (C&S)
endogenous
eukaryotes
exogenous

Gram staining
morphology
MRSA
polymicrobic infections
prokaryotes
selective toxicity
surgical site infections (SSIs)
VRE

REVIEW QUESTIONS

1. What does MRSA stand for? VRE? Why are these important in surgery?
2. Why are antibiotics administered in surgery?
3. Which test is used to identify the organism that causes TB?
4. What does C&S test reveal?
5. Why would a Gram stain be ordered during surgery?
6. How do antibiotics work?
7. What is the difference between bactericidal and bacteriostatic?
8. Why is antimicrobial resistance a problem in surgery?
9. How are antibiotics administered in surgery?
10. Have you served as a scrubbed surgical technologist or in a procedure when an antibiotic was administered? Which antibiotic was used? What category did the agent belong in? How was it administered?

CRITICAL THINKING

Scenario 1

Mrs. Chacon is a 55-year-old woman admitted to surgery for insertion of a venous access catheter. The chart indicates that she has an allergy to cefazolin (Ancef), and the preference card lists a standing order for cephalexin (Keflex) 1 g mixed with 30 mL of saline for topical irrigation.

1. Is this medication order of concern? Explain why or why not.
2. How should you handle this situation to ensure the patient's safety?

Scenario 2

Mr. Fayed is a 33-year-old man who cut his hand while working in the garden 10 days ago. He was initially treated in the emergency department, where the wound was irrigated and closed. He was sent home with a prescription for piperacillin, which he has taken as instructed. The wound remains infected, so he is admitted to surgery for incision and drainage of the wound. Swabs are taken for routine and fungal C&S because the surgeon suspects the infectious agent may be a soil-based fungus.

1. How is a fungus different from bacteria?
2. Why would the antibiotic not work on a fungal infection?

BIBLIOGRAPHY

Bardal S, Waechter J, Martin D: In *Applied pharmacology*, St Louis, 2011, Saunders/Elsevier.

Brink AJ, Coetzee J, Clay CG, et al: Emergence of New Delhi metallo-beta-lactamase (NDM-1) and klebsiella Pneumoniae Carbapenemase (KPC-2) in South Africa, *J Clin Microbiol* 50(2):525–527, 2012.

Damodaran SE, Madhan S: Telavancin: a novel lipoglycopeptide antibiotic, *J Pharmacol Pharmacother* 2(2):135–137, 2011.

Drawz SM, Bonomo RA: Three decades of β-lactamase inhibitors, *Clin Microbiol Rev* 23(1):160–201, 2010.

Fulcher EM, Fulcher RM, Soto CD: *Pharmacology: principles and applications*, ed 3, St Louis, 2012, Saunders/Elsevier.

Gallagher J, MacDougall C: *Antibiotics simplified*, ed 2, Burlington, 2012, Jones & Bartlett Learning.

Goede WJ, Lovely JK, Thompson RL, et al: Assessment of prophylactic antibiotic use in patients with surgical site infections, *Hosp Pharm* 48(7):560–567, 2013.

Gupta N, Limbago BM, Patel JB, et al: Carbapenem-resistant Enterobacteriaceae: epidemiology and prevention, *Clin Infect Dis* 53(1):60–67, 2011.

Holten KB, Onusko EM: Appropriate prescribing of oral beta-lactam antibiotics, *Am Fam Physician* 62(3):611–620, 2000.

Jorgensen JH, Ferraro MJ: Antimicrobial susceptibility testing: a review of general principles and contemporary practices, *Clin Infect Dis* 49(11):1749–1755, 2009.

McHugh SM, Collins CJ, Corrigan MA, et al: The role of topical antibiotics used as prophylaxis in surgical site infection prevention, *J Antimicrob Chemother* 66(4):693–701, 2011.

Nagelhout J, Plaus K: *Handbook of anesthesia*, ed 5, St Louis, 2013, Saunders/Elsevier.

Parry MF, Grant B, Yukna M, et al: Candida osteomyelitis and diskitis after spinal surgery: an outbreak that implicates artificial nail use, *Clin Infect Dis* 32(3):352–357, 2001.

Passaro DJ, Waring L, Armstrong R, et al: Postoperative *Serratia marcescens* wound infections traced to an out-of-hospital source, *J Infect Dis* 175(4):992–995, 1997.

Salkind AR, Rao KC: Antibiotic prophylaxis to prevent surgical site infections, *Am Fam Physician* 83(5):585–590, 2011.

VanMeter KC, VanMeter WG, Hubert RJ: *Microbiology for the healthcare professional*, St Louis, 2013, Mosby/Elsevier.

Zavascki AP, Goldani LZ, Li, J, et al: Polymyxin B for the treatment of multidrug-resistant pathogens: a critical review, *J Antimicrob Chemother* 60(6):1206–1215, 2007.

INTERNET RESOURCES

Centers for Disease Control and Prevention, Antibiotic/antimicrobial resistance, biggest threats: www.cdc.gov/drugresistance/biggest_threats.html.

Centers for Disease Control and Prevention, Carbapenem-resistant Enterobacteriaceae in healthcare settings: www.cdc.gov/HAI/organisms/cre.

Centers for Disease Control and Prevention, Healthcare-associated infections (HAI): www.cdc.gov/hai/.

Centers for Disease Control and Prevention, Interim duodenoscope surveillance protocol: www.cdc.gov/hai/organisms/cre/cre-duodenoscope-surveillance-protocol.html.

Centers for Disease Control and Prevention, Methicillin-resistant Staphylococcus aureus (MRSA) infections: www.cdc.gov/mrsa.

Centers for Disease Control and Prevention, Procedure associated module SSI: www.cdc.gov/nhsn/PDFs/pscManual/9pscSSI current.pdf.

Centers for Disease Control and Prevention, Healthcare-associated infections (HAI), surgical site infection (SSI): www.cdc.gov/HAI/ssi/ssi.html.

Centers for Disease Control and Prevention, Tuberculosis (TB) fact sheet: www.cdc.gov/tb/publications/factsheets/drtb/mdrtb.htm.

Cubicin, Daptomycin information for health professionals: https://www.merck.com/products/#c.

eMedExpert, Cephalosporins: www.emedexpert.com/compare/cephalosporins.shtml.

emedicinehealth, NDM-1 and antibiotic resistance by bacteria: www.emedicinehealth.com/ndm-1/article_em.htm.

Leinum C.J., Boeser K.D., Ceftaroline fosamil: a new FDA-approved anti-MRSA cephalosporin antibiotic: www.healio.com/infectious-disease/vaccine-preventable-diseases/news/print/infectious-disease-news/%7B82e25871-ce14-43f9-8eab-d66aa4a85570%7D/ceftaroline-fosamil-a-new-fda-approved-anti-mrsa-cephalosporin-antibiotic.

Pfizer Products, Clindamycin (Cleocin) prescribing information: www.pfizerpro.com/pfizer-products.

Pfizer Products, Quinupristin/dalfopristin (Synercid) prescribing information: https://www.pfizermedicalinformation.com/en-us/cleocin-t.

RxList Vibativ, Telavancin: www.rxlist.com/vibativ-drug.htm.

The Joint Commission, Surgical Care Improvement Project: www.jointcommission.org/surgical_care_improvement_project.

World Health Organization, Patient safety, safe surgery saves lives: https://www.who.int/news/item/24-06-2008-new-checklist-to-help-make-surgery-safer.

KEY TERMS

HAI
peak and trough
sepsis

superbugs
superinfection

ANTIBIOTIC THERAPY

Advanced practitioners functioning as surgical first assistants will encounter the use of antibiotic therapy for the treatment and prevention of infections in the surgical patient. Preoperative, intraoperative, and postoperative care of the surgical patient has expanded from the hospital setting to include outpatient facilities, surgery centers, specialty clinics, nursing homes, and even long-care facilities. Thus, the term for a hospital-acquired infection (nosocomial) has been expanded to *healthcare-associated infection (HAI)*. HAI is defined by the Centers for Disease Control and Prevention (CDC) as a localized or systemic condition that results from an adverse reaction to infection (infectious agents or toxins), and was not present, or incubating, at the time of admission. So, an infection is considered an HAI if it is not related to the admitting diagnosis or develops within 48 hours after admission. This is described in the National Nosocomial Infections Surveillance System established by the CDC to track, investigate, and help prevent nosocomial infections. Antibiotics are administered for treatment of sepsis, prevention of surgical site infections (SSIs), intraoperative wound irrigation, and postoperative infection control. Because there are many classifications of antibiotics, the selection of the appropriate medication relies on several factors. For any specific infection, however, there is usually one antibiotic that research determines to be superior. Some of the factors for medication selection include patient allergy, inability of the antibiotic to reach the site of infection, patient susceptibility to the medication's toxicity, medication efficacy, and the medication's spectrum. Although the physician selects the appropriate antibiotic, the surgical first assistant must have knowledge of antibiotic use and actions to ensure that the patient receives the correct dosage of antibiotic at the right time. The surgical first assistant acts as another line of defense against medication errors and adverse reactions caused by antibiotic therapy, as discussed in Chapter 4.

ASSISTANT ADVICE

The surgical first assistant involved in postoperative patient care should note that patients who are given clear explanations and instructions of why the antibiotic(s) is (are) being given are more likely to comply and complete the full course of the prescribed medications.

ANTIBIOTIC RESISTANCE

The main reason for the development of drug-resistant bacteria is the misuse of antimicrobial agents. This misuse includes inept prescribing and inappropriate use, failure to complete the full course of medication, administering antibacterial agents to treat viral infections (such as influenza), antibiotics in the food chain, and not following all guidelines established to prevent the spread of infections in patient care settings. Microbial resistance is bacteria's ability to overcome the bactericidal effects of an antibiotic. Resistance traits are encoded into the bacteria's genes and can be transmitted to other bacteria. Microorganisms can proliferate and mutate rapidly and adapt to new environments and hosts. Because of these abilities, microorganisms can "learn" to withstand the effects of antibiotics, and new superbugs emerge. Multidrug resistance is a serious problem that has spread out of the hospital environment and into the community. This acquired resistance can render currently effective antibiotics useless. In 2008 these resistant pathogens were dubbed the "ESKAPE" bacteria and include *Enterococcus faecium, Staphylococcus aureus, Klebsiella pneumoniae, Acinetobacter baumannii, Pseudomonas aeruginosa,* and *Enterobacter* species. Added to this list are *Escherichia coli* and *Mycobacterium tuberculosis*. These pathogens currently cause most of the US hospital infections and effectively "escape" the effects of antibacterial drug treatment. Unfortunately, there is an ever-widening gap between the number of these deadly antibiotic-resistant microorganisms and new, effective drugs to treat them. Few of the right type of new antibiotics are completing the drug development requirements of the US Food and Drug Administration, and added to this, companies are not spending the money to develop antibiotics that are used short term and are expensive to produce. This is unlikely to change in the near future, and the result is antibiotic development not keeping pace with microbial resistance.

As discussed in this chapter, another example of a lethal microorganism is carbapenem-resistant *Enterobacteriaceae* (CRE). The usual form of enterobacteria is present within the body as normal flora (*E. coli*) and causes no problems. Once it gets into the bloodstream, bladder, or other such areas, though, it becomes very dangerous to the patient. Some of these pathogens have developed defenses to fight most antibiotics; thus, it is considered highly resistant and has earned it the name "killer bacteria" and "nightmare bacteria." This superbug is spreading throughout the United States and is found in hospitals, long-term acute care facilities, and nursing homes. CRE's mortality rate is between 40% and 50% for patients who have severe infections from it. The literature suggests aggressive "detect and protect" actions, such as intensive infection prevention (aseptic technique) and antibiotic prescribing changes.

A *superinfection* is an additional infection that appears during the course of antibiotic treatment of a primary infection. An example is a yeast infection that occurs during treatment of bacterial pneumonia with penicillin. Broad-spectrum antibiotics (such as tetracyclines and penicillins) kill off more normal flora and so set the stage for superinfections. They may occur if the antibiotic dosage was too large for the patient (i.e., patient's size/weight) or by the drug's inhibition or alteration of the normal flora within the body, which allows the secondary infection to occur.

PEAK AND TROUGH

Antibiotic medications rely on their ability to penetrate the bacteria cell wall and bind with sufficient concentration levels to be effective. The concentration levels depend on the half-life and elimination of the medication. When maintaining a therapeutic

dosage of antibiotics (as described in the Advanced Practices section of Chapter 4), it is important to understand peak and trough levels. The time when the medication is at the highest plasma concentration is referred to as its *peak level*. This peak level depends on the absorption rate and the route of administration. Intravenously administered medications take much less time to reach peak levels than oral medications. The point of time when the medication is at the lowest level of plasma concentration is referred to as the *trough level*. Ideally, to maintain a therapeutic response, an antibiotic would be redosed before it reaches trough level.

SEPSIS

Antibiotic therapy is essential for the treatment of sepsis. Every year, severe sepsis attacks more than one million Americans. Sepsis is defined as a systemic inflammatory response to the presence of pus-forming bacteria or their toxins in the blood or tissues. It is a life-threatening syndrome that is the leading cause of death in intensive care units, usually resulting from an overwhelming infection. The patient's response to sepsis may be low and short term, to critical and long term or demise. Sepsis can be divided into several categories according to symptoms and certain criteria. Each category has an associated mortality rate (Table 5.A). The clinical management of sepsis is a multifocal approach that includes resuscitation, organ system support, and control of the infection. The control of infection combines the use of antibiotics in addition to drainage or debridement of involved tissues. Septic patients will be on an antibiotic therapy, and it is imperative that therapy be continued throughout the surgical procedure, as the source of the infection is removed.

ASSISTANT ADVICE

Check the dosage and timing of the antibiotic ordered for the patient. Be sure the next doses are available in the surgical suite if required during the procedure. Also check with the surgeon concerning any extra bolus of medication that may be needed and have it available.

TABLE 5.A	**Associated Mortality Rates of Sepsis**	
Definition	**Symptoms and Criteria**	**Mortality Rate**
Systemic inflammatory response syndrome (SIRS)	Two or more of the following: Temperature <36°C or >38°C Heart rate >90 beats per min Respiration >20 breaths per min or $Paco_2$ <32 mm Hg WBC count >12,000 or <4000 or 10% immature cells	3%–17% depending on the number of symptoms
Sepsis	SIRS with addition of an infection site confirmed by culture (positive blood culture not necessary) and no ongoing sign of organ failure	15%–30% Note: for newborns and pediatric patients with sepsis—9%–36%
Severe sepsis	Sepsis plus organ dysfunction and tissue hypoperfusion or hypotension	28%–50%
Septic shock	Hypotension induced by sepsis despite fluid bolus organ and tissue hypoperfusion	40%–60%

Paco_2, partial pressure of carbon dioxide in arterial blood; *WBC*, white blood cell.

PREOPERATIVE ANTIBIOTIC PROPHYLAXIS

The use of prophylactic antibiotics to prevent SSIs has proved beneficial in certain procedures. However, in other situations these antibiotics have no benefit to the patient. Prophylactic antibiotics may be beneficial when used before implant procedures and clean-contaminated (surgical wound classification category 3) surgical wounds (category IA). They have no benefit in clean surgical wounds (incised, noninfected) or contaminated wounds. They may be used on a patient with congenital or valvular heart disease or who has had rheumatic fever. This is to reduce the amount of normal flora, thus decreasing the chance of endocarditis from bacteria. Another indication for preoperative antibiotics is neutropenia (low neutrophil counts) that could increase the risk of infection. The risk of side effects, creating superinfections, and adverse reactions must be carefully weighed against the advantages of administering prophylactic antibiotics in each patient. Infants and the elderly have metabolisms and excretion that differ from typical adult patients, so this puts them at higher risk of drug toxicity because antibiotics can accumulate to toxic levels in their blood. Women who are pregnant or lactating pose problems with antibiotic therapy because some drugs can cross the placenta and enter breast milk.

Errors that occur most during prophylactic antibiotic therapy concern the timing of administration and the duration of the therapy. In general, preoperative antibiotics should be administered within 30 minutes before incision and be continued not more than 24 hours postoperatively.

The administration of the initial dose of preoperative antibiotics presents a challenge to healthcare providers in today's fast-paced systems. Patients may arrive at the facility within 1 hour of their scheduled procedure. Most facilities will have a standard protocol for starting preoperative antibiotics. The surgical first assistant must be familiar with the protocol and make sure that it is followed at all times. Many surgeons are requiring the administration of the antibiotic when patients arrive in the surgical suite to ensure proper timing of antiinfective coverage. Antibiotic name, dosage, and time of administration are being included in the "time out" taken before the surgical procedure begins. The choice of antibiotic will depend on the type, classification, and site of the procedure. The medication will cover against any natural flora in the surgical field. *S. aureus* and *Staphylococcus epidermidis* cause most surgical wound infections. Administering a first-generation cephalosporin, such as cefazolin, can cover these microorganisms. Another indicator of antibiotic choice is any allergies the patient may have. In patients with an allergy to penicillin, the surgeon may prescribe clindamycin or, in some cases, vancomycin.

INTRAOPERATIVE ANTIBIOTIC WOUND IRRIGATION

Many surgeons choose to use an antibiotic agent in the irrigation fluid to help to prevent SSIs. This usually will be the final irrigation before closure of the wound. The antibiotic of choice, such as Ancef, is mixed in the appropriate volume of irrigation fluid (usually 500 mL). To prevent the irrigation solution from cooling, this should not be mixed in advance. When the irrigation solution is placed into the wound, it should remain for a short period of time to allow the antibiotic to absorb into the tissues. (Refer to Chapter 11 for more information on irrigation fluids.)

ANTIVIRALS AND ANTIFUNGALS

Antibacterials (antibiotics) are the more commonly used antimicrobial agents in surgery. However, the surgical first assistant should have a basic knowledge of other types of antimicrobials. Two of these are antivirals and antifungals. The identification of viral infections, including those that affect the surgical team members, has brought about the development of new drugs. Antivirals are a class of drugs that specifically treat viral infections, and like antibiotics, specific antivirals are used to treat specific infections. They work by inhibiting the pathogen's ability to reproduce, rather than destroying it. Viruses use the host's cells to replicate, and this makes it difficult to develop drugs that will harm the virus without harming the host. Viral infections include human immunodeficiency virus (HIV), the herpes virus, hepatitis B and C, and influenza B and C. (Viral drugs used for treatment of HIV can be found in the section on federal agencies in Chapter 2.) A breakthrough in using antivirals for cancer treatment has been established with the human papillomavirus vaccine for cervical cancer. Many cancers could have a viral origin, but research is just now finding the few that have been implicated as actually causing human cancers.

> **! CAUTION**
> Cool temperature irrigation fluid may adversely affect the patient's core body temperature.

Antifungals are drugs used to treat fungal infections, such as athlete's foot, candidiasis (thrush), and types of dermatophyte infections, such as ringworm. Both fungal and human cells are eukaryotes and similar on the molecular level. This makes it difficult to develop antifungals that will not harm the host cells. Antifungal drugs have the potential for serious side effects, such as liver damage and anaphylaxis, if not used properly.

ADVANCED PRACTICES: REVIEW QUESTIONS

1. List three factors to consider when choosing an appropriate antibiotic.
2. The time when a medication is at the highest plasma concentration is referred to as the _____ _____.
3. The decay and putrefaction of living tissue from an overwhelming infection is called:
   a. Dehydration
   b. Sepsis
   c. Sciatica
   d. Antibiotic resistance

4. How long before a surgical procedure should preoperative prophylactic antibiotics be administered?
   a. 10 minutes
   b. 30 minutes
   c. 1 hour
   d. 2 hours
5. An antibiotic commonly used within the sterile field is _____.

ADVANCED PRACTICES: BIBLIOGRAPHY

Fulcher EM, Fulcher RM, Soto CD: *Pharmacology: principles and applications,* ed 3, St Louis, 2012, Saunders/Elsevier.

Kee JL, Hayes ER, McCuistion LE: *Pharmacology: a patient-centered nursing process approach*, ed 8, St Louis, Saunders/Elsevier.

ADVANCED PRACTICES: INTERNET RESOURCES

Al-Khafaji AH, Sharma S, Eschun G: *Multiple organ dysfunction syndrome in sepsis*, Medscape: http://emedicine.medscape.com/article/169640-overview.

Answers.com, Antiviral Drugs: www.answers.com/topic/antiviral-drug.

Boucher HW, Talbot GH, Bradley JS, et al: Bad bugs, no drugs, no ESKAPE! An update from the Infectious Diseases Society of America, *Clin Infect Dis* 48(1):1–12, 2009.

CNBC, Deadly 'superbug' is spreading in US hospitals: www.cnbc.com/2014/07/24/cre-one-of-the-deadliest-superbugs-is-spreading-in-us-hospitals.html.

LiveScience, CRE infection: causes, symptoms & treatment: www.livescience.com/50041-cre-symptoms-treatment.html.

Medscape, Prevent hospital-acquired infections: the NNIS System: http://www.medscape.com/viewarticle/414409_7.

Medscape, Systemic Inflammatory Response Syndrome: http://emedicine.medscape.com/article/168943-overview.

6

Diagnostic Agents

OBJECTIVES

After completing this chapter, you should be able to do the following:

1. Define terms and abbreviations related to diagnostic agents.
2. Explain the use of radiographic contrast media in surgery and provide examples.
3. Explain the use of dyes in surgery and provide examples.
4. Explain the use of staining agents in surgery and provide examples.

OUTLINE

Surgery is a discipline that depends on visualizing the anatomy and the physiological functioning of body organs and systems. It is very dependent on techniques that give insight into the position, activity, and health of these structures. Since the discovery of x-rays at the turn of the 19th century by Carl Roentgen, imaging (or radiographic testing) has played a central role in the management of patients, and this guidance is used for both diagnosis and treatment. Pharmacological agents called *radiopaque contrast media* (ROCM) are used in certain diagnostic radiographic tests. For these tests to be performed, a contrast medium is injected into the circulatory system or instilled into a body cavity; then a radiograph (commonly called an *x-ray*) is taken. Many contrast media contain iodine or barium, which are radiopaque, the opposite of *radiotransparent*. Radiopaque means the substance does not permit the x-rays to pass through. Thus, anatomic structures that take up iodine or barium appear opaque on radiographic examination; this means that such pathological conditions as tumors, stones, or blockages become visible.

> **! CAUTION**
>
> In surgery, ROCM are often referred to incorrectly as "dyes." Do not become confused! ROCM are an entirely different category of diagnostic agents used for very different purposes.

Dyes are solutions that color or mark tissue for identification. Dyes may be used to mark skin incisions, delineate normal tissue planes, or enhance visualization of certain anatomic structures during a surgical procedure. Dyes may be applied topically, injected into the bloodstream, or instilled into a body cavity.

Staining agents are used in surgery to help visually identify abnormal cells, most frequently in procedures on the cervix. Staining agents are chemicals in solution that react differently with abnormal cells from the way they react with normal cells.

CONTRAST MEDIA

Contrast media are high-density pharmacological agents (Fig. 6.1) used to visualize low-contrast body tissues that include vascular structures, the urinary bladder, kidneys, the gastrointestinal tract, and the biliary tree. Although these agents are primarily used in the diagnostic imaging department of healthcare facilities, some diagnostic imaging procedures are performed in surgery. Many different contrast media are available for various diagnostic examinations, several of which are provided in Table 6.1 as examples. ROCM are classified into two main categories: ionic (molecules that break apart into ions when dissolved in water) and nonionic (do not break apart when dissolved in water).

All contrast media used in surgery contain iodine; therefore, a thorough patient history of allergies or reactions to iodine

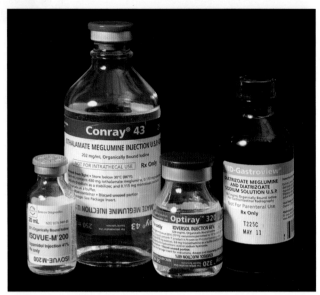

Fig. 6.1 Various iodinated contrast agents. (From Adler AM, Carlton RR: *Introduction to radiologic and imaging sciences and patient care*, ed 6, St Louis, 2016, Elsevier.)

TABLE 6.1   Examples of Radiopaque Contrast Media

Trade Name	Generic Name
Hypaque-76	diatrizoate meglumine 66% and diatrizoate sodium 10%
Hypaque-Cysto	diatrizoate meglumine
Cystografin	diatrizoate meglumine
Renografin-60	diatrizoate meglumine and diatrizoate sodium
Conray 43	iothalamate meglumine
Omnipaque	iohexol
Isovue	iopamidol
Cholografin	iodipamide meglumine
Optiray	ioversol
Ultravist	iopromide
Visipaque	iodixanol

must be obtained and noted in the chart (this includes shell-fish allergies). The circulator will also check for a history of patient allergies or reactions to iodine during the preoperative assessment.

! CAUTION

If the patient has a sensitivity to iodine, a facility may require a premedication protocol of prednisone and diphenhydramine (Benadryl) before using any ROCM containing iodine.

If the patient has a positive history for iodine reaction and use of contrast media is anticipated during the surgical procedure, the anesthesia care provider and the surgeon should be alerted before patient transport to the operating room. The surgical technologist should prepare for these patients by having a selection of nonionic contrast agents available in the operating room.

Most reactions to ROCM are mild and limited, requiring little or no treatment. However, severe allergic reactions can result in a life-threatening condition called *anaphylaxis* (see Chapter 15), which requires a rapid and definitive treatment protocol.

The use of ROCM provides an excellent example of pharmacokinetics in action.

? QUICK QUESTION

What does the term "pharmacokinetics" mean, and what are the four processes involved in pharmacokinetics? See Chapter 1 to check your answers.

When administered intravenously, a contrast agent is absorbed immediately because it directly enters the circulatory system for distribution. The agent is diluted by the circulating volume of blood as it continues to be distributed. Most ROCM are not highly bound to circulating plasma proteins and do not undergo significant biotransformation in the liver. Thus, ROCM molecules are excreted virtually unchanged through renal glomerular filtration. The presence of active ROCM in the urinary system enables visualization of the kidneys, ureters, and bladder with intravenous urography (IVU). Intraarterial administration of ROCM (e.g., as seen in surgery during placement of aortic endostent grafts or femoral embolectomy) enables immediate visualization of intended blood vessels on an arteriogram.

As a surgical technologist, you must exercise caution when preparing these agents because they are clear in color and may easily be confused with other medications on the sterile back table. As per your facility policy, all containers and syringes (including those containing contrast media) must be clearly labeled to avoid administration errors (see Chapter 4). Most contrast media are sensitive to light, so they should be kept covered and away from direct lighting when in storage. These agents may be safely exposed to light when on the sterile back table during a procedure, though, because the duration of exposure is not sufficient to cause damage to the contrast media. Four contrast media agents frequently used in surgery are discussed here as examples.

Hypaque

Diatrizoate meglumine 66% and diatrizoate sodium 10% (Hypaque-76) is a first-generation ROCM. The percentage given in the names refers to the amount of meglumine or sodium per 100 mL of solution, not the amount of iodine. (Hypaque is also available in other concentrations and forms, including a powder for oral administration.) It is supplied in glass vials of 50 mL. Hypaque is an ionic agent, also categorized as a high-osmolar contrast medium (HOCM). Adverse effects, such as hypersensitivity, are more common with intravascular administration of HOCM, so the use of agents such as Hypaque is limited. One formulation, Hypaque-Cysto 30% (diatrizoate meglumine), is intended for urologic administration. It can be used for retrograde urography, a diagnostic procedure often performed in surgery. For example, Hypaque-Cysto may be administered from the sterile back table during ureteroscopy for stone extraction. A cystoscopy is performed, and a ureteral catheter is advanced into the affected ureter. A contrast agent is injected through the catheter to enable radiographic imaging of the ureter and renal

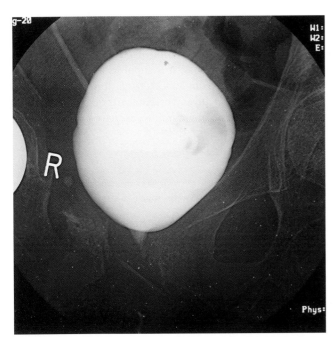

Fig. 6.2 Postoperative cystogram showing no leak from the urinary bladder. (From Muthukumar N, Smith RM, McCaskie AW, et al.: A rare presentation of pelvic fracture as haematuria, *Injury* 34(7):540–542, 2003.)

pelvis, visualizing the location of a urinary stone. Hypaque-Cysto may also be instilled directly into the urinary bladder through a urethral catheter. The bladder is then filled (distended) with the contrast, and a radiograph is taken (Fig. 6.2).

> **! CAUTION**
>
> Hypaque-76 is *not* intended for intrathecal (into the lumbar subarachnoid space) administration and should not be injected directly into the carotid artery.

Omnipaque

Iohexol (Omnipaque) is a water-soluble, iodine-based radiographic contrast medium containing approximately 45% iodine. It is nonionic and is classified as a second generation of contrast media, lower in osmolality than first-generation agents, such as Hypaque. Lower-osmolar contrast media (LOCM) are associated with fewer adverse reactions than HOCM. Omnipaque is available in various strengths (140, 180, 240, 300, and 350), expressed as milligrams of iodine per milliliter (mgI/mL). It is packaged in glass vials or polymer (polypropylene plastic) bottles ranging in size from 10 mL to 500 mL, depending on concentration. Omnipaque is currently one of only a few ROCM that are approved by the US Food and Drug Administration (FDA) for intrathecal use but *only* in concentrations of 180, 240, and 300 mgI/mL.

> **! CAUTION**
>
> Omnipaque in concentrations of 140 and 350 mgI/mL are intended for intravascular injection *only* because severe adverse reactions have been reported when these concentrations have been injected intrathecally. Always verify that the correct concentration is used for an intended purpose.

Intrathecal (into the lumbar subarachnoid space) injection of Omnipaque in concentrations of 180, 240, or 300 mgI/mL is used for contrast enhancement of computed tomography (CECT) myelography to visualize the spinal cord and nerve roots. When administered intrathecally, this agent diffuses throughout the cerebral spinal fluid, where it gradually reaches systemic circulation to be transported to the kidneys for excretion.

When injected into a blood vessel, Omnipaque will opacify (make opaque) that blood vessel—and all other vessels in the path of flow—on radiographic examination (angiography). Angiography is used to demonstrate blockages or anatomic abnormalities of the vascular system. Variations of angiography include angiocardiography, aortography, and peripheral arteriography.

> **? MAKE IT SIMPLE**
>
> Use medical terminology word-building techniques to better understand the language of diagnostic radiography. The suffix "-graphy" means "the process of recording." Thus, angiography is the process of recording vessels, and angiocardiography is the process of recording vessels of the heart. The term *arteriography* is more specific, indicating the process of recording an artery—remember that not all vessels are arteries. The suffix "-gram" indicates a record or writing, such as the digital image that results from the process of recording a structure. Thus, angio*graphy* is required to produce the image called an angio*gram*.

Angiography may be performed on vessels of the head, neck, abdomen, or kidneys, as well as on peripheral blood vessels. Omnipaque may be used for intraoperative arteriography. For example, it may be used to confirm removal of a blockage in a peripheral vessel, such as after a femoral embolectomy. It may also be used during placement of an aortic stent graft (endograft) to confirm the graft position. IVU may be performed with intravenous (IV) injection of Omnipaque. Following the processes of pharmacokinetics, the agent will travel to the kidneys, and a urogram will be taken to visualize renal structures or detect possible blockage. Omnipaque is also used for cholangiography (Insight 6.1).

Omnipaque is contraindicated for use in patients with known hypersensitivity to iodine without proper premedication protocols.

> **? QUICK QUESTION**
>
> What does it mean to say that a medication is *contraindicated* in a patient with known *hypersensitivity*? See Chapter 1 to check your answers.

Isovue

Iopamidol (Isovue) is another second-generation, nonionic ROCM. It is an LOCM used for intravascular and body cavity administration for radiographic procedures. It should be used immediately after opening, and any remaining in the bottle should be discarded. Isovue comes in concentrations of 200, 250, 300, and 370 mg of organically bound iodine per milliliter. It is packaged in vials and bottles ranging in size from 30 to 200 mL. It

Various radiopaque contrast media (ROCM) are used in surgery for operative cholangiography (open or laparoscopic) to determine the presence of stones in the common bile duct (Figure). Often the contrast medium is diluted at the sterile back table with equal parts of normal saline solution before administration. To perform operative cholangiography, the common bile duct is identified, and a cholangiogram catheter is advanced into the common bile duct and secured. A labeled, 30-mL syringe filled with ROCM solution is connected to the cholangiogram catheter. The agent is injected, and a radiograph is taken.

A less-invasive technique, endoscopic retrograde cholangiopancreatography, may be used to identify and extract common bile duct stones, so intraoperative cholangiography is less frequently performed.

Figure Cholangiogram: (A) normal; (B) calculus.

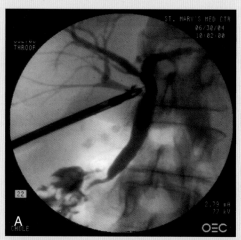

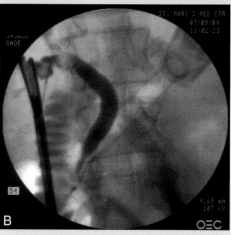

is used for cerebral angiography, peripheral arteriography, venography, urography, arthrography, computed tomography (CT) enhancement, and CECT head and body imaging. Isovue-M (also containing tromethamine and edetate calcium disodium) is the only formulation of Isovue approved for intrathecal administration, but only in concentrations of 200 and 300 mg/mL.

Visipaque

Iodixanol (Visipaque) is a third-generation, nonionic ROCM. In addition, it is the only contrast medium that has the same osmolarity as blood—called *isomolar*. It is available in concentrations of 270 and 320 mg of organically bound iodine per milliliter for intravascular injection. It has many of the same properties as Omnipaque—for example, when injected into a blood vessel, it opacifies that vessel and others in the path of flow for radiographic examination. However, Visipaque is *not* approved for intrathecal use. It is supplied in glass and plastic bottles ranging in size from 50 to 200 mL. It is used in cardiography; peripheral, visceral, and cerebral arteriography; CECT of the head and body; cholangiography; excretory urography; and peripheral venography.

DYES

Dyes are solutions that color or mark tissue or enhance direct observation of a structure. Dyes have varied uses in surgery. They are used to mark skin incisions and structural positioning of normal body anatomy and for visual identification of organ injury or disease. Four of the most common dyes used in surgery are discussed here, with examples of practical applications (Table 6.2).

Methylene Blue

Methylene blue USP is available in a 1% solution (10 mg/mL of water), packaged in 1-mL and 10-mL vials or 5-mL ampules. It is most often used in surgery during procedures on the urinary bladder, uterus, or fallopian tubes. Methylene blue is added to a fluid, such as normal saline, to give a deep blue color to the solution. For the detection of possible bladder injury during hysterectomy, the solution is instilled into the bladder through an indwelling urinary catheter. If the bladder has a leak or tear, blue solution will be obvious in the pelvis and will be visible as it flows out of the damaged area. Methylene blue can be given intravenously and, following the processes of pharmacokinetics, is excreted in urine. This allows the surgeon to check the urinary tract for leaks or fistulas.

In gynecology, a methylene blue solution is used to demonstrate patency of the fallopian tubes. During a procedure called a *tubal dye study*, or chromotubation, a laparoscope is used to observe the fimbria (ends of the uterine tubes), while methylene blue solution is instilled into the uterus through a special cervical cannula (see Fig. 1.11 and Fig. 6.3). Methylene blue solution enters the fallopian tubes and is observed exiting into the pelvic cavity, verifying patent tubes. If the tubes are blocked, often because of pelvic inflammatory disease, methylene blue solution will not be evident in the pelvis.

TABLE 6.2	**Dyes Used in Surgery**
Name	**Purpose**
Methylene blue	Pelvic surgery: detect bladder injury
	Tubal dye studies: verify patency of uterine tubes
	Lymphadenectomy: identify lymph nodes for biopsy
Lymphazurin	Sentinel node biopsy: identify sentinel node for excision
Indigo carmine	Kidney or bladder procedures: detect injury to urinary structures
	Verify kidney function during any surgical procedure: colored urine will be excreted
	Cystoscopy: identify ureteral orifices
Gentian violet	Skin marking

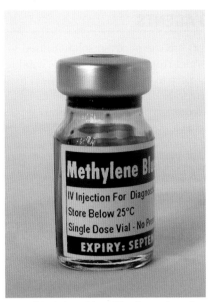

Fig. 6.3 Methylene blue. (iStock.com/czardases)

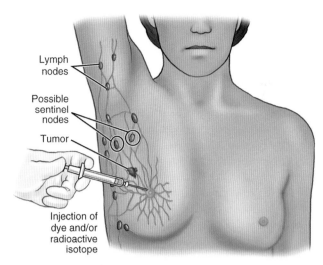

Lymph nodes

Possible sentinel nodes

Tumor

Injection of dye and/or radioactive isotope

Fig. 6.4 Sentinel lymph node biopsy. (From Brooks ML, Brooks DL: *Exploring medical language*, ed 9, St Louis, 2014, Elsevier.)

INSIGHT 6.2 Marking the Skin for Breast Surgery

In the surgical procedure of reduction mammoplasty, measurements and markings are made for removing excess breast tissue and skin and transposing the nipple-areola complexes. The marks with a skin-marking pen are made immediately preoperatively by the surgeon with the patient standing or sitting upright because this is the natural position of the breasts. It is important for the circulator not to remove these markings with the skin preparation. Once the patient is positioned on the table and anesthetized, additional markings may be made with a 25-gauge needle dipped into methylene blue and used to "tattoo" breast tissue as additional guides for the surgeon during the procedure.

INSIGHT 6.3 Sentinel Lymph Node Biopsy

Sentinel lymph node biopsy is performed following a diagnosis of breast cancer. Within a few hours of the procedure, the patient is taken to the radiology and nuclear medicine departments. The radiologist places a localization wire into the tumor to pinpoint its location. Then the patient goes to nuclear medicine for a mapping of the lymphatic system. This is accomplished with a radioactive isotope (called a *tracer*), technetium-99, which is injected at or around the tumor site. The tracer enters the lymphatic system and travels to the regional basin and settles in the first, or sentinel, lymph node. The radiologist will use a gamma, or scintillation, camera to map this drainage path, and a scan, such as a radiograph, is taken and sent to surgery. This is called *lymphoscintigraphy.*

The patient is taken to surgery, where the surgeon injects 3 to 5 mL of isosulfan blue (Lymphazurin 1%) or methylene blue approximately 5 minutes before the incision is made. The dye travels through the lymphatic system just as the tracer did. The surgeon may use a gamma probe, which is covered with a sterile sleeve, to find the radioactive "hot spots" and then mark the skin with a skin-marking pen at the site of the sentinel node. The incision is made, and the surgeon follows the Lymphazurin blue path to excise the node, which is sent to the pathology department for examination. If the pathology report comes back negative for cancer, the breast cancer is considered to have not spread, or metastasized, to the lymph nodes. If the report comes back showing cancer in the node, further lymph node dissection is carried out, with more of the specimen sent to pathology for diagnosis.

In endoscopic polypectomy, methylene blue can be injected into the submucosa, under the polyp, to determine tissue planes. It can also be used to verify complete removal of a polyp or to check for perforation. Methylene blue is also used in lymphadenectomy procedures to identify a sufficient number of lymph nodes for excision and pathological examination.

Although less frequent in current practice, methylene blue may also be used immediately before the surgical procedure to outline, or mark, normal body anatomy or position, such as when a tissue flap or graft is measured, marked, "cut," and then transferred to fill a defect on the body (Insight 6.2). Commercially available sterile skin-marking pens have largely replaced the use of methylene blue for this purpose.

Isosulfan Blue (Lymphazurin 1%)

Lymphazurin is a sterile, aqueous solution for the delineation of lymphatic vessels. It is administered subcutaneously and is selectively picked up by lymphatic vessels that drain the region of the injection site, making them a bright blue color. This makes the vessels easily discernible from the surrounding tissue. It is primarily excreted via the biliary route and should not be used on patients with known hypersensitivity to the medication or related compounds. Lymphazurin is supplied as 5-mL, single-dose vials.

Lymphazurin is used as an adjunct to lymphography to diagnose primary and secondary lymphedema of the extremities, lymph node involvement by primary or secondary neoplasm, and lymph node response to therapeutic modalities. Lymphazurin is most commonly used in the surgical setting for sentinel node biopsy for breast tumors (Fig. 6.4). The surgeon injects 3 mL to 5 mL of the medication before the skin preparation. This allows approximately 5 minutes' time before the first incision is made, allowing the medication to be carried by the lymphatic system. The surgeon follows the blue path of lymphatic drainage from the breast tumor to the first node of the axillary basin, or sentinel node, which is then dissected for pathological examination (Insight 6.3).

Indigo Carmine

Indigo carmine is a blue dye that is usually given intravenously to color urine for verification of bladder integrity or kidney function. Each 5 mL of indigo carmine contains 40 mg of indigotindisulfonate sodium in water. When administered intravenously, it is immediately delivered (absorbed) into the circulatory system and distributed throughout the body. Indigo carmine is not metabolized by the liver, so it is excreted by the kidneys unchanged into urine. This entire pharmacokinetic process usually takes approximately 10 minutes after IV administration. Because it retains its blue color in urine, rapid identification of leaks or damage to the ureters or bladder is possible. In addition, this technique can be used to demonstrate kidney function during procedures near the kidney or renal vessels. An indwelling urinary catheter is inserted preoperatively and when indigo carmine is administered intravenously, excreted urine will appear bluish-green in the urinary drainage bag. IV injection of indigo carmine during cystoscopy may be used to help to identify the location of ureteral openings. Indigo carmine is packaged in 5-mL glass ampules and when stored should be protected from light.

Gentian Violet

Gentian violet is a purple dye most frequently used in surgery to mark incision lines. Sterile marking pens containing gentian violet are available from various manufacturers. These pens are particularly useful for plastic and reconstructive procedures involving complicated incisions, such as Z-plasty, tissue flaps, or grafts. Sterile marking pens may be used to label containers of medications (Fig. 6.5).

> **NOTE:** Gentian violet is also an antifungal agent, so it is classified in two medication categories: dyes and antifungals. Although not a surgical use, it is applied topically to treat types of fungal infections inside the mouth (thrush) and vagina (yeast infection) and of the skin.

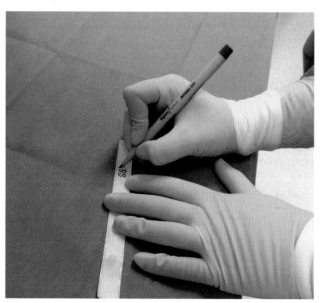

Fig. 6.5 Use of a commercial marking pen to identify medications on the back table.

STAINING AGENTS

Staining agents are chemicals in solution used to visually differentiate normal from abnormal tissue. Staining agents may be used in surgery to help identify abnormal tissue for biopsy or excision. Because of differences in cell metabolism between normal and abnormal cells, some chemicals applied to the suspect area react in a way that more clearly demonstrates the location of tissue changes. In surgery, staining techniques are most often used by gynecologists to locate areas of cervical dysplasia for biopsy or excisional conization.

Lugol Solution

Lugol solution is a strong iodine mixture used to perform Schiller tests on cervical tissue (Fig. 6.6). For a Schiller test, Lugol solution is applied topically to the external cervical os with a sponge stick or large cotton-tipped applicator. Abnormal cells will not take up the brown iodine stain as readily as normal cells, visually demonstrating the area of cervical dysplasia to be biopsied. Lugol solution is contraindicated for use in patients with a history of hypersensitivity to iodine. Lugol solution is also used medically to treat overactive thyroid gland function, iodine deficiency, and to protect the thyroid gland from the effects of radiation, as a result of radiation therapy treatments with radioactive iodine (see Chapter 8).

> **! CAUTION**
>
> Lugol iodine solution is packed in a container identical to Monsel solution. It is important to always correctly identify medications with their labels and not take the type of container for granted. Monsel solution is a chemical hemostatic (see Chapter 9), which may be used to cauterize the cervical surface after biopsy. If Monsel solution is mistakenly applied at the beginning of the procedure instead of Lugol solution, the tissue to be biopsied may be damaged and thus less able to provide definitive diagnosis.

Acetic Acid

Acetic acid (commonly known as *vinegar*) may also be used to help identify areas of cervical dysplasia (see Fig. 6.6). Although it is not specifically a colored staining agent, acetic acid causes abnormal tissue to appear whiter than surrounding healthy tissue. Acetic acid may be used as a staining agent when a laser is used to excise dysplasia. Laser energy is absorbed by different colors in the spectrum, and tissue stained brown with an iodine solution may interact less effectively with the laser.

> **KEY CONCEPTS**
>
> - Different agents, such as contrast media, dyes, and staining agents, are used in surgery to facilitate diagnosis of various pathological conditions.
> - ROCM are used to demonstrate anatomic structures or abnormalities under radiographic examination.
> - Dyes are used to mark (color) tissue or structures for direct visualization.
> - Staining agents are used to provide visual contrast between normal and abnormal tissue.

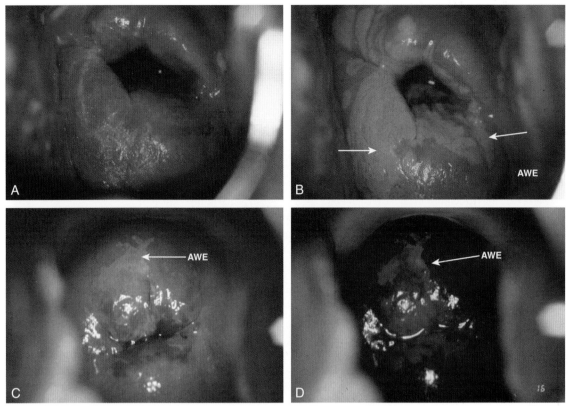

Fig. 6.6 (A) Cervix before application of acetic acid. (B) Cervix after application of acetic acid, showing acetowhite epithelium (AWE) extending into cervical canal. (C) AWE lesion before application of Lugol solution. (D) After application of Lugol solution, the same AWE is now iodine negative. (From Pfenninger JL, Fowler GC: *Pfenninger & Fowler's procedures for primary care*, ed 3, St Louis, 2011, Elsevier.)

LEARNING THE LANGUAGE (KEY TERMS)

Using your textbook or a standard medical dictionary, look up and write the definitions of each item.

dyes
intrathecal
radiopaque
radiopaque contrast media (ROCM)
staining agents

REVIEW QUESTIONS

1. What is the difference between contrast media and dyes?
2. Why should the patient's medical history for allergies be considered before a contrast medium is administered?
3. How does isosulfan blue (Lymphazurin) help the surgeon to find the sentinel node?
4. How is methylene blue used in a Tubal Dye Study (TDS)?
5. Why would acetic acid be used instead of Lugol solution for cervical biopsy?

CRITICAL THINKING

1. What types of ROCM should be available in the operating room as alternatives in patients with a history of allergies to iodine?
2. Explain the importance of sentinel lymph node biopsy for breast cancer diagnosis.
3. Outline the process of pharmacokinetics as it applies to contrast media.
4. Name a procedure that uses methylene blue placed into the bladder.

Scenario

Nancy Cho is scheduled for a cervical cone biopsy. You have two brown iodine-based solutions on your back table—Lugol solution and Monsel solution.

1. What category is Lugol solution, and what is its purpose in this procedure?
2. What category is Monsel solution, and what is its purpose in this procedure?
3. Which solution is used first? Why?
4. What would happen if these solutions were switched, and the wrong solution was administered instead of the intended solution?

BIBLIOGRAPHY

Blessing WD, Stolier AJ, Teng SC, et al: A comparison of methylene blue and lymphazurin in breast cancer sentinel node mapping, Am J Surg 184(4):341–345, 2002.

Maddox TG: Adverse reactions to contrast material: recognition, prevention, and treatment, Am Fam Physician 66(7):1229–1235, 2002.

Widmark JM: Imaging-related medications: a class overview, Proc (Bayl Univ Med Cent) 20(4):408–417, 2007.

INTERNET RESOURCES

Drugs.com, Professionals, Isovue: https://www.drugs.com/dosage/isovue-250.html.

Drugs.com, Professionals, *Hypaque-76*: https://www.drugs.com/pro/hypaque.html#s-34089-3.

Drugs.com, Professionals, *Hypaque-Cysto*: https://www.drugs.com/cons/hypaque-cysto.html.

Drugs.com, Professionals, *Visipaque:* www.drugs.com/pro/visipaque.html.

GE Healthcare, *Omnipaque*: https://www.gehealthcare.com/products/contrast-media#omnipaque.

Siddiqi NH, Contrast medium reactions, *Medscape*: http://emedicine.medscape.com/article/422855-overview.

KEY TERMS

acute renal failure (ARF)
diaphoresis
hydration

iodinated
nanotechnology
urticarial

RADIOPAQUE CONTRAST MEDIA

As previously defined in this chapter, radiopaque contrast media (ROCM) are high-density pharmacologic substances administered to the patient to visualize low-contrast body tissues. ROCM are available in parenteral, enteral, ionic, nonionic, high-osmolality, and low-osmolality forms. The most-often used ROCM are iodine and barium. Both of these substances have a higher atomic mass number (iodine is 53, barium is 56) and mass density than the lower-contrast tissues being examined. These tissues include vasculature, kidneys, gastrointestinal (GI) tract, and the biliary tree. When one of these iodinated compounds fills a blood vessel or when barium fills a section of the GI tract, these internal structures become visible on radiographs. Serum iodine concentrations must be within the range of 280 to 370 mg/mL for a normal x-ray film to show a vascular lumen. It must be injected intravascularly, at a rate equal to or greater than the patient's blood flow. If the ROCM is injected too slowly, the cardiovascular system will dilute its iodine concentration before imaging can be achieved. Intravascular ROCM do not cross cellular membranes well and are distributed into the bloodstream, where they enhance visibility of veins and arteries. When administered intravenously into the heart chambers, the ROCM will enhance visibility to the heart and major thoracic vessels. The urinary tract can be visualized within 15 minutes of a rapid intravenous (IV) injection and within 30 minutes of a slow IV infusion in patients with normal renal function. Urinary tract visibility will be delayed or not occur in patients with renal dysfunction or failure. Intravascular ROCM are excreted mainly by the kidneys. In normal renal function, up to 100% of the intravascular dose is excreted in 24 hours. A very small percentage may be passed through the intestines via the hepatic-biliary system. For patients with renal dysfunction, several days may be required to completely excrete the ROCM.

RISK FACTORS FOR IODINATED CONTRAST MEDIA

In recent years, there has been a dramatic increase in the use of diagnostic agents in the surgical setting, especially iodinated contrast media used for radiologic imaging. The advanced practitioner performing as the surgical first assistant should be aware of patient risk factors before administration of these agents. Risk factors have been identified that may add to the susceptibility of an adverse reaction. An estimated one of every 20,000 to 40,000 patients receiving ROCM dies as a result of adverse effects. One factor is the route of administration. The risk of reaction from intravascular administration of contrast media occurs more often than extravascular administration (through the GI tract). Reactions occurring through intravascular administration are usually mild and self-limiting, and those from extravascular administration are rare. However, either route can produce serious, and at times life-threatening, reactions. Other risk factors include advanced age and class IV congestive heart failure, because these can increase the likelihood of renal failure, following administration of the contrast media. Patients who have had a previous reaction to contrast materials are understandably at higher risk, although reactions do not recur in all patients. Patients with chronic renal insufficiency, asthma, and diabetes mellitus must have these diseases addressed and treated before the administration of any contrast media.

ADVERSE REACTIONS

As already stated, the identification of allergies is essential before administering any radiographic contrast agents. Symptoms for reactions are categorized according to their severity (Table 6.A). However, the degree of severity and type of onset are patient dependent. It should be noted that reactions can occur 20 to 30 minutes after injection of the agent and up to 7 days after the procedure. In addition to allergic reactions, an adverse effect of special importance is nephrotoxicity resulting in acute renal failure (ARF). Renal insufficiency is caused by a dosage-related toxic injury to the renal tubules. Patients should be assessed for risk factors that may contribute to ARF (Table 6.B). The assessment should also include renal function studies before contrast is administered by obtaining a blood urea nitrogen and creatinine laboratory tests. These are the best indicators of renal function, and the results must be available before the procedure.

TABLE 6.A   Symptoms of Adverse Reactions for Contrast Media

Mild	Moderate	Severe
Scattered urticaria	Persistent vomiting	Cardiac arrhythmia
Nausea	Headache	Hypotension
Vomiting	Facial edema	Severe bronchospasm
Diaphoresis	Mild bronchospasm	Laryngeal edema
Coughing	Dyspnea	Seizures
Dizziness	Palpitations	Pulmonary edema

TABLE 6.B   Risk Factors for Contrast-Induced Nephropathy

Patient Factors	Procedural Factors
Preexisting renal conditions	High volume of contrast administered
Diabetes	Failure to verify renal laboratory function tests
Dehydration	Failure to aggressively hydrate
Advanced age	Failure to obtain medical history
Nephrotoxic medications	Failure to space procedures at least 5 days apart
Congestive heart failure Liver disease	Failure to get appropriate medications preoperatively

Current treatment to reduce nephrotoxicity is hydration to keep the kidneys flushing during the procedure and to minimize the volume of contrast media administered. The patient's hydration status should also be monitored after the procedure. ROCM can also cause vasodilation with flushing experienced by some patients, and osmotic fluid shifts that can result in acute heart failure in patients with chronic congestive heart failure. High-osmolar ROCM are referred to as *high-osmolar contrast media* (HOCM). They dissociate into active particles in the bloodstream and can cause some anticoagulation, which may result in bleeding and bruising in the patient. These are also associated with higher rates of adverse reactions when given intravenously. For this reason, HOCM are being replaced by nonionic monomers with water-soluble molecules that do not dissociate in solution. These monomers are called *lower-osmolar contrast media* (LOCM). LOCM have fewer adverse reactions and are tolerated better for intravascular use; HOCMs are used with nonvascular procedures, such as retrograde cystourethrography.

ASSISTANT ADVICE

A crash cart should be available for all radiographic procedures.

MEDICATIONS

Current studies suggest the administration of acetylcysteine, an antioxidant, may reduce the incidence of contrast-induced ARF. Patients may be given acetylcysteine the day before, the day of, and 2 days after the procedure. Other medications used to reduce the incidence of adverse reactions to contrast media include methylprednisolone (Medrol) and prednisolone (Omnipred),

which are corticosteroids; diphenhydramine (Benadryl), which is an antihistamine used to treat allergic symptoms; hydroxyzine (Vistaril) to relieve itching, nausea, and vomiting caused by allergies; and histamine H_2 receptor blockers, such as cimetidine (Tagamet), or famotidine (Pepcid).

Many factors must be considered before any medications are given to the patient receiving contrast media for radiologic imaging. The surgical first assistant must assist the physician in providing the best patient care by identifying patient risk factors, understanding and minimizing adverse effects, and managing reactions of contrast agents.

NEW DIAGNOSTIC IMAGING PROCEDURES

New diagnostic approaches for whole-body imaging are using quantum dots, or nanocrystals, as fluorescent and bioluminescent reporters (or tags) that are genetically encoded. These "glowing" tags can provide information for better understanding of human biology, and to help develop treatments for diseases, such as cancer, infection, and cardiovascular disease.

One example of this new imaging technology used to diagnose cardiovascular disease and malfunction is an ultrasound contrast agent that consists of millions of tiny bubbles. These ultrasound microbubbles scatter light and allow the physician to see which part of the heart muscle is not functioning properly. The ultrasound component of this technology is highly sensitive and produces a characteristic transient effect for better diagnosis. Other applications include imaging systems to obtain and process information on the molecular and cellular levels of our bodies, models to track neurologic damage and repair the central nervous system, and radiodiagnostic agents to label white blood cells without the need to remove and reinject blood into patients. Research is ongoing for these and many more applications using molecular imaging.

An example of newer processes using an established dye is fluorescein. There are many fluorescein derivatives, and fluorescein sodium has been traditionally applied to the cornea to detect abrasions (see Chapter 10). This dye is used intravenously for angiography to diagnose and categorize vascular disorders of the eye, such as macular degeneration, diabetic retinopathy, and intraocular tumors. Fluorescein is also used during craniotomy to assist with guided resection of brain tumors.

Nanotechnology is making a significant impact on many medical fronts, including diagnostic imaging. Researchers are using nanoscale manipulations to improve the sensitivity, biocompatibility, and biodistribution of contrast materials. One of the challenges to nanoparticle systems is to modify them for prolonged circulation time, while maintaining their biocompatibility. Then they must be broken down and removed from circulation when their goal has been accomplished. A goal of nanotechnology is targeting. This is the ability to identify tissues of interest and then selectively accumulate inside them. Through targeting, nanotechnology can assist contrast materials in providing more useful and detailed information. This would include tissue types, margins, and the ability to distinguish malignant or abnormal tissues much earlier than can be accomplished by giving the contrast material systemically.

Targeting contrast materials to a specific tissue could allow for lower doses. This would save money and reduce the exposure of the patient to potentially toxic materials. Because there is a lesser amount of the contrast material used, less is floating freely in the body, so the resulting image can be improved.

ADVANCED PRACTICES: REVIEW QUESTIONS

1. Which route of administration for iodinated contrast media is more likely to cause an adverse reaction?
   a. Oral
   b. Intravascular
   c. Extravascular
   d. Rectal

2. Name three risk factors that may contribute to acute renal failure after administration of contrast media.

3. Which is the current treatment to reduce nephrotoxicity after the administration of contrast media?
   a. Antibiotic therapy
   b. Administration of a vasodilator
   c. Hydration
   d. Dehydration

4. Name three symptoms of an adverse reaction to contrast media.

5. A new ultrasonic diagnostic contrast agent used to study the heart consists of millions of _____.

ADVANCED PRACTICES: BIBLIOGRAPHY

Fulcher EM, Fulcher RM, Soto CD: *Pharmacology: principles and applications*, ed 3St Louis, 2012, Saunders/Elsevier.

Kee JL, Hayes ER, McCuistion LE: *Pharmacology: a patient-centered nursing process approach*, ed 4St Louis, 2015, Saunders/Elsevier.

Kiessling F, Fokong S, Koczera P, et al: Ultrasound microbubbles for molecular diagnosis, therapy, and theranostics, *J Nucl Med* 53(3):345–348, 2012.

Lee KH: Quantum dots: a quantum jump for molecular imaging? *J Nucl Med* 48(9):1408–1410, 2007. Accessed at www.ncbi.nlm.nih.gov/pubmed/22393225 Accessed August 7, 2015

Pogue BW, Gibbs-Strauss S, Valdés PA, et al: Review of neurosurgical fluorescence imaging methodologies, *IEEE J Sel Top Quantum Electron* 16(3):493–505, 2010. Available at www.ncbi.nlm.nih.gov/pmc/articles/PMC2910912/ Accessed August 7, 2015

Rosen JE, Yoffe S, Meerasa A, et al: Nanotechnology and diagnostic imaging: new advances in contrast agent technology, *J Nanomed Nanotechnol* 2:115, 2011.

Schutt EG, Klein DH, Mattrey RM, et al: Injectable microbubbles as contrast agents for diagnostic ultrasound imaging: the key role of perfluorochemicals, *Angew Chem Int Ed Engl* 42(28):3218–3235, 2003.

ADVANCED PRACTICES: INTERNET RESOURCES

MedlinePlus, Drugs, herbs and supplements: www.nlm.nih.gov/medlineplus/druginformation.html.

MedlinePlus, Medical encyclopedia, Fluorescein angiography: www.nlm.nih.gov/medlineplus/ency/article/003846.html.

Medscape, eMedicine, Contrast medium reactions, recognition and treatment: http://emedicine.medscape.com/article/422855-overview.

7

Diuretics

This category of medications is not routinely administered from the sterile back table, but the effects of these agents do affect the surgical technologist's daily practice, both preoperatively and intraoperatively. *Diuretics* are medications administered to reduce body fluids by preventing reabsorption of sodium and water by the kidneys. As a result, the patient excretes large amounts of dilute urine known as *diuresis*. Various subcategories of diuretics are used in the management of several chronic medical conditions, such as hypertension (high blood pressure), congestive heart failure (CHF) (a condition in which the heart muscle is too weak to pump effectively), and glaucoma (a group of ocular diseases characterized by increased intraocular pressure).

 TECH TIP

The only diuretic administered from the sterile back table is mannitol, which is contained in the ophthalmic medication Miochol-E (see Chapter 10).

For a better understanding of how diuretics work, it may be helpful to review the basic physiology of body fluids and electrolytes. Electrolytes are minerals made up of electrically charged particles held together by ionic bonds. Ionic bonds are easily broken when dissolved in water, causing the particles to separate into positive and negative ions. For example, sodium chloride (NaCl) breaks into sodium (Na+) and chloride (Cl−) in body fluid. The major body electrolytes include sodium,

potassium, calcium, chloride, magnesium, and phosphorus. Electrolytes are found inside and outside cells and are acquired through food and water.

Because diuretics cause the excretion of fluid in the form of dilute urine, most diuretics also cause excretion of electrolytes, primarily sodium (Na+). Other critical electrolytes, including potassium (K+) and calcium (Ca2+), are also excreted in the fluid.

 MAKE IT SIMPLE

A simple statement about the physiology of fluid and electrolyte balance is this principle: where the fluid goes, so go the electrolytes, and where the electrolytes go, so goes the fluid.

Diuretics help to lower blood pressure by increasing the elimination of fluids (and associated electrolytes) from the body, causing a decrease in the blood volume. When there is less blood volume circulating, there is less pressure on the blood vessels and the heart does not pump as forcefully or fast (which reduces cardiac output, the volume of blood pumped by the heart per minute). This concept can be compared to a water balloon. When it is full (has a high volume of water), the pressure of the water pushing on the walls of the balloon is high. When some of the water is removed (lowering of the volume), the pressure is lessened (lower).

For further understanding of the action of diuretics, it is also necessary to briefly review the renal process of excretion. Consult your physiology textbook for additional information on fluids, electrolytes, and renal function.

RENAL PROCESS OF EXCRETION

The primary function of the renal (urinary) system is to maintain homeostasis, and one way the kidneys maintain the body's equilibrium is by balancing levels of fluids and electrolytes. This balance is achieved by filtering blood and removing excess water and dissolved substances, or *solutes*, such as sodium and potassium. The nephron (Fig. 7.1) is a microscopic filtering unit that removes water and waste solutes. Millions of nephrons are present within the kidneys. Blood is brought to the nephron through the afferent arteriole into the glomerulus (a cluster of capillaries within the Bowman capsule), where filtration occurs. Filtration is the process of forcing fluids and solutes through a membrane by pressure. Filtered blood then returns to the circulatory system via the efferent arteriole. The remaining fluid, or *filtrate*—which contains all the substances present in blood, except formed elements and most proteins—then undergoes tubular reabsorption. Only specific amounts of needed substances, including water, are reabsorbed. Tubular reabsorption takes place in the proximal convoluted tubule and the ascending and descending limbs of the loop of the nephron (loop of Henle).

The next part of the renal excretion process is tubular secretion, which involves the active transport of substances, such as potassium ions, hydrogen ions, creatinine (a waste product resulting from muscle metabolism), and urea (a waste product resulting from protein metabolism), from blood surrounding the tubule into the filtrate. Tubular secretion, which takes place in the distal convoluted tubule, eliminates waste products and controls blood pH. Additional water is reabsorbed when the filtrate proceeds to the collecting ducts. The filtrate is emptied from collecting ducts into the renal pelvis to the ureter and bladder and is excreted as urine.

PREOPERATIVE AND INTRAOPERATIVE IMPLICATIONS OF DIURETIC THERAPY

The surgical technologist should be aware of the potential impact of long-term diuretic therapy on a patient scheduled for surgery. A key electrolyte, potassium, may be seriously depleted in patients taking certain diuretics. When the level of potassium in the blood is low, the condition is called *hypokalemia*. If patients undergoing long-term diuretic therapy require surgery, preoperative blood chemistry tests are performed to determine serum potassium levels. An average potassium level is considered to be between 3.5 and 5.0 mEq/L. Potassium levels that are either too low or too high (hyperkalemia) may cause cardiac arrhythmias (absence of normal heart rhythm) under anesthesia (Insight 7.1). Cardiac arrhythmias, such as premature ventricular contractions, increase the potential risk of cardiac

---

QUICK QUESTION

The renal process of excretion is also part of how the body processes medications. What is the term used to indicate how the body processes drugs? See Chapter 1 to check your answer.

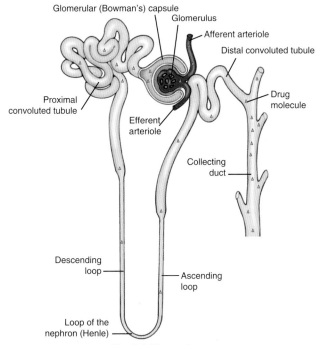

Fig. 7.1 The nephron.

INSIGHT 7.1   Physiology Insight: The Importance of Potassium in Cardiac Function

Potassium (K+), a mineral element, is the primary intracellular electrolyte in the body. It plays a vital role in many body functions, such as nerve impulse conduction, acid-base balance, and promotion of carbohydrate and protein metabolism. Every body cell, especially muscle tissue, requires a high potassium content to function. It facilitates contraction of both skeletal and smooth muscles—including myocardial (heart muscle) contraction. Potassium levels in the body have a very narrow normal range (3.5–5.0 mEq/L), and even a slight deviation in either direction can cause problems. An excess of potassium (*hyper*kalemia) alters the normal polarized state of cardiac muscle fibers. This results in a decrease in the rate and force of the heart's contractions. Very high potassium levels can block conduction of cardiac impulses. This results in rapid heart rate (tachycardia) initially and slow heart rate (bradycardia) later. If potassium levels are too low (*hypo*kalemia), the heart can develop an abnormal rhythm (dysrhythmia). Both hyperkalemia and hypokalemia can lead to muscle weakness and flaccid paralysis. Abnormal potassium levels can diminish excitability and the conduction rate of the heart muscle and may lead to cardiac arrest. The cause of abnormal levels is usually not dietary deficiency. Many foods contain potassium, including meats, milk, peanut butter, potatoes, bananas, apples, carrots, tomatoes, and dark-green leafy vegetables. Instead, hypokalemia can result from excessive vomiting and diarrhea, severe trauma (such as burns), chronic renal disease, excessive doses of cortisone, or long-term diuretic therapy for chronic conditions (such as hypertension [high blood pressure]). Hyperkalemia results from renal dysfunction, such as the kidneys' inability to excrete excess amounts of potassium, or when there is decreased urine output or renal failure.

arrest, so the patient's potassium level is carefully evaluated before the administration of general anesthesia. Hypokalemia may cause muscle weakness, which makes muscles more sensitive to muscle relaxants used for general anesthesia (see Chapter 14). Patients with significant hypokalemia may require administration of intravenous potassium before nonemergency surgery. Potassium infusion should not be administered rapidly, so a nonemergency procedure may be delayed or canceled and rescheduled. The operating room staff should be mindful of such possibilities. Long-term diuretic therapy is most frequently seen in elderly patients with systemic fluid management conditions, such as hypertension or heart or liver failure.

 TECH TIP

If there is any question about the patient's potassium level before nonemergency surgery, prepare for the surgical procedure as scheduled, but do not open the sterile field until the anesthesia care provider has determined if it is safe to proceed with the operation.

Surgical technologists should also understand the purposes for *intraoperative* use of diuretics and how that differs from long-term diuretic therapy. Intraoperative administration of diuretics is considered to be short-term therapy, and it is usually indicated when a condition requires a rapid but temporary reduction in fluid volume. In these cases, the anesthesia care provider will administer a diuretic intravenously. Diuretics may be used during surgery to reduce intraocular pressure, reduce intracranial pressure, or to protect kidney function. During intraocular surgery, such as retinal detachment, a diuretic may be given to prevent the accumulation of fluid caused by the inflammatory response to tissue manipulation. Diuretics may be administered during craniotomy to reduce brain swelling, especially when the tissue has been damaged by traumatic injury. During vascular procedures on the aorta (especially those near the kidney), diuretics may be given to keep fluid flowing through the kidneys, thus providing a measure of continued kidney function. Note that the risk of hypokalemia is significantly reduced when diuretics are used for short-term treatment of such specific temporary conditions.

Although diuretics are rarely administered from the sterile back table, it is important that surgical technologists understand how the intraoperative use of diuretics affects the surgical patient. Because diuretics reduce fluid by causing the excretion of large amounts of dilute urine, it is necessary to insert an indwelling urinary catheter in the patient before surgery. A urinary drainage bag with an accurate measuring device is used to record urinary output at regular intervals.

 TECH TIP

The surgical technologist should anticipate the need for an indwelling urinary catheter and drainage bag when preparing for surgical procedures in which diuretics may be administered.

CATEGORIES OF DIURETIC AGENTS

Different types of diuretics exert effects at different locations along the nephron. Diuretics are classified by site of action and the mechanism by which the solute is altered (Table 7.1).

Loop Diuretics

Loop diuretics are highly potent diuretics used to remove fluid arising from renal, hepatic, or cardiac dysfunction and to treat acute pulmonary edema. Hepatic dysfunction may be caused by cirrhosis or liver failure. The most common cardiac dysfunction requiring treatment with diuretics is CHF (Insight 7.2). Loop diuretics work by decreasing the reabsorption of sodium (Na+) in the ascending loop of Henle, which in turn affects the ability of the *distal* tubule to reabsorb sodium. These diuretics exert a potent effect because the site of action is so broad. They inhibit the reabsorption of 20% to 30% of the sodium load. When sodium is not reabsorbed into the body, fluid passively follows sodium out of the body taking chloride and potassium out as well. Examples of loop diuretics are furosemide (Lasix), bumetanide, and torsemide. Furosemide is the oldest and most commonly used agent in this category. In surgery, furosemide is particularly useful in intracranial procedures. Furosemide decreases intracranial pressure by quickly removing fluid that accumulates in response to the trauma of intracranial procedures or injuries. When furosemide is administered intravenously, the onset of diuresis can be expected within 5 to 15 minutes and will continue for approximately 2 hours.

Thiazide Diuretics

Thiazide diuretics are low-potency diuretics used as first-line treatment for hypertension and mild chronic edema. Thiazides

TABLE 7.1	**Diuretics by Classification**	
Class	**Generic Name**	**Trade Name**
Loop diuretics	bumetanide	N/A
	furosemide	Lasix
	torsemide	N/A
Thiazide diuretics	chlorothiazide	Diuril
	hydrochlorothiazide	Microzide
	chlorthalidone	N/A
Potassium-sparing diuretics	amiloride	N/A
	eplerenone	Inspra
	spironolactone	Aldactone
	triamterene	Dyrenium
Carbonic anhydrase inhibitors	acetazolamide	N/A
	brinzolamide	Azopt
	dorzolamide	Trusopt
	methazolamide	Neptazane
Osmotic diuretics	mannitol	Osmitrol

work by inhibiting the reabsorption of sodium ions in the distal convoluted tubule. Because of the limited site of action, thiazides exert a weaker effect, inhibiting the reabsorption of only approximately 5% of the sodium load. These agents are administered orally, so they are not used intraoperatively. Examples of thiazide diuretics include chlorothiazide (Diuril) and hydrochlorothiazide (Micozide).

Potassium-Sparing Diuretics

Potassium-sparing diuretics are low-potency diuretics commonly used to treat edema and hypertension and to help restore potassium levels in hypokalemic patients. Potassium-sparing diuretics prevent the reabsorption of sodium by acting on the sodium channels in the cells of the distal convoluted tubules. The specific site of action prevents potassium loss. Potassium-sparing diuretics exert a mild diuretic effect because only a small amount of the glomerular filtrate ever reaches the distal convoluted tubule. They inhibit only 1% to 3% of the sodium load. Potassium-sparing diuretics are usually administered in combination with other diuretics, such as thiazides and loop diuretics, to minimize potassium loss in patients with hypertension or CHF. These diuretics are not administered intraoperatively. Common agents in this category include amiloride, eplerenone (Inspra), spironolactone (Aldactone), and triamterene

(Dyrenium). Adverse effects can include hyperkalemia, which can affect surgical intervention as previously discussed.

Carbonic Anhydrase Inhibitors

Carbonic anhydrase inhibitors (CAIs) are low-potency diuretics specifically used to treat mild, acute closed-angle glaucoma and chronic open-angle glaucoma (see Chapter 10). These diuretics act on the proximal convoluted tubule, so urine output is not significantly affected. The carbonic anhydrase enzyme is also active in formation of aqueous humor in the eye. By inhibiting carbonic anhydrase, these drugs decrease production of aqueous humor, thus lowering intraocular pressure. The most commonly used CAI is acetazolamide. Acetazolamide may be given orally to cataract patients after surgery because pressure may build up in the eye as a response to manipulation of tissues. Other CAIs include brinzolamide (Azopt) and dorzolamide (Trusopt), which are administered as topical drops (see Chapter 10), and methazolamide (Neptazane), which is administered orally.

Osmotic Diuretics

Osmotic diuretics are highly potent agents administered intravenously. Osmotic diuretics are *not* used for management of chronic conditions, such as CHF. Osmotic diuretics are used to prevent acute renal failure after cardiac surgery, to treat increased intracranial pressure and cerebral edema, and to reduce intraocular pressure in open-globe procedures of the eye, such as retinal detachment. The mechanism of action of osmotic diuretics is unlike that of any diuretics previously described. Osmotic diuretics increase blood pressure and volume by drawing fluid out of tissues and into the circulatory system rapidly (Fig. 7.2). Thus, osmotic diuretics are contraindicated in patients with hypertension and edema.

As the name implies, these drugs exert their effects through the process of osmosis. Remember, osmosis is the process of

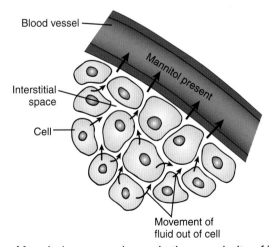

Fig. 7.2 Mannitol causes a change in the osmolarity of blood, drawing interstitial and intracellular fluid into the bloodstream. This action eventually increases the amount of fluid excreted by the kidneys.

water moving through a semipermeable membrane from an area of lesser concentration of solute (e.g., sodium) to an area of greater concentration of solute. Water moves toward the diuretic agent present in the glomerulus, thus preventing the water from being reabsorbed. Water and nearly all the associated electrolytes are then excreted with the diuretic agent in the urine.

The most commonly used osmotic diuretic is mannitol (Osmitrol). Mannitol may be used to provide a rapid reduction in intraocular pressure in patients experiencing acute angle-closure glaucoma. It is administered intravenously, warmed, through a filter to trap crystals that may form. Mannitol may also be given during some neurosurgical procedures to reduce intracranial pressure. In vascular procedures, particularly on the aorta, mannitol may be used to protect kidney function by increasing the volume of fluid entering the kidneys. Mannitol is also used in the treatment of malignant hyperthermia, a condition associated with administration of some general anesthetic agents (see Chapter 15).

KEY CONCEPTS

- Diuretics are agents administered to reduce the amount of fluid accumulating in patients with renal, hepatic, or cardiac dysfunction, as well as to relieve excessive intracranial or intraocular pressure. Excess fluid is removed through excretion of urine.
- Patients receiving long-term diuretic therapy have an increased risk of hypokalemia. If a surgical patient is hypokalemic, potential exists for cardiac arrhythmias when under general anesthesia. For detection of hypokalemia, blood chemistry analysis is performed preoperatively for all surgical patients taking diuretics. The sterile field should not be opened until the potassium levels are verified.
- Some surgical procedures require short-term intraoperative administration of diuretics. Diuretics are given intravenously in surgery during some ophthalmic, intracranial, and vascular procedures. An indwelling urinary catheter must be inserted on all surgical patients who may receive diuretics intraoperatively.
- The most common diuretics administered during surgery are mannitol (Osmitrol) and furosemide (Lasix).

LEARNING THE LANGUAGE (KEY TERMS)

Using your textbook or a standard medical dictionary, look up and write the definitions of each item.

arrhythmia
congestive heart failure (CHF)
diuresis
electrolyte
efferent arteriole

glaucoma
hyperkalemia
hypertension
hypokalemia
nephron

REVIEW QUESTIONS

1. How does the nephron work to eliminate waste products and excess water?
2. How do diuretics work?
3. Which structures of the nephron are affected by diuretics?
4. Why would a diuretic be prescribed for long-term use?

5. What is a common adverse effect of long-term diuretic therapy on a patient? How does that condition affect the administration of a general anesthetic?
6. What type of patient may come to surgery on long-term diuretic therapy?
7. Why are diuretics used intraoperatively?
8. Which diuretics are used intraoperatively?

CRITICAL THINKING

Scenario 1

Mrs. Hernandez is an 85-year-old woman admitted to surgery for insertion of a hip prosthesis to treat a hip fracture. The surgical technologist assigned to transport the patient to the preoperative holding area performed a routine review of the patient's medical chart in the emergency department. The medical chart indicates that Mrs. Hernandez is being treated for chronic hypertension.

1. Knowing that she has a concurrent diagnosis of hypertension, which additional related items should be checked on her chart?

2. How might this situation affect the preparations going on in the surgery department?
3. What action or actions should the surgical technologist take before bringing the patient to preoperative holding?

Scenario 2

Mr. Van Nguyen is a 47-year-old man admitted to surgery for repair of a retinal detachment under general anesthesia.

1. Which diuretic may be administered intraoperatively?
2. What items should the surgical technologist have available for preoperative preparation of the patient specific to this situation?

BIBLIOGRAPHY

Bardal S, Waechter J, Martin D: *Applied pharmacology*, St Louis, 2011, Saunders/Elsevier.

Duke JC, Keech BM, editors: *Duke's anesthesia secrets*, ed 5, Philadelphia, 2016, Elsevier.

Fulcher EM, Fulcher RM, Soto CD: *Pharmacology: principles and applications*, ed 3, St Louis, 2012, Saunders/Elsevier.

Key JL, Hayes ER, McCuistion LE: *Pharmacology: a patient-centered nursing process approach*, ed 8, St Louis, 2015, Saunders/Elsevier.

Nagelhout JJ, Plaus KL: *Handbook of anesthesia*, ed 5, Maryland Heights, 2014, Saunders/Elsevier.

INTERNET RESOURCES

Cardiovascular Pharmacology Concepts, General pharmacology, Renal handling of sodium and water: www.cvpharmacology.com/diuretic/diuretics.

LiverTox, Drug Record, Loop diuretics: http://livertox.nih.gov/LoopDiuretics.htm.

Advanced Practices for the Surgical First Assistant
Chapter 7—Diuretics

KEY TERMS

diuresis

hypokalemia

As discussed in the chapter, diuretics are administered for the management of several medical conditions: to decrease hypertension, to decrease edema (peripheral and pulmonary) in congestive heart failure (CHF), to decrease edema in renal or liver disorders, and to treat glaucoma. Diuretics achieve their treatment goals by bringing about a negative fluid balance, mobilizing excessive extracellular fluid, and reducing excess fluid volume. When the patient receiving diuretics is scheduled for surgery, preoperative evaluations are required. The surgical first assistant must understand the physiologic effects on the body and any possible surgical complications that may arise from these medications. Hypokalemia, depletion of potassium in the blood serum, is often caused by the effects of diuretics on the kidneys. Thiazide and loop diuretics cause the highest rate of potassium loss. Diuretics increase the body's flow of urine (diuresis). Although water and sodium are excreted from the body by the kidneys, other electrolytes, such as potassium, are also excreted. Potassium is one of the essential minerals needed by the body to maintain homeostasis. It helps to regulate normal heart rhythm, blood pressure, and nerve connections. Potassium is also needed to convert blood sugar into glycogen for energy that can be stored in the muscles. Next to calcium and phosphorus, potassium is the most abundant mineral found in the body. Potassium cannot be produced by the body and must be replaced through diet or supplements. See Box 7.1. A for a list of foods rich in potassium. Nearly 98% of the total potassium is found inside the cells, with the remaining 2% in the blood serum. Small fluctuations in the blood serum potassium may have adverse effects in the functions of the heart, nerves, and muscles. All patients on diuretic therapy are routinely tested preoperatively for blood serum potassium levels. Abnormal levels should be corrected before any elective surgical procedure.

POTASSIUM LEVELS

Potassium levels in the blood serum are identified through analysis of a blood sample. In most cases, the test is part of a routine chemical analysis that also includes other minerals. A normal level of potassium is 3.5 to 5.0 mEq/L. A level of 3.0 mEq/L with

BOX 7.1 Foods High in Potassium Content	
• Apricots	• Potatoes
• Avocados	• Poultry
• Bananas	• Prunes
• Beans	• Pumpkin
• Cantaloupe	• Raisins
• Chocolate	• Spinach
• Fish	• Squash
• Honeydew	• Sunflower seeds
• Kiwi fruit	• Sweet potatoes
• Lima beans	• Tomatoes
• Meats	• Vegetable juice
• Milk	• Whole grains
• Mushrooms	• Winter squash
• Oranges and juice	• Yogurt
• Peaches	

symptoms or of 2.5 mEq/L with or without symptoms is considered severe hypokalemia and requires aggressive inpatient treatment. Patients with levels between 3.0 and 3.5 mEq/L are considered mildly hypokalemic and are usually treated on an outpatient basis with diet or oral supplements.

ASSISTANT ADVICE
Some sources give normal potassium levels at 3.6–5.2 mEq/L.

TREATMENT OF HYPOKALEMIA

Treatment of hypokalemia involves replacing the potassium with diet or a supplement to obtain and maintain a normal serum potassium level. Treatment by oral intake or a supplement is adequate for minor depletion of potassium and can be performed at home over a period of time. Because of the slow release of potassium into the system, oral replacement treatment is by far the best method for replacement without any serious side effects. Acute hypokalemia (level <2.5 mEq/L) is a serious life-threatening condition and needs to be replaced by intravenous administration of potassium, such as potassium chloride, as an inpatient procedure. Cardiac monitoring is necessary because of possible arrhythmia caused by the fluctuations of potassium levels. Dosage required for correction is based on the accepted formula that 10 mEq/L of potassium chloride will increase the blood serum level by 0.1 mEq/L. Intravenous administration of 10 mEq/h not exceeding 200 mEq/L is usually recommended for severe hypokalemia. Decisions for the treatment of hypokalemia are patient-specific and depend upon many factors, including patient diagnosis, the illness and its circumstances, the patient's ability to tolerate fluids, and the patient's ability to take oral medications.

ALDOSTERONE

Although not technically a diuretic, aldosterone does affect kidney function. Aldosterone is a mineralocorticoid hormone produced by the adrenal cortex (see Chapter 8). It increases the reabsorption of sodium and water and the secretion of potassium in the kidneys. Aldosterone's action increases blood volume and thus blood pressure. Medications that interfere with aldosterone's action are used to treat hypertension. An example is spironolactone (Aldactone), which blocks the aldosterone receptor and so lowers blood pressure.

ADVANCED PRACTICES: REVIEW QUESTIONS

1. The term to describe a depletion of potassium in the blood serum is
   a. Hypovolemia
   b. Hypocalcemia
   c. Hypothermia
   d. Hypokalemia
2. Normal level of potassium in blood serum is _____ mEq/L.
3. Describe the treatment for chronic and acute hypokalemia.

4. Which category of medication causes the highest rate of potassium depletion?
   a. Antibiotics
   b. Analgesics
   c. Diuretics
   d. Steroids
5. Name two food sources that are high in potassium.
6. How does aldosterone affect blood pressure?

ADVANCED PRACTICES: BIBLIOGRAPHY

Fulcher EM, Fulcher RM, Soto CD: *Pharmacology: principles and applications*, ed 3, St Louis, 2012, Saunders/Elsevier.
Kee JL, Hayes ER, McCuistion LE: *Pharmacology: a patient-centered nursing process approach*, ed 8, St Louis, 2015, Saunders/Elsevier.

ADVANCED PRACTICES: INTERNET RESOURCES

Answers.com, Diuretics: www.answers.com/topic/diuretics.
Drugs.com, *Potassium content of food list*, High potassium food list: www.drugs.com/cg/potassium-content-of-foods-list.html.

Mayo Clinic, Symptoms, *Low potassium (hypokalemia), Definition*: www.mayoclinic.org/symptoms/low-potassium/basics/definition/sym-20050632.
MedicineNet, *Low potassium (hypokalemia) index, What is low potassium?*: www.medicinenet.com/low_potassium_hypokalemia/index.htm.
You & Your Hormones, *Hormones, Aldosterone*: www.yourhormones.info/Hormones/Aldosterone.aspx.

8

Hormones

OBJECTIVES

After completing this chapter, you should be able to do the following:

1. Define terms and abbreviations related to hormones and the endocrine system.
2. Discuss the endocrine system and the four main groups of hormonal action effects on the body.
3. Discuss the structure, function, and importance of the pituitary gland, thyroid gland, parathyroid glands, and adrenal glands.
4. Explain why epinephrine is of particular interest to the surgical technologist and identify safety practices regarding the use of epinephrine from the sterile field.
5. Identify the two major groups of adrenal cortex hormones and the purposes of each.
6. Discuss the structure, function, and importance of the pancreas.
7. State medical and surgical uses for various hormones in relation to the ovaries.
8. State medical and surgical uses for various hormones in relation to the testes.

OUTLINE

Hormones are chemicals released by endocrine glands into the bloodstream (Fig. 8.1). These diverse substances maintain homeostasis (relatively constant conditions in the body) by altering the activities of specific target cells. Functions regulated by hormones include reproduction, growth and development, and metabolism. Hormones have a wide range of actions and effects, and each hormone has a specific function at a specific location in the body. In addition to naturally occurring hormones, several synthetic hormones have been developed. Most hormones are administered as replacement therapy in the medical rather than in the surgical setting, but some hormones are used in surgery and may be administered from the sterile back table during the course of a procedure.

ENDOCRINE SYSTEM REVIEW

The endocrine system works with the nervous system to relay messages to maintain homeostasis. The endocrine system communicates by sending chemical messengers (hormones) to target cells located all over the body. Hormones are produced by endocrine glands and secreted into the extracellular space. They enter capillaries and are carried by the bloodstream to target cells. Hormones bind to receptor sites on cells and cause a change in cell physiology. Chemical messages take longer to work than those relayed by the nervous system, but effects generally last longer. Hormonal effects are many and varied, but actions on the body may be categorized into the following four main groups:

- Regulation of internal chemical balance and volume
- Response to environmental changes, including stress, trauma, and temperature changes
- Growth and development
- Reproduction

Hormones can be classified as steroid and nonsteroid. Steroid hormones are derived from cholesterol. In cellular mitochondria, enzymes convert cholesterol into pregnenolone, which is not a hormone but the immediate precursor molecule to the synthesis of all steroid hormones.

Steroid hormones are classified as glucocorticoids (primarily cortisol), mineralocorticoids (primarily aldosterone), estrogens, progestogens (progesterone), and androgens (male sex hormones; primarily testosterone). Nonsteroid hormones are synthesized from amino acids. The simplest hormones are amines, derived from a single amino acid. Amine hormones include epinephrine, norepinephrine, thyroxine (T_4), and triiodothyronine (T_3). Hormones made of short chains of amino acids are called *peptide hormones*. Antidiuretic hormone (ADH) and oxytocin are examples of peptide hormones. Protein hormones are longer, folded chains of amino acids. Examples of

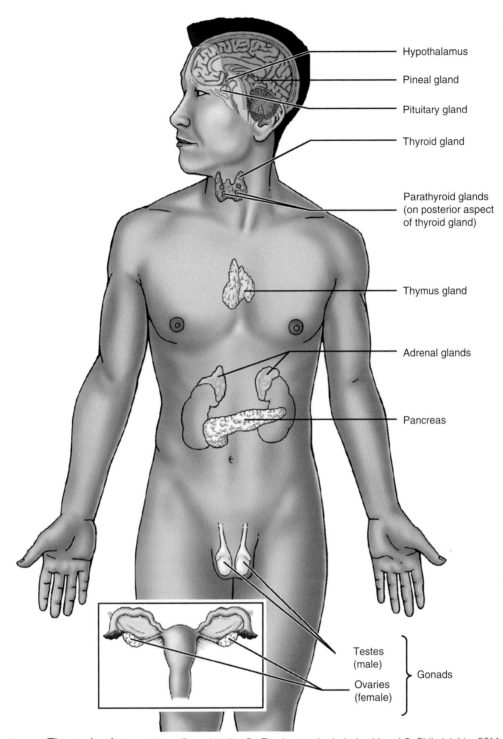

Fig. 8.1 The endocrine system. (From Herlihy B: *The human body in health*, ed 5, Philadelphia, 2014, Elsevier.)

Labels: Hypothalamus, Pineal gland, Pituitary gland, Thyroid gland, Parathyroid glands (on posterior aspect of thyroid gland), Thymus gland, Adrenal glands, Pancreas, Testes (male), Ovaries (female), Gonads

protein hormones are growth hormone (GH), parathyroid hormone (PTH), insulin, and glucagon (Box 8.1).

The majority of endocrine disorders are caused by either hyposecretion or hypersecretion of hormones. Treatment for hyposecretion may include administration of hormones for supplement or replacement. Hypersecretion may be treated medically with drugs to reduce secretion or surgically by gland removal, depending on indications.

ENDOCRINE GLANDS

Pituitary Gland

The pituitary gland, known as the *master gland*, has a vital role in reproduction and growth, and it regulates the function of the renal system and thyroid gland. The pituitary gland is connected to the hypothalamus by a stalk called the *infundibulum*. It is divided into two lobes: the anterior (or adenohypophysis)

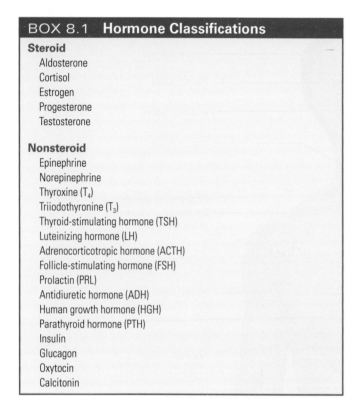

BOX 8.1 Hormone Classifications

Steroid
Aldosterone
Cortisol
Estrogen
Progesterone
Testosterone

Nonsteroid
Epinephrine
Norepinephrine
Thyroxine (T_4)
Triiodothyronine (T_3)
Thyroid-stimulating hormone (TSH)
Luteinizing hormone (LH)
Adrenocorticotropic hormone (ACTH)
Follicle-stimulating hormone (FSH)
Prolactin (PRL)
Antidiuretic hormone (ADH)
Human growth hormone (HGH)
Parathyroid hormone (PTH)
Insulin
Glucagon
Oxytocin
Calcitonin

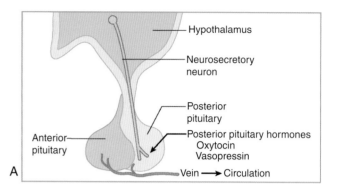

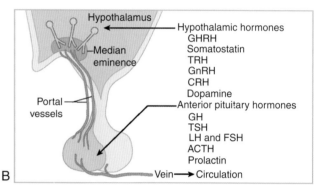

Fig. 8.2 The pituitary gland is divided into two lobes: anterior (adenohypophysis) and posterior (neurohypophysis). (A) The posterior lobe releases hormones that are produced by the hypothalamus (oxytocin and vasopressin). (B) The anterior lobe releases hormones, such as growth hormone (*GH*) and thyroid-stimulating hormone (*TSH*), in response to signals from the hypothalamus. *ACTH*, Adrenocorticotropic hormone; *CRH*, corticotropin-releasing hormone; *FSH*, follicle-stimulating hormone; *GHRH*, growth hormone-releasing hormone; *GnRH*, gonadotropin-releasing hormone; *LH*, luteinizing hormone; *TRH*, thyrotropin-releasing hormone. (From Kester M, Karpa K, Quraishi S, et al: *Elsevier's integrated review pharmacology*, ed 2, St Louis, 2012, Elsevier.)

and the posterior (or neurohypophysis). The adenohypophysis communicates with the hypothalamus through factors released into the blood supply (Fig. 8.2). Hormones secreted by the adenohypophysis include human growth hormone (Insight 8.1), thyroid-stimulating hormone (TSH), adrenocorticotropic hormone, prolactin, dopamine, and gonadotropic hormones, which include follicle-stimulating hormone and luteinizing hormone. The hypothalamus synthesizes oxytocin and vasopressin (also known as *ADH*) and transports those hormones to the neurohypophysis, where they are released.

A pituitary hormone of particular importance to the surgical technologist is oxytocin. Oxytocin stimulates the uterine contractions necessary for normal labor and delivery. If a patient is unable to produce sufficient oxytocin naturally, it may be administered intravenously to induce labor. The amount of oxytocin given is individualized and can be adjusted as needed depending upon the uterine and fetal response. Its goal is to establish uterine contractions that promote the progress of labor. The patient should be continually monitored to avoid overstimulation of the uterus.

After delivery of the infant, the uterus must continue to contract to expel the placenta and to stop postpartum bleeding from the placental attachment site. After a cesarean section delivery oxytocin is administered intravenously by the anesthesia provider to supplement natural uterine contractions and slow postpartum bleeding. If uterine contractions are not firm enough, oxytocin may be injected directly into the uterine muscle. The scrubbed surgical technologist uses a syringe and a large-bore hypodermic needle (such as 18 gauge) to draw up the desired dose of oxytocin from a properly identified vial held by the circulator, changes needles, labels the syringe, and then passes the medication to the surgeon. Oxytocin is also available as Pitocin (Insight 8.2).

QUICK QUESTION

Insight 8.2 talks about medications given to newborns for *prophylaxis*. Do you know what this means? See Chapter 5 for the answer.

Thyroid Gland

The thyroid gland is a vascular structure consisting of two lobes joined by an isthmus (Fig. 8.3). The largest of the endocrine glands, the thyroid, is located below the larynx, on both sides of the trachea in the anterior neck. It sets the rate of body metabolism. In children, an underfunctioning thyroid (hypothyroidism) can stunt growth and delay mental development. Lack of thyroid hormones slows metabolism. An adult with hypothyroidism is sleepy, tires easily, is less mentally alert, has reduced endurance, and has a slow heart rate (bradycardia). Overfunctioning of the thyroid (hyperthyroidism) causes restlessness, nervousness, sweating, and tachycardia (rapid heart rate). The most common cause of hyperthyroidism is Graves' disease, an autoimmune disorder in which the body attacks the thyroid gland, causing it to overproduce thyroxine.

INSIGHT 8.1 Biotechnology or Recombinant Deoxyribonucleic Acid Technology

Human growth hormone is used for long-term treatment of children with growth failure caused by hyposecretion of growth hormone (GH). GH obtained from domestic mammals, such as cows and pigs, does not work for humans. For many years, the only source for GH therapy was that extracted from the glands of human cadavers; however, this practice was terminated when several patients died from a rare neurologic disease attributed to contaminated glands. Thus, another source had to be found. That source is biotechnology or recombinant deoxyribonucleic acid (DNA) technology (see Chapter 1). This is defined as several techniques for cutting apart and splicing together different pieces of DNA. Segments of foreign DNA are transferred to another cell or organism, and the substances the DNA carries the code for are produced. Thus, these cells or organisms become factories to produce the substances coded for by the inserted DNA.

For example, this process is carried out to make human insulin. Although bovine and porcine insulin is similar to human insulin, the composition is slightly different. This difference can cause problems for a number of diabetic patients' immune systems, which produce antibodies against it. Thus, researchers inserted the human insulin gene into a suitable vector (*Escherichia coli* bacterial cell) to produce an insulin that is chemically identical to what is produced in humans.

Another hormone that is produced using recombinant DNA technology is parathyroid hormone. This medication has a special side effect: when given in daily injections, it promotes strong bones. Thus, it has also been approved as a treatment for osteoporosis.

Recombinant DNA technology has also made possible human clotting factor (factor IX) production. Before this achievement, clotting factors were extracted from donated blood, which carried the risk of human immunodeficiency virus/acquired immunodeficiency syndrome. Factor IX is the first to be produced and used in the treatment of patients with hemophilia.

INSIGHT 8.2 Medications Used in Labor and Delivery

Many surgical technologists work in labor and delivery departments, where medications are different from those used in surgery. These include medications for the mothers-to-be and the newborns. Sometimes they are needed to induce and help labor to progress. These medications are called *uterotropic drugs* and include oxytocin (which is described in this chapter). Oxytocin facilitates uterine smooth muscle contractions and is prepared in synthetic form as Pitocin. Other uterotropics are hormone-like lipid compounds called *prostaglandins*. An example is dinoprostone, a naturally occurring prostaglandin E_2 (PGE_2) marketed as Prepidil or Cervidil. Prepidil is a gel that comes in prefilled syringes (0.5 mg) and is inserted into the cervical os. Cervidil is a timed-release (10 mg) insert left in place for 12 hours.

Shortly after babies are born, they receive medications for prophylaxis. These include an injection of vitamin K to combat the possibility of vitamin K deficiency bleeding. This is a serious disorder caused by the lack of vitamin K needed to clot the blood. Newborns also receive 0.5% erythromycin ophthalmic ointment as prophylaxis for neonatal conjunctivitis caused by *Neisseria gonorrhoeae* or *Chlamydia trachomatis* from the mother. One example of this ointment is Ilotycin. Babies may also receive the first dose of the hepatitis B vaccine.

Another medication, RhO(D) immune globulin (human), is used to prevent certain blood problems that could occur during pregnancy. This medication is marketed as RhoGAM and given to the mother-to-be in cases of Rh incompatibility. This occurs when the mother is Rh negative and the baby is Rh positive (the baby's red blood cells have a substance called the *Rh factor*, and the mother's blood does not). If the baby's blood leaks into the mother's circulatory system, the mother's body could produce antibodies to the Rh factor. This is called *sensitization*. These antibodies can cross the placenta and destroy the unborn baby's red blood cells. To prevent this, an injection of RhoGAM is given to the mother at approximately week 28 of the pregnancy and again within 72 hours after delivery. Normally the mother is not exposed to the baby's blood cells until after birth, so the first baby would not be affected. However, subsequent pregnancies are at risk.

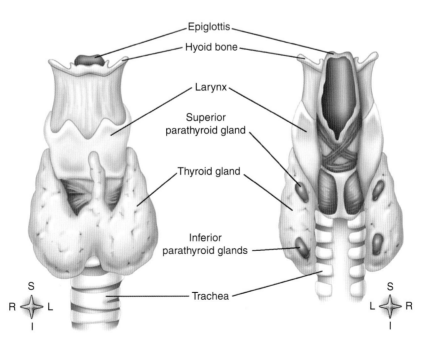

Fig. 8.3 Thyroid and parathyroid glands. (From Eisenberg RL and Johnson NM: *Comprehensive radiographic pathology*, ed 6, St Louis, 2016, Elsevier.)

The thyroid secretes three important hormones: T_4, T_3, and calcitonin. T_4 and T_3 are regulated by TSH, which is produced in the anterior lobe of the pituitary gland (adenohypophysis). These hormones are essential for normal growth and development; they also help regulate metabolism of carbohydrates, lipids, and proteins. Both T_3 and T_4 require iodine salts for production. Iodine salts are obtained from foods after absorption through the intestines. Then iodine salts are transported by the bloodstream to the thyroid for use in hormone production. Calcitonin helps to control calcium and phosphate concentrations in the blood, and it is regulated by blood levels of these ions. Calcitonin can affect calcium and phosphate levels by inhibiting the rate of release from bone, increasing the rate of incorporation of these ions into bone, and increasing excretion of these ions by the kidneys.

Thyroid hormones are administered to treat hypothyroidism caused by disease or surgical removal of the thyroid gland. Naturally occurring thyroid hormone has been extracted from the thyroid gland of pigs (porcine) and is labeled as desiccated thyroid (Thyroid USP, Armour). Types of synthetic thyroid hormone available include levothyroxine (Synthroid) and liothyronine (T_3, Triostat). Hypothyroidism is treated in the medical rather than surgical setting, so thyroid hormones are not administered from the sterile back table.

Antithyroid medications may be used to treat hyperthyroidism. Antithyroid medications are *not* hormones but agents that interfere with the synthesis of thyroid hormones. A common antithyroid agent is methimazole, which may be used in the medical setting before surgery to reduce the size of a thyroid tumor or to inactivate thyroid tissue.

? MAKE IT SIMPLE

Use medical terminology to apply the terms "hyper-" and "hypo-" to words in this chapter. "Hyper-" is a prefix that refers to excessive or above, and "hypo-" refers to below or less than normal. Hence, hyperthyroidism refers to excessive or overfunctioning of the thyroid gland, and hypothyroidism is underfunctioning.

Parathyroid Glands

The parathyroid glands are small, yellowish-brown ovals, approximately 6 mm in length, and frequently covered with adipose tissue (see Fig. 8.3). The superior parathyroid glands are usually found embedded in the posterolateral surface of the thyroid gland's superior pole. The inferior parathyroid glands vary more in their position but are often found in the lower pole of the thyroid. The number of parathyroid glands may vary from 2 to 12, with 90% of patients having four: two on each side of the thyroid gland. They produce PTH, which monitors circulating concentrations of calcium ions in the blood. PTH has four major functions: to stimulate osteoclasts, accelerating mineral turnover and the release of calcium from bone; to inhibit osteoblasts, reducing the rate of calcium deposition in bone; to enhance the reabsorption of calcium at the kidneys, reducing its loss via urine; and to stimulate the formation and secretion of calcitriol at the kidneys, for the enhancement of calcium and phosphate absorption by the digestive tract. Inadequate amounts of PTH result in low calcium concentrations and hypoparathyroidism. This can cause a condition called *tetany*, characterized by prolonged muscle spasms involving the face and extremities. An example of a PTH is teriparatide (Forteo), which is a synthetic version produced by biotechnology (recombinant deoxyribonucleic acid [DNA] technology). Because hypoparathyroidism is treated medically, PTHs are not administered in surgery from the sterile back table.

If calcium concentrations become too high, hyperparathyroidism results. In this condition, bones can grow thin and brittle, skeletal muscles weaken, and the central nervous system is depressed. Surgical removal of parathyroid tissue may be indicated to treat hyperparathyroidism.

Adrenal Glands

The adrenal glands are pyramid-shaped glands positioned on top of each kidney. The adrenals are highly vascular and consist of a central portion (the medulla) and an outer portion (the cortex) (Fig. 8.4). The adrenal medulla produces, stores, and secretes the hormones epinephrine (adrenaline), norepinephrine (noradrenaline), and dopamine, collectively called *catecholamines*.

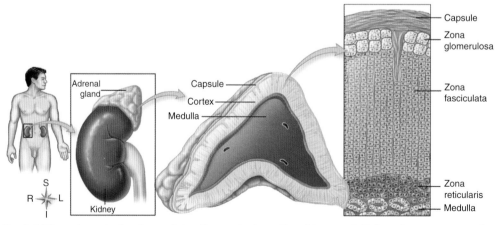

Fig. 8.4 The adrenal gland consists of a central portion (the medulla) and an outer portion (the cortex). The medulla secretes epinephrine, norepinephrine, and dopamine. The adrenal cortex secretes glucocorticoid and mineralocorticoid hormones, collectively referred to as the *steroid hormones*. (From Patton KT, Thibodeau GA: *Anatomy & physiology*, ed 7, St Louis, 2010, Mosby/Elsevier.)

The catecholamines are *sympathomimetic*, meaning they mimic effects of the sympathetic portion of the autonomic nervous system. Epinephrine and norepinephrine work with the sympathetic nervous system to prepare the body for the fight-or-flight response to stress. Effects of these hormones include increased heart rate, increased force of cardiac muscle contraction, vasoconstriction, elevated blood pressure, increased respiratory rate, and decreased digestive system activity.

Epinephrine

Epinephrine is of particular interest to the surgical technologist because it is used frequently in surgery. Epinephrine is often used in combination with local anesthetics, such as lidocaine and bupivacaine, to prolong anesthesia. When injected in dilute amounts (1:100,000 or 1:200,000), epinephrine causes local vasoconstriction; this means it reduces blood flow, so it reduces the absorption rate of the anesthetic (i.e., the local effect lasts longer).

⚠ CAUTION

Epinephrine in local anesthetics is contraindicated for injection in areas of limited blood supply, such as fingers or toes. A local anesthetic agent containing epinephrine may have a red image on the label or red printing noting its concentration. The color red is used to provide a visual "alert," an additional safety measure, to help prevent inadvertent use of epinephrine when contraindicated (see Chapter 13).

 MAKE IT SIMPLE

An easy phrase to remember when to avoid use of epinephrine in a local anesthetic is, "Don't use on penis, toes, fingers, or tip of nose."

INSIGHT 8.3 Immunosuppressant Agents

Organ transplantation is the replacement of a diseased organ with a healthy donor organ. This procedure introduces foreign tissue into the recipient's system and will trigger the immune response, which can result in the destruction of the transplanted tissue. Thus, tissue must be matched between donor and recipient to avoid rejection. Even with careful tissue matching, though, some incompatibilities will exist (except in cases of identical twins or autotransplantation). Glucocorticoids are used to prevent or alleviate the effects of the immune response when the response is detrimental. For transplant patients, the medication therapy will be lifelong or as long as the transplanted tissue is in place.

Glucocorticoids act by inhibiting synthesis of chemical mediators, such as histamines, and so reduce swelling, redness, warmth, and pain. They also suppress the infiltration of phagocytes to decrease lysosomal enzyme damage and suppress the proliferation of lymphocytes to reduce the immune component of inflammation.

When the immune system is suppressed with glucocorticoids, infectious organisms have the opportunity to multiply. Minor infections may become clinically significant after such therapy, so use in some patients, such as those with fungal or herpes infections, must be avoided. Glucocorticoids should be used cautiously in patients with diabetes mellitus, peptic ulcers, inflammatory bowel disorders, hypertension, congestive heart failure, or renal problems.

Concentrated epinephrine 1 mg/mL (1:1000) may be applied topically for hemostasis in limited areas. For example, in middle ear procedures tiny pledgets of Gelfoam (a gelatin sponge for hemostasis discussed in Chapter 9) are typically dipped in epinephrine (1:1000) and applied to very small areas of capillary bleeding. In ear surgery, epinephrine 1 mg/mL (1:1000) is used *only* for topical application—*never* injection. If epinephrine 1 mg/mL (1:1000) is mistakenly injected, deadly tachycardia and hypertension may result. Refer to Insight 4.1 in Chapter 4 for epinephrine information.

NOTE: Epinephrine is a vasoconstrictor and not a local anesthetic.

Steroids

Adrenal cortex hormones are classified into two major groups—glucocorticoids and mineralocorticoids—collectively known as *steroids*. The most important mineralocorticoid is aldosterone, which maintains homeostatic levels of sodium and potassium in the blood. Most significant to the surgical technologist are the glucocorticoids, which are used alone or in combination to reduce or inhibit the inflammatory response after surgical procedures, such as shoulder arthroscopy or cataract extraction, as discussed in Chapter 10. The combination of Kenalog-40 and dexamethasone is an example of glucocorticoids that might be used intraoperatively in orthopedic surgery.

Glucocorticoids are used medically to help prevent rejection of donated organs (Insight 8.3), to reduce the inflammatory response in patients with arthritis, and with aldosterone as replacement therapy for Addison's disease (Insight 8.4). They are also used for the treatment of autoimmune disorders, to suppress hypersensitivity reactions, and to alleviate cerebral edema. Glucocorticoids are used intraoperatively and postoperatively on orthopedic procedures to treat bursitis, synovitis, and epicondylitis. When administered for diseases, such as arthritis, they are used as palliatives. Palliative drugs relieve symptoms, but they do not cure the condition or disease.

INSIGHT 8.4 Pathology Insight: Addison's Disease

Addison's disease, also known as *adrenocortical hypofunction* or *adrenal insufficiency*, occurs when the adrenal cortex does not secrete adequate amounts of steroid hormone. The disorder was first described by Thomas Addison in 1855, when the primary cause was tuberculosis. However, autoimmune disease is currently the most common cause. Why? Because the body's circulating antibodies react specifically against adrenal tissue to destroy it. Tumors or hemorrhage of the adrenal glands can also cause the disorder, as can hypopituitarism—decreasing adrenocorticotropic hormone secretion—or abrupt withdrawal of long-term corticosteroid treatment. The disorder can occur at any age, even infancy, and is found in both males and females. Medical treatment involves replacement hormones, such as prednisone or hydrocortisone and fludrocortisone. John F. Kennedy had Addison's disease. He had almost no adrenal tissue, but by taking replacement hormones, he was able to function in one of the world's most demanding jobs—the presidency of the United States (1960–1963).

Glucocorticoids may be administered orally, topically, intramuscularly, intraarticularly, intravenously, or by inhalation. These hormones may be long- or short-acting, depending on the agent used. Naturally occurring steroids include cortisone, hydrocortisone, aldosterone, and deoxycorticosterone. Many synthetic glucocorticoids have been produced. A partial list of synthetic steroid hormones includes synthetic cortisone acetate, synthetic hydrocortisone (cortisol, Solu-Cortef), prednisone, prednisolone (Delta-Cortef), methylprednisolone (Medrol, Depo-Medrol, Solu-Medrol), triamcinolone (Kenalog-40), fluticasone (Flonase, Flovent), dexamethasone, and betamethasone (Celestone Soluspan).

Pancreas

The pancreas, which is posterior to the stomach and behind the parietal peritoneum, is divided into three anatomic areas: the head (which lies within the loop of the duodenum), body, and tail (Fig. 8.5). A unique feature of the pancreas is that it functions as an exocrine gland for digestion and as an endocrine gland for release of hormones. The exocrine pancreas is the primary source for the vital digestive enzymes amylase, lipase, and proteinase. A duct from the gland—the pancreatic duct—transports these digestive enzymes to the duodenum.

The endocrine portion of the pancreas is closely associated with blood vessels, which facilitate the transport of pancreatic hormones to the body. Pancreatic hormones are produced by clusters of cells called *pancreatic islets* or the *islets of Langerhans.*

Pancreatic alpha (α) cells secrete glucagon, and pancreatic beta (β) cells secrete insulin. Both pancreatic hormones, insulin and glucagon, regulate metabolism of glucose, a simple sugar used as an energy source. Glucagon is a protein; it stimulates the liver to break down glycogen into glucose, thus increasing blood glucose levels. Insulin, also a protein, stimulates the liver to form glycogen from glucose, thus lowering blood glucose levels.

Diabetes mellitus is the inability to effectively regulate glucose. There are two major types of diabetes: type 1 and type 2. Type 1 diabetes is caused by an autoimmune disorder in which the body attacks its own pancreatic beta (β) cells. As a result, the body fails to produce insulin, so an outside source must be provided. Insulin was first obtained from animals, but human insulin is now produced via biotechnology. In type 2 diabetes the body's tissues fail to respond to the action of insulin on target cells. Type 2 diabetes may be effectively managed with diet and exercise or administration of oral antidiabetic drugs, which include glyburide, pioglitazone (Actos), sitagliptin (Januvia), and metformin. Medications used to treat diabetes are not administered from the sterile back table.

Ovaries

The ovaries, located in the pelvic cavity, are paired glands that produce estrogen and progesterone (Fig. 8.6). Estrogen and progesterone are critical to the development and maintenance of female sex characteristics, including the menstrual

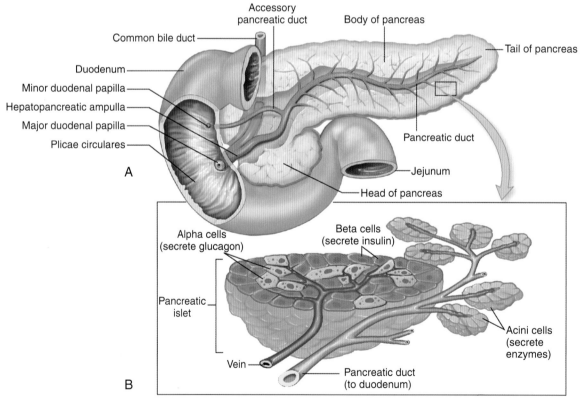

Fig. 8.5 (A) The pancreas is divided into three anatomic areas: the head (which lies within the loop of the duodenum), body, and tail. (B) The exocrine cells of the pancreas secrete digestive enzymes into the pancreatic duct, which leads to the duodenum. The endocrine cells of the pancreas secrete hormones into the bloodstream. Pancreatic alpha (α) cells secrete glucagon and pancreatic beta (β) cells secrete insulin. (From Patton KT, Thibodeau GA: *Anatomy & physiology*, ed 7, St Louis, 2010, Mosby.)

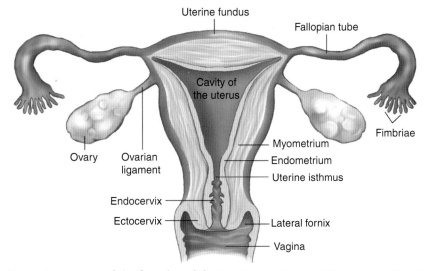

Fig. 8.6 Normal anatomy of the female pelvis. Note the relationship of the ovaries to the lateral walls of the uterus and the position of the fallopian tubes to the ovaries. (From Hagen-Ansert SL: *Textbook of diagnostic sonography*, ed 7, St Louis, 2012, Elsevier.)

INSIGHT 8.5 Pathology Insight: The Role of Estrogen in Osteoporosis

Osteoporosis is a disorder in which the skeletal system loses too much mineralized bone volume. Normal bones are remodeled throughout life. Until approximately age 30 years, bone formation exceeds bone resorption. Bone resorption later outpaces formation, though, and the result is a net bone loss of approximately 0.5% per year after age 30 years. After menopause, bone resorption is accelerated in women because estrogen production decreases. Bone tissue needs estrogen to absorb calcium. Estrogen also increases vitamin D metabolism—a process necessary for calcium absorption from the intestines. Without proper levels of estrogen in the body, the amount of calcium stored in bones is diminished and bones become more porous (i.e., osteoporotic). The skeleton weakens, so it is less able to support body weight. Osteoporotic bone can be seen on routine spine radiographs. The shape of the bone is the same, but the image is less distinct; this suggests porous, or weaker, bone.

A more sensitive test is a bone-density scan known as *dual-energy x-ray absorptiometry*. Many times, however, the first indication of osteoporosis is a fracture—in the femur at the hip, in the radius near the wrist, or as compression fractures of the vertebrae. Over time, osteoporotic symptoms include loss of height, stooped posture, and back pain. Estrogen replacement, also known as *hormone replacement therapy* (HRT), to treat osteoporosis is controversial. The Women's Health Initiative demonstrated that HRT reduces the risk of hip fractures, but presents significant risk for stroke and blood clots, especially in older women. As a result, HRT is not recommended for most postmenopausal women solely to improve bone density.

outside the uterus, such as in the pelvic cavity. Birth control hormones may also be used to treat symptoms of fibrocystic breast changes. Approximately 50% of women experience fibrocystic changes in their breasts—fluid-filled sacs surrounded by fibrous tissue that may become swollen and painful during the menstrual cycle.

Estrogens are also used for palliative treatment of advanced androgen-dependent prostate cancer and metastatic breast cancer. Common estrogens available are conjugated estrogens (Premarin), synthetic conjugated estrogens, and estradiol (Estrace). One type of synthetic progesterone (progestin) available is medroxyprogesterone (Provera). Provera may be used in the treatment of secondary amenorrhea or abnormal uterine bleeding caused by hormonal imbalances.

Estrogen and progesterone deficiencies are treated in the medical setting rather than the surgical setting, so they are not routinely administered from the sterile back table. A rare exception is a cream form of estrogen, which might be used on vaginal packing placed after vaginal hysterectomy.

Testes

The testes are paired glands located in the scrotum (Fig. 8.7). Endocrine cells are distributed throughout the testes and produce male sex hormones called *androgens*. Androgens, primarily testosterone, are critical for the development of male sex organs and maintenance of secondary sex characteristics. Androgens, especially testosterone (Depo-Testosterone), are administered if replacement therapy is indicated, as seen in hypogonadism. Testosterone may also be used to treat some types of advanced breast cancer in females. The androgen danazol may be used to treat diseases in females, such as endometriosis. In addition, patients scheduled for an endometrial ablation may be placed on danazol therapy a few weeks before surgery to reduce the volume of the endometrial layer. Androgens are used in the medical setting rather than the surgical setting, so these hormones are not administered from the sterile back table.

cycle, pregnancy, and lactation. These hormones are available in several forms—tablets, capsules, and oil (intramuscular use only)—and are administered to treat amenorrhea, dysmenorrhea, and the side effects of menopause. Estrogen and progesterone derivatives are used as oral contraceptives (birth control hormones) and may be used for hormone replacement therapy after menopause or oophorectomy (Insight 8.5). Birth control hormones may also be used to treat symptomatic endometriosis if pregnancy is not desired. Endometriosis is an abnormal condition in which functional endometrial tissue is found situated

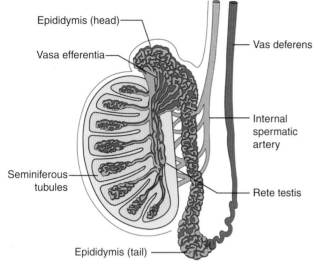

Epididymis (head)

Vasa efferentia

Vas deferens

Internal spermatic artery

Seminiferous tubules

Rete testis

Epididymis (tail)

Fig. 8.7 Normal anatomy of the testes. (From Hudson CN, Setchell ME: *Shaw's textbook of operative gynaecology*, ed 7, St Louis, 2011, Elsevier.)

KEY CONCEPTS

- The endocrine system works with the nervous system to relay chemical messages called *hormones.*
- Hormones maintain homeostasis by altering activities of specific target cells.
- Hormones' activities include regulation of internal chemical balance and volume, response to environmental changes, growth and development, and reproduction.
- Most endocrine disorders are caused by hyposecretion or hypersecretion of hormones and are treated with medications administered from the medical setting.
- Some hormones are synthesized by biotechnology, also called *recombinant DNA technology.*
- Hormones most commonly administered in surgery are oxytocin, epinephrine, and the glucocorticoids.
- Additional caution must be used when handling concentrated epinephrine at the sterile back table to avoid inadvertent injection.

LEARNING THE LANGUAGE (KEY TERMS)

Using your textbook or a standard medical dictionary, look up and write the definition of each term.

androgens
endometriosis

fibrocystic breast changes
palliatives

REVIEW QUESTIONS

1. What is the general purpose of the endocrine system?
2. For what purpose are the following hormones administered?
   a. Thyroid hormones
   b. Cortisone
   c. Testosterone
   d. Insulin
   e. Estrogen
   f. Oxytocin
3. Why would a male receive a female hormone? Why would a female receive a male hormone?
4. What is the purpose of Pitocin?
5. Which surgical procedures may involve the administration of hormones from the sterile back table?
   a. Which hormones may be administered?
   b. How will each of those hormones be administered?
   c. What is the purpose of each of those hormones?
6. What is the purpose for administration of epinephrine 1 mg/mL (1:1000)? Which route is used?
7. What safety measures must be used when epinephrine is administered from the sterile back table?

CRITICAL THINKING

1. Can you think of other medications that are given for palliative purposes?
2. What are the strengths of epinephrine normally encountered in the surgical setting?

Scenario

Joseph Goldstein is a 55-year-old man scheduled for a total thyroidectomy. His diagnosis is carcinoma of the thyroid gland.

Answer the following questions as they relate to Mr. Goldstein's procedure.
1. What other endocrine glands would be involved in this procedure?
2. Where are these other glands located?
3. How will the removal of the thyroid and these other glands affect the patient postoperatively?
4. What can be done to correct any imbalances caused by removing the thyroid glands?

BIBLIOGRAPHY

Fulcher EM, Fulcher RM, Soto CD: *Pharmacology: principles and applications*, ed 3, St Louis, 2012, Elsevier.

Kee JL, Hayes ER, McCuistion LE: *Pharmacology: a patient-centered nursing process approach*, ed 8, St Louis, 2015, Saunders/Elsevier.

Skidmore-Roth L: *Mosby's drug guide for nursing students*, ed 11, St Louis, 2015, Mosby/Elsevier.

INTERNET RESOURCES

Biotech Articles, Recombinant DNA Technology and Production of Hormones: www.biotecharticles.com/Genetics-Article/Recombinant-DNA-Technology-and-Production-of-Hormones-145.html.

Drugs.com: www.drugs.com.

Drugs.com, Conditions, Hyperthyroidism, Methimazole: www.drugs.com/cdi/methimazole.html.

Drugs.com, Conditions, Levothyroxine, Uses, dosage, side effects: www.drugs.com/levothyroxine.html.

Drugs.com, Dexamethasone: www.drugs.com/dexamethasone.html.

Drugs.com, Glucophage: www.drugs.com/glucophage.html.

Drugs.com, Kenalog: www.drugs.com/kenalog.html.

Drugs.com, Liothyronine: www.drugs.com/cdi/liothyronine.html.

Drugs.com, Professionals, Medfacts, Thyroid, Desiccated (Thyroid USP), Information on drugs: https://www.drugs.com/monograph/thyroid.html.

Encyclopedia.com, Immunosuppressant Drugs: www.encyclopedia.com/topic/immunosuppressive_drug.aspx.

Healthline, Reference Library, Glucocorticoids: www.healthline.com/health/glucocorticoids#Overview1.

Healthline, Reference Library, Immunosuppressant Drugs: www.healthline.com/health/immunosuppressant-drugs#Overview1.

MedicineNet.com: http://MedicineNet.com.

Medline Plus, Drugs, Herbs and Supplements, Dexamethasone: www.nlm.nih.gov/medlineplus/druginfo/meds/a682792.html.

New Hampshire National Health Clinic, About Armour™ Thyroid: www.webmd.com/drugs/2/drug-3694/armour-thyroid-oral/details.

RxList Oxycontin: www.rxlist.com/oxycontin-drug.htm.

The Free Dictionary, hyper: www.medical-dictionary.thefreedictionary.com/hyper.

The Free Dictionary, hypo: www.thefreedictionary.com/hypo.

WebMD, Fitness & Exercise, Human Growth Hormone (HGH): www.webMD.com/fitness-exercise/human-growth-hormone-hgh.

You & Your Hormones, Society for Endocrinology: www.yourhormones.info.

CLASSIFICATION OF HORMONES

Hormones are classified by the following characteristics: their target site (as thyroid-stimulating hormone); whether they are steroid or nonsteroid in chemical composition; and whether they are water soluble and can cross the cell's plasma membrane (hydrophilic) or not (hydrophobic). Hydrophilic hormones are derived from amino acids, peptides, and proteins. Hydrophobic hormones include steroids, which are derived from cholesterol. The more common classification is into steroid and nonsteroid categories. Steroid hormones include cortisol, aldosterone, estrogen, progesterone, and testosterone. Note that estrogen, progesterone, and testosterone are also sex hormones. Nonsteroid hormones include the remainder of those as described and listed in this chapter. Hormones that are not used completely are inactivated by enzymes in the blood or in intracellular spaces and excreted primarily in the urine, with some found in bile. Most have short half-lives of approximately 10 to 20 minutes and so exert their effects rapidly. Some, though, have effects that last for several hours for prolonged stimulation of an organ.

TREATMENT OPTIONS

The thyroid and the parathyroid glands are among the most common glands of the endocrine system to be affected by a disorder and/or a disease. Treatment usually requires both drug therapy and surgery. The hormones secreted by these glands are essential for homeostasis; therefore, any abnormal secretion must be corrected. The medical therapy is usually directed by an endocrinologist, whereas surgical removal requires an endocrine surgeon (general or head and neck surgeon). The advanced practitioner acting as a surgical first assistant may be exposed to only the surgical aspect, but should also have knowledge of the medical component. It is important to understand how each affects the other.

THYROID GLAND

As previously described in the chapter, the thyroid consists of two lobes connected by the isthmus and secretes hormones.

Ideally, it is important for the surgical patient to be euthyroid before any procedure. If the patient is hyperthyroid (an overfunctioning of the gland and thus overproduction of thyroid hormones), medical management with antithyroid agents or radioactive iodine ablation is indicated. If the patient is not managed, a condition called *thyroid storm*, or *hyperthyroid crisis*, could occur. This is a failure of the body to tolerate increased thyroid hormones in response to a stressor (such as surgery). Thyroid storm is defined as an acute, life-threatening, thyroid hormone–induced hypermetabolic state, also referred to as *thyrotoxicosis*. Specifically, thyroid storm is a decompensated state of thyrotoxicosis that can cause death unless recognized early and treated aggressively. It is precipitated when the metabolic, thermoregulatory, and cardiovascular mechanisms that compensate for thyrotoxicosis fail. Symptoms include hyperpyrexia, cardiac arrhythmias, mental status changes, congestive heart failure, diaphoresis, agitation, and hemodynamic instability. If left untreated, thyroid storm can lead to congestive heart failure, cardiovascular collapse, coma, and death within 24 hours. In the past, thyroid storm occurred intraoperatively and postoperatively from thyroid surgery in patients with Graves' disease and, in some cases, in patients with toxic nodular goiter. It can also occur after administration of iodine-rich contrast media during radiologic studies. Currently, thyroid storm is rare because of prompt recognition, appropriate medical workup, and preoperative treatment (Table 8.A). If the patient is hypothyroid (underfunctioning of the gland), medical management with thyroid hormone replacement therapy is indicated before surgery. This condition, in its advanced stage known as *myxedema*, is characterized by hypothermia, carbon dioxide retention, and bradycardia. There may be emergency situations in which the patient must have surgery and is not euthyroid. When this occurs, the surgeon and anesthesia personnel will decide the best medications and treatment plan preoperatively and intraoperatively.

PARATHYROID GLANDS

Parathyroid glands are located in the neck, usually posterior to the thyroid gland. The glands may be found within the thyroid gland, in adipose tissue under the thyroid gland, or in the mediastinum. Incidentally, it is possible for the patient to have

TABLE 8.A   Medical Treatment of Thyroid Disease

Medicine	Treatment of	Action	Therapeutic Dosage	Side Effects
methimazole	Hyperthyroidism	Inhibits thyroid hormone synthesis	Initially: 15–60 mg/day in 1–3 divided doses, PO Maintenance: 5–15 mg/day	Rash, urticaria, headache, GI tract symptoms
PTU	Hyperthyroidism	Inhibits conversion of T_3 and T_4 hormones	Initially: 100 mg q8h Maintenance: 100–150 mg/day, PO	Rash, hair loss, GI symptoms, loss of taste, drowsiness, decreased white blood cells, decreased platelets
SSKI	Hyperthyroidism	To reduce thyroid gland size and vascularity	Preoperatively: 50–250 mg, tid for 10–14 days, PO	Dilute with water and take after meals
Synthetic Thyroid Replacement Medications				
levothyroxine sodium (Synthroid)	Hypothyroidism	Increases metabolic rate, replaces thyroid hormones (T_4)	Initially: 25–50 mcg/day, PO Maintenance: 50–200 mcg/day, PO	Nausea, vomiting, diarrhea, cramps, tremors, nervousness, insomnia, headache, weight loss
liothyronine (Cytomel, Triostat)	Hypothyroidism	Replaces thyroid hormones (T_3)	Initially: 5–25 mcg/day, PO Maintenance: 25–75 mcg/day, PO	Cardiac side effects
thyroid (Armour Thyroid)	Hypothyroidism	Reduces goiter size	Initially: 15–30 mg/day, PO Maintenance: 60–120 mg/day, PO	Tachycardia, irritability, nervousness, insomnia, weight loss

GI, Gastrointestinal; PO, by mouth (per os); PTU, propylthiouracil; q8h, every 8 hours; SSKI, saturated solution of potassium iodide; T_3, triiodothyronine; T_4, thyroxine; tid, three times a day (ter in die).

TABLE 8.B   Medical Treatment of Parathyroid Disease

Medicine	Condition	Action	Therapeutic Dosage	Side Effects
calcitriol (Rocaltrol)	Hypoparathyroidism, hypocalcemia	Enhancement of calcium deposits in bones	0.25–0.50 mcg/day, PO	Lethargy, headache, nausea, vomiting, dry mouth, drowsiness
calcium (combined with vitamin D)	Hypoparathyroidism	Replaces calcium	500 mg bid, PO after meals	
teriparatide (Forteo)	Osteoporosis, for those at high risk of fractures	Increases the number and action of osteoblasts	20 mcg/day, SC	Dizziness, headache, depression, hypertension, vomiting, diarrhea

bid, twice a day (bis in die); PO, By mouth (per os); SC, subcutaneous.

anywhere from 2 to 12 parathyroid glands. As stated in the chapter, they secrete parathyroid hormone (PTH), which is responsible for regulating calcium levels in the body. Overfunctioning of the parathyroid glands causes the secretion of too much PTH. Hyperparathyroidism is the most common disorder causing the patient's blood calcium level to be elevated. Hypoparathyroidism is responsible for low levels of calcium and develops in 1% to 2% of patients after total thyroidectomy. Both conditions may be treated with medication therapy (Table 8.B); however, most cases of hyperparathyroidism are treated surgically. Parathyroid glands weigh approximately 30 mg and are 3 to 6 mm in size, ranging from approximately the size of a grain of rice to the size of a pea. Therefore, finding them in the tissue can be a challenge. Radiologic studies may be helpful, but another method to assist in finding the overactive gland(s) is for the patient to have a sestamibi scan. This involves an injection of technetium-99 administered in nuclear medicine preoperatively. It is absorbed by the overactive parathyroid gland, and the surgeon will then use a probe to locate and surgically remove the affected gland.

BLOOD SERUM CALCIUM LEVELS

Calcium is the most abundant and important mineral in the body. It is responsible for building and repairing bones and teeth, and for helping nerve function. It is necessary for muscle contraction, blood clotting, and proper function of the heart. Maintaining a normal level of calcium is essential for homeostasis, and it must be replaced continuously by diet or supplemental agents. Ninety-nine percent of calcium is stored in the bones with the remaining 1% found in the blood. The normal laboratory value of calcium is 8.5 to 10.2 mg/dL (milligrams per deciliter) but may vary somewhat from laboratory to laboratory. A patient with a laboratory value lower than the normal is considered to have hypocalcemia, whereas patients with values higher than normal have hypercalcemia. Hypocalcemia may be caused by radical surgery in the central neck, including total thyroidectomy and radical neck dissection. Patients undergoing any central neck procedure will need to have calcium levels tested immediately postoperatively. A drop in the serum calcium level to less than 7.0 mg/dL may be treated with calcium gluconate administrated intravenously. The usual initial intravenous dose for hypocalcemia is 100 to 300 mg of elemental calcium (10 mL of calcium gluconate contains 90 mg of elemental calcium) intravenous in 50 to 100 mL of normal saline or D5W (5% dextrose in water) over 5 to 10 minutes. Faster infusions may result in cardiac dysfunction or cardiac arrest. Hypercalcemia may be caused by overfunctioning of one or more parathyroid glands. This is usually treated with surgical intervention, as described later.

HYPERPARATHYROIDISM

Hyperparathyroidism is described as an oversecretion of PTH, causing high calcium levels (hypercalcemia) in patients. There are two basic types of hyperparathyroidism: primary and secondary. Primary hyperparathyroidism, the most common disorder, is often caused by at least one diseased gland (usually adenoma) that overstimulates the secretion of PTH. Surgical removal of the affected gland is usually required. The most common procedure today is minimally invasive excision of the affected gland with rapid PTH study. As previously described, the gland is localized with the use of a sestamibi scan performed preoperatively in the nuclear medicine department. At the beginning of the procedure, a blood sample is drawn and processed to identify the amount of serum PTH. A small incision is made over the location of the affected gland, and the gland is surgically removed. The half-life of PTH is approximately 10 minutes; therefore, after this time a second blood sample is drawn and processed in the same manner as the first. If the results reveal that the serum PTH level has dropped by at least

50%, it is accepted that only one gland was affected, and the surgical procedure is concluded. Postoperative calcium levels are closely monitored for 24 hours.

Secondary hyperparathyroidism is a result of renal failure, which stimulates the parathyroid glands to secrete more PTH. This condition, when treated with hypocalcemic or vitamin D analogue medicine, produces limited results. Surgical management is still the most effective treatment. The surgical procedure requires that all but one half of the parathyroid glands are removed. With only one half of the gland functioning, the PTH level is reduced dramatically. Some surgeons will choose to transplant the remaining half gland in the sternocleidomastoid muscle for easy access if more gland needs to be removed at a later date.

HYPOPARATHYROIDISM

Hypoparathyroidism is a condition in which the parathyroid glands do not secrete an adequate amount of PTH, rendering the patient hypocalcemic. This condition is caused by inadvertent excision of all parathyroid tissue during a total thyroidectomy and is referred to as *true hypoparathyroidism*, found in 3% to 5% of total thyroidectomy. Postoperative calcium levels are monitored after total thyroidectomy to determine any functioning parathyroid tissue. If levels are low, replacement PTH is prescribed. Another type of hypoparathyroidism, termed *pseudohypoparathyroidism*, is a rare, inherited familiar disorder. Females are twice as likely to inherit the condition as males. Both disorders are treated with a hypercalcemic medicine to regulate the calcium levels. There is no surgical procedure to correct this disorder.

ADVANCED PRACTICES: REVIEW QUESTIONS

1. What two endocrine glands are most commonly affected by a disorder or disease?
2. At the time of any thyroid surgery, it is best for the patient to be in the state of _____.
   a. Hyperthyroid
   b. Hypothyroid
   c. Euthyroid
   d. Thyrotoxicosis
3. List three symptoms of thyroid storm.

4. Which is the most common disorder of the endocrine system that may cause a patient's blood calcium to be elevated?
   a. Hyperthyroidism
   b. Hyperparathyroidism
   c. Hypothyroidism
   d. Hypoparathyroidism
5. Describe the common causes of primary and secondary hyperparathyroidism.
6. What is the most common cause of hypoparathyroidism?
7. What happens to hormones that are not used completely in the body?

ADVANCED PRACTICES: BIBLIOGRAPHY

Fulcher EM, Fulcher RM, Soto CD: *Pharmacology: principles and applications*, ed 3, St Louis, 2012, Saunders/Elsevier.

Kee JL, Hayes ER, McCuistion LE: *Pharmacology: a patient-centered nursing process approach*, ed 8, St Louis, 2015, Saunders/Elsevier.

Skidmore-Roth L: *Mosby's drug guide for nursing students*, ed 11, St Louis, 2015, Mosby/Elsevier.

ADVANCED PRACTICES: INTERNET RESOURCES

Medline Plus, Calcium Blood Test: www.nlm.nih.gov/medlineplus/ency/article/003477.htm.

Cleveland Clinic, Center for Continuing Education, Disease Management, Endocrinology: www.clevelandclinicmeded.com/medicalpubs/diseasemanagement/endocrinology/.

Drugs.com, Calcitonin Nasal: www.drugs.com/mtm/calcitonin-nasal.html.

Drugs.com, Condition, Underactive Thyroid (Hypothyroidism) Medications: www.drugs.com/condition/hypothyroidism.html.

Drugs.com, Drug Classes, Hormones: https://www.drugs.com/drug-class/hormones.html.

Drugs.com, Propylthiouracil: www.drugs.com/pro/propylthiouracil.html.

endocrineweb: www.endocrineweb.com.

endocrineweb, Parathyroid Function: www.endocrineweb.com/function.html.

HealthCentral: http://healthcentral.com.

Mayo Clinic, Diseases and Conditions, Hyperthyroidism (Overactive Thyroid), Definition: www.mayoclinic.org/diseases-conditions/hyperthyroidism/basics/definition/con-20020986.

Mayo Clinic, Diseases and Conditions, Hypothyroidism (Underactive Thyroid), Definition: www.mayoclinic.org/diseases-conditions/hypothyroidism/basics/definition/con-20021179?reDate=10082015.

MedicineNet, Calcitonin Nasal Spray: www.medicinenet.com/calcitonin_nasal_spray/article.htm.

MedicineNet.com, Liothyronine: www.medicinenet.com/liothyronine_sodium/article.htm.

MedlinePlus, Parathyroid Gland Removal: www.nlm.nih.gov/medlineplus/ency/article/002931.htm.

Misra M., Singhal A., Campbell D.E.: Thyroid storm, Medscape: http://emedicine.medscape.com/article/925147-overview.

New York Thyroid Center, Surgical Procedures, Thyroid Surgery: www.columbiasurgery.org/thyroid/.

Norman J.: Introduction to endocrinology & endocrine surgery, endocrineweb: www.endocrineweb.com/whatisendo.html.

parathyroid.com, Sestamibi Scan for Hyperparathyroidism (Parathyroid Problems): http://parathyroid.com/sestamibi.htm.

PathologyOutlines.com, Parathyroid Gland: www.pathologyoutlines.com/parathyroidpf.html.

RxList, RxList, Forteo: www.rxlist.com/forteo-drug.htm.

RxList, Rocaltrol: www.rxlist.com/rocaltrol-drug.htm.

WebMD: www.webmd.com.

9

Medications That Affect Coagulation

OBJECTIVES

After completing this chapter, you should be able to do the following:

1. Define terms and abbreviations related to blood coagulation and medications that affect coagulation.
2. Describe the physiology of blood clot formation.
3. Define coagulants and describe the two major categories of coagulants.
4. Discuss various types of hemostatic agents, including uses, side effects, contraindications, and administration routes.
5. Discuss various types of systemic coagulants, including uses, side effects, contraindications, and administration routes.
6. Discuss various types of anticoagulants, including uses, onset, side effects, contraindications, and administration routes.
7. Discuss safety considerations for heparin dosing from the sterile field.

OUTLINE

Blood naturally contains both coagulants, which promote clotting, and anticoagulants, which inhibit clotting. Normally anticoagulants are dominant; they keep blood in liquid form. When damage occurs to blood vessels, the body's coagulation mechanism begins clot formation to prevent excessive blood loss. At times, it becomes necessary to enhance or assist natural coagulation. During surgical intervention, the blood supply to an area may be disrupted, causing blood loss. Intraoperatively, damaged blood vessels are controlled with the use of thermal hemostasis (electrosurgical unit) or mechanical hemostasis (such as ligatures or hemostatic clips). The natural coagulation process usually works effectively on damaged capillaries, arterioles, and venules, but this process may be assisted. Topical hemostatics are coagulants used on areas of capillary bleeding as an adjunct to natural hemostasis, and when natural coagulation factors are absent or insufficient, systemic coagulants are used to restore or enhance the coagulation process. Although systemic coagulants are usually administered in the medical setting, they may be given immediately preoperatively or intraoperatively.

Conversely, blood coagulation may also be undesirable. Systemic *anti*coagulants are used to prevent or delay the onset of the coagulation sequence during surgical procedures performed on blood vessels, for example. Heparin is one such systemic anticoagulant. It is routinely administered intravenously by the anesthesia care provider and topically from the sterile back table during peripheral and cardiovascular surgical procedures to prevent adverse clotting. Most other systemic anticoagulants are administered in the medical setting to prevent conditions such as deep vein thrombosis (DVT) or pulmonary embolism (PE), which can be postoperative complications. Patients on long-term anticoagulation require special consideration when undergoing an invasive surgical procedure because of their delayed coagulation time.

When a blood clot, or thrombus, forms within an intact blood vessel, a mechanism in the blood acts to dissolve the clot naturally. If the natural anticoagulation process is inadequate, thrombolytics may be administered to speed clot breakdown. Thrombolytics are agents used to help to speed the breakdown of existing blood clots, as seen in conditions such as DVT, PE, coronary artery thrombosis, and myocardial infarction (MI).

MAKE IT SIMPLE

Use medical terminology word-building skills to help you understand the terms *coagulation*, *anticoagulation*, and *hemostasis*. First, the word *coagulation* in medicine means the clotting of blood, and the prefix "anti-" means against. Thus coagulation means blood clotting, and anticoagulation signifies a substance that inhibits clotting. You will see more terms in this chapter with "anti-" as a prefix. *Hemostasis* can be broken down into *heme*, the Greek word for blood, and *stasis*, which means "to halt," so hemostasis means to halt or arrest the flow of blood.

QUICK QUESTION

What is the definition of the term *systemic*? For your answer, refer to Drug Administration Routes in Chapter 1.

PHYSIOLOGY OF CLOT FORMATION

The body's coagulation mechanism prevents blood loss because of trauma or damage to small blood vessels. (However, trauma to large blood vessels requires surgical intervention—thermal or mechanical hemostasis—to control blood loss.) Damage to a small blood vessel results in spasm and tissue damage, which causes a series of reactions. These reactions produce a protein called *fibrin*. Fibrin sticks to damaged blood vessels, which causes a platelet plug to form; this leads to coagulation. In fact, blood clot formation is a cascade of events occurring in three basic stages. See Fig. 9.1 for a simplified version of this clotting cascade.

Stage 1: Thromboplastin (also known as *prothrombin activator*) is formed.

Stage 2: Thromboplastin converts prothrombin (known as *factor II*) into thrombin.

Stage 3: Thrombin converts fibrinogen (known as *factor I*) to fibrin.

Fibrin is a mesh of protein threads—a net that traps blood cells to form a clot (Fig. 9.2).

Stage 1 involves two different mechanisms for the formation of thromboplastin—the extrinsic pathway and intrinsic pathway. These two meet at a specific point in the process called the *common pathway*. The *extrinsic* pathway is initiated by factors outside the blood. It is triggered by a clotting factor released from damaged tissue (i.e., tissue thromboplastin, or factor III). The extrinsic pathway is a very rapid process that produces a clot in seconds. Tissue thromboplastin (factor III) combines with antihemophilic factor (AHF) VIII and calcium to activate the Stuart-Prower factor. When activated, factor X reacts with proaccelerin (factor V) and calcium to form thromboplastin.

The *intrinsic* pathway is initiated by substances contained in the blood. This pathway is more complex and takes several minutes. When a blood vessel is damaged, the Hageman factor (factor XII) is activated. Factor XII then activates plasma thromboplastin antecedent (PTA; factor XI), which activates

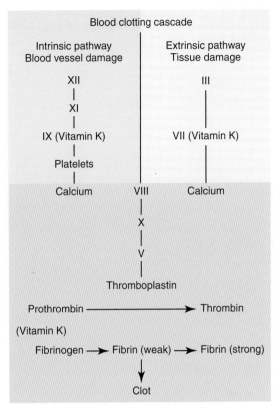

Fig. 9.1 Blood coagulation pathways.

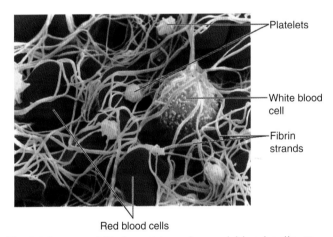

Fig. 9.2 Image of fibrin net trapping red blood cells. (From Waugh A, Grant A: *Ross and Wilson anatomy and physiology in health and illness*, ed 11, St Louis, 2010, Elsevier.)

plasma thromboplastin component (PTC; factor IX). Then as in the extrinsic pathway, activated factor IX combines with AHF and calcium to activate factor X, and factor X reacts with proaccelerin (factor V) and calcium to form thromboplastin. Note the intrinsic and extrinsic pathways come together at activated factor X.

The clotting cascade requires calcium at all stages (i.e., calcium enables many of the steps). Vitamin K also plays a vital role in coagulation. For example, it is required to synthesize prothrombin (factor II), proconvertin (factor VII), PTC (factor IX), and the Stuart-Prower factor. See Table 9.1 for a summary of blood coagulation factors and their pathways.

TABLE 9.1   Blood Coagulation Factors

Factor	Name	Function	Pathways
I	Fibrinogen	Converted to fibrin	Both
II	Prothrombin	Converted to thrombin	Both
III	Tissue factor thromboplastin	Triggers extrinsic pathway	Extrinsic
IV	Calcium	Essential in all three stages of clotting	Both
V	Proaccelerin	Accelerates conversion of prothrombin to thrombin	Both
VI		Factor VI is no longer believed to be involved in blood coagulation. Considered to be the same as factor V	
VII	Proconvertin	Essential for extrinsic pathway	Extrinsic
VIII	Antihemophilic factor	Accelerates activation of factor X	Intrinsic
IX	Plasma thromboplastin component (Christmas factor)	Essential for intrinsic pathway; accelerates activation of factor X	Intrinsic
X	Stuart-Prower factor	Essential for intrinsic and extrinsic pathways	Both
XI	Plasma thromboplastin antecedent	Essential for intrinsic pathway; accelerates activation of factor IX	Intrinsic
XII	Hageman factor	Essential for intrinsic pathway	Intrinsic
XIII	Fibrin-stabilizing factor	Strengthens fibrin clot	Both

Occasionally, clotting may take place within an unbroken blood vessel; this abnormal clotting is called *thrombosis*. If it forms in an artery, such a clot (thrombus) may cut off blood supply to an area. If a thrombus forms in a vein, it may inhibit return of blood to systemic circulation, or a venous clot may break off and become an embolus—traveling to the heart, brain, or lungs—causing severe complications, even death. Blood clots may dissolve naturally; the reason is that blood normally contains a clot-dissolving enzyme, fibrinolysin. If the body's natural declotting mechanism is inadequate, medical or surgical intervention may be required. For example, arterial embolectomy may be necessary when blood clots form in the femoral, popliteal, or tibial artery. If a blood clot forms in a vein, medical treatment may be sufficient. With bed rest and administration of a thrombolytic agent, such a clot may dissolve.

Coagulants

Coagulants are drugs that promote, accelerate, or make possible blood coagulation. There are two major categories of coagulants: hemostatics and systemic coagulants. Hemostatics are topical agents used almost exclusively in the surgical setting. Systemic coagulants are generally used in the medical setting.

Hemostatics

Hemostatics are agents that enhance or accelerate blood clotting at a surgical site. These agents serve as adjuncts to natural coagulation, which controls minor capillary bleeding. Thus traditional hemostatics are not effective against arterial or major venous bleeding. Hemostatic agents, such as QuikClot, have been developed to treat severe traumatic bleeding on the battlefield, in trauma situations by emergency responders, and by law enforcement. These agents are not intended for use in the routine surgical setting.

Hemostatics used in surgery are applied topically in the form of films, powders, sponges, or solutions. Several different types of hemostatic agents are available (Box 9.1), and each is supplied in sterile packaging for delivery to the sterile field.

BOX 9.1   Topical Hemostatics by Category

Absorbable Gelatin
FloSeal
Gelfilm
Gelfoam powder
Gelfoam sponge
Gelita-Spon
Surgiflo
Surgifoam

Microfibrillar Collagen Hemostat
Arista Absorbable Hemostat
Avitene Microfibrillar Collagen Hemostat (MCH)
Instat MCH

Oxidized Cellulose
Gelita-Cel
Oxycel
Surgicel
Surgicel Fibrillar
Surgicel Nu-Knit
Surgicel Structured Non-Woven material (SNoW)

Absorbable Collagen Sponge
Helistat
Helitene

Thrombin (see Table 9.4)
Miscellaneous Agents
Bone wax
Chemical hemostatics
Tannic acid
Silver nitrate
Monsel's solution

ABSORBABLE GELATIN

Absorbable gelatin hemostatics are animal in origin, made from purified porcine skin gelatin USP. Applied topically with pressure to bleeding sites, these agents are thought to be mechanical rather than chemical in their mode of action. Gelatin hemostatics are absorbed completely in 4 to 6 weeks, depending on such factors as the amount used and the surgical site. Gelatin hemostatics may be used dry or moistened with saline; however, they should not be used in the presence of infection, and they should never be placed intravascularly. Examples of gelatin hemostatics include Gelfilm, Gelfoam powder and sponges, Surgifoam, and Gelita-Spon. Dry Gelfilm has the consistency of stiff cellophane; moistened, it becomes pliable. As a pliable film, it can be cut into desired shapes and sizes. It is approved for use in neurosurgery and thoracic and ocular surgery. Gelfoam powder can be made into a paste by mixing with saline. The powder form promotes granulation tissue, so it may be used on areas of skin ulceration. Gelfoam sponges are also available. They come in several sizes (Table 9.2) for various applications and may be cut into desired shapes, as shown in Fig. 9.3. Gelfoam is commonly used in orthopedic, general, otolaryngology, neurosurgical, and dental procedures. An example is Gelfoam used in otologic surgery, such as tympanoplasty. It is cut into tiny pieces called *pledgets*, which may be used to pack the area around a tympanic graft or to apply a very small amount of epinephrine (topically) on bleeding surfaces inside the middle ear (see Chapter 4).

Gelfoam is also available in a kit, combined with human thrombin, sterile saline, and a 10-mL syringe with needle, marketed as Gelfoam Plus. A Gelfoam sponge contained in the kit is moistened with a thrombin solution containing 125 units/mL and applied to a bleeding surface.

Gelita-Spon sponge induces hemostasis through its porous structure and absorbs more than 40 times its weight in blood and fluids. As the sponge fills with blood, it helps stop bleeding by forming a clot and induces platelet aggregation (clumping together) through surface contact. It is absorbed by the body in less than 4 weeks.

Absorbable gelatin is also available in "flowable" form, which conforms to uneven bleeding surfaces. It enables clot formation by providing a matrix for blood platelets to adhere and aggregate, which initiates the body's natural hemostatic cascade. Flowable gelatins include Floseal and Surgiflo. Floseal Hemostatic Matrix is a combination of gelatin granules (the gelatin matrix) and topical human thrombin. These are contained

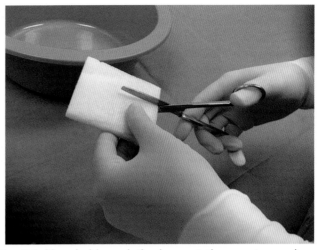

Fig. 9.3 Absorbable gelatin hemostatic agents, such as Gelfoam sponge, may be cut into desired shapes and sizes. (Gelfoam Copyright Pfizer Inc. All rights reserved. Gelfoam is a registered trademark of Pharmacia & Upjohn Company LLC, and indirectly wholly owned subsidiary of Pfizer Inc.)

in a kit that includes a syringe of injectable 0.9% sodium chloride used to reconstitute the vial of thrombin. Also included are a bowl and adapters to assist in mixing the thrombin and gelatin matrix, which is labeled and passed to the surgeon. Once mixed, Floseal should be used within 4 hours. Go to www.floseal.com, and select *Instructions for Use* to view a video on its preparation. Surgiflo Hemostatic Matrix is supplied in a prefilled syringe to be mixed with saline or thrombin. It absorbs within approximately 4 to 6 weeks with little tissue reaction. Both Floseal and Surgiflo kits contain a needle-free vial adapter to assist in eliminating needle sticks during preparation.

> **! CAUTION**
>
> Consult package inserts for detailed information and directions for the appropriate preparation and use of flowable gelatins. The scrubbed surgical technologist must become familiar with each new hemostatic product developed, so that it can be properly prepared for use.

ABSORBABLE COLLAGEN SPONGE

Absorbable collagen sponges are made from purified bovine collagen. The sponge is cut to a desired shape and applied with pressure to a bleeding site. When applied to bleeding surfaces, the sponge promotes platelet aggregation. Collagen may reduce the bonding strength of methyl methacrylate (bone cement), so it should not be applied to bone before placement of a prosthesis requiring cement fixation. Some collagens are not used in genitourinary or ophthalmic procedures. Examples of absorbable collagen sponges are Helistat and Helitene.

MICROFIBRILLAR COLLAGEN HEMOSTAT

Avitene Microfibrillar Collagen Hemostat (MCH) is a dry, fibrous preparation of purified bovine corium collagen (Fig. 9.4).

TABLE 9.2	Gelfoam Sponge Sizes
Manufacturer's Code	**Actual Size**
4ᵃ	2 cm × 2 cm
12.7	2 cm × 6 cm (12 cm²)
50	8 cm × 6.25 cm (50 cm²)
100	8 cm × 12.5 cm (100 cm²)
200	8 cm × 25 cm (200 cm²)

ᵃSize 4 is used in dental procedures.

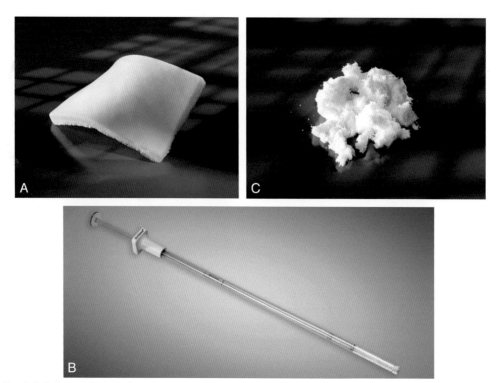

Fig. 9.4 Avitene Microfibrillar Collagen Hemostat is a microfibrillar collagen hemostatic agent, which comes in various forms. (A) Avitene ultrafoam; (B) Endo-Avitene; (C) Avitene flour. (Copyright © 2019 BD. All rights reserved. Used with the permission of BD.)

Direct application to bleeding surfaces attracts platelets to the substance, thus triggering further platelet aggregation, leading to formation of a fibrin clot. Avitene should be applied with dry instruments only because it will adhere to wet surfaces. Wetting also decreases its hemostatic efficiency. In addition, contact with nonbleeding surfaces must be avoided because adhesions may result. Excess Avitene should be removed by irrigation within a few minutes. Avitene is available in powder form (called "*flour*") in amounts of 0.5, 1, and 5 g, in preloaded 1-g syringes (called *Syringe-Avitene*), in sheets that can be cut to desired size and shape, and in a sponge (called *Avitene Ultrafoam*). Avitene is also packaged in delivery devices for endoscopic (Endo-Avitene) and specialty applications.

Instat MCH is derived from bovine deep flexor tendon, a source of pure collagen. The microfibrillar form allows the surgeon to grasp only the amount needed with a forceps, and it can be applied to irregularly shaped bleeding surfaces. Instat causes platelet aggregation, resulting in a clot formation. Onset of action is 2 to 4 minutes. Instat MCH is absorbable, but removal is recommended. It is available in 0.5- and 1-g containers.

Arista Absorbable Hemostat is a plant-based, absorbable powder derived from purified plant starch. It contains microporous polysaccharide hemospheres. These spheres act as a molecular sieve for blood clotting when mechanical methods are not effective or practical. Arista contains no thrombin and is typically absorbed by the body in 24 to 48 hours. It comes in the form of a fine, dry white powder in its own applicator. Excess blood or fluids (including any irrigation) should be removed from the bleeding tissue before Arista is applied. Once hemostasis is achieved,

excess Arista should be removed by irrigation. It should not be used in neurosurgical or ophthalmic procedures.

OXIDIZED CELLULOSE

The hemostatic action of oxidized cellulose is not clearly understood. When applied to bleeding surfaces, oxidized cellulose swells, becoming a gelatinous mass that serves as a nucleus for clotting. Oxidized regenerated cellulose (ORC) is the newer version, manufactured by dissolving cellulose and extruding it as a continuous fiber. ORC is absorbable, but removal is recommended after hemostasis is achieved. It is available in knitted gauze strips or fiber form and is best applied when dry. The fiber form can be grasped with dry tissue forceps in the specific amount needed. The gauze form may be cut to desired shape and size. ORC is commonly used in neurosurgery and otolaryngology. Examples of ORC include Surgicel gauze, Surgicel Nu-Knit (a knitted fabric), Surgicel Fibrillar, and Surgicel Structured Non-Woven material (SNoW), all available in multiple sizes (Table 9.3). Surgicel absorbable hemostat is also bactericidal and effective against a wide range of gram-positive and gram-negative microorganisms. ORC has a low pH and should not be used with any agent containing bovine or human thrombin.

Gelita-Cel is made of 100% organic, oxidized cellulose extracted from cotton. It adapts to the wound surface and turns into a gelatinous mass, which acts as a nucleus for clotting. This provides a strong matrix for platelet adhesion and aggregation. Gelita-Cel is absorbed by the body in less than 4 weeks.

TABLE 9.3	Surgicel, Surgicel Nu-Knit, and Surgicel Fibrillar Sizes		
Surgicel (in inches)	Surgicel Nu-Knit (in inches)	Surgicel Fibrillar (in inches)	Surgicel SNoW (in inches)
0.5 × 2		1 × 2	1 × 1
2 × 3		2 × 4	2 × 4
2 × 14	3 × 4	4 × 4	4 × 4
4 × 8	6 × 9		

SNoW, Structured Non-Woven material.

THROMBIN

In the body, thrombin is an enzyme that assists in the conversion of fibrinogen to fibrin in the blood-clotting cascade. As a medication, it comes as a topical liquid hemostatic agent that was initially of bovine origin (Thrombin-JMI). Some patients developed antibodies against bovine thrombin, which resulted in a US Food and Drug Administration (FDA) "boxed" warning (formerly known as "black box" warnings). Because of this, human-derived thrombin (2007) and recombinant human thrombin (2008) were developed. Thrombin may come prepared in a spray bottle kit or in a powder form that must be reconstituted with sterile water or saline. Thrombin should be used immediately after preparation, or it should be refrigerated and used immediately after reconstituting. As previously stated, thrombin works by catalyzing the conversion of fibrinogen to fibrin, thus increasing the speed of the natural clotting mechanism. Thrombin may be applied topically in solution, as a powder, or in combination with a gelatin sponge. Thrombi-Gel is a combination of bovine thrombin and calcium chloride freeze-dried into a gelatin sponge, also available in a nonwoven gauze form (Thrombi-Pad).

> ### ! CAUTION
> Thrombin must *never* be introduced into large blood vessels because significant intravascular clotting and death may result. In addition, to avoid inadvertent injection, thrombin should *never* be kept on the sterile back table in a syringe.

Thrombin is measured in units rather than milligrams and comes in strengths, depending upon the type used, from 800 to 20,000 units for different applications. The speed of thrombin's clotting action depends on the concentration used (e.g., 100 units/mL—1000 units of thrombin with 10 mL of diluent). Concentrations as high as 2000 units/mL may be used if needed. Areas of profuse bleeding, as in liver trauma, may require the highest concentration of thrombin.

Thrombin derived from humans is available as topical human thrombin (Evithrom) from human plasma and the first recombinant form, topical recombinant thrombin (Recothrom). Topical human thrombin (Evithrom) comes in a frozen solution that must be thawed before topical administration. It is available in vials of 2, 5, or 20 mL containing 800 to 1200 units/mL of human thrombin and is approved for use in combination with gelatin sponges. Recothrom is supplied in 5000- and 20,000-unit vials of powder, which must be reconstituted with sterile saline to make a solution of 1000 units of thrombin per milliliter. It is approved for use with gelatin sponges. It is contraindicated for use in patients with known hypersensitivity to hamster or snake proteins.

In addition, thrombin is used in combination with other agents to form fibrin sealants. Fibrin sealant (Tisseel) contains human thrombin, human fibrinogen, and a synthetic fibrinolysis inhibitor. It is available in a freeze-dried kit that requires reconstituting before use and also in a frozen prefilled syringe that requires thawing before administration. Both forms are supplied in 2-, 4-, and 10-mL volume sizes. Fibrin sealant (Evicel) is supplied in a kit of two syringes containing human fibrinogen (BAC2) and human thrombin in frozen solutions. These agents must be thawed before use. A spray applicator is included in the kit, and it is available in 2-, 4-, and 10-mL total volumes with syringes containing equal volumes of fibrinogen and thrombin.

Thrombin (freeze-dried) is also mixed with a flowable gelatin matrix to form a paste and used as a topical hemostatic agent (Surgiflo, Floseal) in surgical procedures, other than ophthalmics. These agents are absorbable, and each comes in a kit containing prefilled syringes of the gelatin matrix: 2000 International Units (IU) of topical thrombin (human) in Surgiflo, 500 units/mL in Floseal; and other mixing supplies to prepare the mixtures for application. See Table 9.4 for a list of hemostatics containing thrombin.

Tissue sealants are agents related to fibrin sealants but are used for different purposes (Insight 9.1).

> ### ? QUICK QUESTION
> One form of thrombin must be reconstituted. How would this be done? Refer to Drug Forms and Preparations in Chapter 1 for the answer.

MISCELLANEOUS AGENTS USED AS HEMOSTATICS

Bone Wax

Bone wax is a topical hemostatic agent made from beeswax. It comes packaged for sterile delivery in a foil-type wrapper inside a peel-back package (Fig. 9.5). Bone wax is used primarily in orthopedics and neurosurgery to control bleeding on bone

TABLE 9.4   Hemostatic Agents Containing Topical Thrombin

Generic Name	Brand Name
thrombin, topical (bovine)	Thrombin-JMI
thrombin (bovine) gelatin sponge	Thrombi-Gel
thrombin (bovine) nonwoven gauze	Thrombi-Pad
thrombin, topical (human)	Evithrom
thrombin, topical (recombinant)	Recothrom
fibrin sealant	Tisseel, Evicel
thrombin, topical (human) and gelatin matrix	FloSeal, Surgiflo

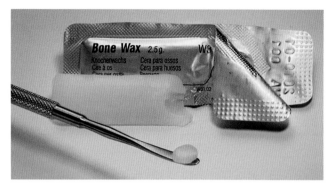

Fig. 9.5 Bone wax comes packaged for sterile delivery in a foil-type wrapper inside a peel-back package. It may be applied in small amounts to bone with an elevator, such as a freer. (Courtesy Frank Pronesti T/A heirloomstudio.com.)

INSIGHT 9.1   Tissue Sealants and Biologics Prepared From the Back Table

Tissue sealants are sometimes confused with the hemostatic purpose of fibrin sealants. Tissue sealants are most often used to seal the small perforations left after suturing a tissue layer, such as a blood vessel or the dura. Tissue sealants can be from a natural source or a synthetic source. BioGlue is a natural protein-binding agent made from purified bovine serum albumin and glutaraldehyde. It is supplied in a dual-chambered syringe with a special applicator tip in volumes of 2, 5, and 10 mL. It may be used in cardiovascular surgery.

Synthetic tissue sealants include CoSeal and DuraSeal, hydrogels made from polyethylene glycol. CoSeal may be used in vascular surgery. It swells up to 4 times its volume in 24 hours and is available in dual-syringe kits in volumes of 2, 4, and 8 mL. DuraSeal is used as an adjunct to closure of the dura. It is also supplied in a dual-syringe system. It is unique in that it is colored blue for easy identification during application.

Dermabond is a synthetic agent, cyanoacrylate, used to close small skin incisions, such as those used for laparoscopic cholecystectomy. It comes in a handheld sterile applicator.

In addition, there are many biologics that are prepared on the sterile back table that include bone morphogenic protein, bone graft substitutes, autologous platelet systems for platelet-rich plasma therapy, and pleural air leak sealants. These products come in kits with syringes, dual syringes, and/or mixing supplies that require preparation by the surgical technologist before use. Some require reconstituting, as discussed in Chapter 1. An example is an orthobiologic implant (Restore) derived from porcine small intestine submucosa that has been processed, disinfected, and sterilized. It is designed as a tissue scaffold that is reabsorbable by the body. The implant helps to reinforce weakened or damaged soft tissue and is a less invasive alternative to allograft. Examples of surgical procedures that may use an orthobiologic implant are rotator cuff repair and Achilles tendon repair. The implant must be kept refrigerated until needed and then soaked for 7 to 10 minutes (or reconstituted) in sterile saline/buffer or water before use.

It is easy to get so many different agents confused, so the surgical technologist must stay current with the introduction of new products in surgery, their purposes, uses, and unique preparation directions on the sterile field.

when kept outside the foil package for extended periods of time. There have been reports of complications, including chronic inflammation and granuloma formation, attributed to the use of bone wax.

TECH TIP

To keep bone wax softened and ready for use by the surgeon, the scrubbed surgical technologist can break off small pieces of wax, roll each into a small, rounded shape, and place in between and at the base of two (gloved) fingers of the nondominant hand. This helps to keep the bone wax warm and pliable yet should not interfere with handling instruments and supplies.

Chemical Hemostatics

Some hemostatic agents, such as tannic acid and silver nitrate, chemically cauterize bleeding surfaces. Tannic acid is a powder made from an astringent plant. Applied topically to mucous membranes, it helps to stop capillary bleeding. Tannic acid may be used after tonsillectomy in combination with other agents, such as 1% Neo-Synephrine (phenylephrine, a vasoconstrictor). Another example is mixing tannic acid with a combination of agents (which include glycerin, propylene glycol, Zephiran [benzalkonium] chloride, ephedrine sulfate, and phenylephrine solution) to form Simiele solution. A tonsil sponge is saturated with the tannic acid and Neo-Synephrine mixture or the Simiele solution and applied to the tonsillar fossa to control minor bleeding.

Silver nitrate is another cauterizing agent, especially when mixed with potassium nitrate. This combination is molded onto applicator sticks (which come in 6- and 12-inch lengths) and is used to cauterize wounds. It can also remove granulation tissue or warts. Silver nitrate sticks also come in 18-inch lengths for use with a sigmoidoscope. The applicator tips are moistened with water and applied to the desired area for treatment. Silver nitrate has a caustic effect and should not be used around eyes. It may also discolor the treatment site with repeated application.

Another chemical hemostatic agent is Monsel's solution, a deep brown mixture of ferrous sulfate, sulfuric acid, and nitric acid diluted with water or available as a paste. Monsel's solution

surfaces. It acts as a mechanical barrier rather than as a matrix for clotting. Bone wax is a pliable, opaque, waxy substance that can be separated and shaped to different sizes (usually small spheres). It is sparingly applied directly onto bone with the gloved finger or on an elevator, such as a freer. It may harden

may be applied to the bleeding surface remaining after a cervical cone biopsy.

> **! CAUTION**
>
> Monsel's solution may be easily confused with another brown-colored solution on the back table for cervical cone biopsy, Lugol's solution (see Chapter 6). Lugol's solution is a mild iodine solution used to stain the cervix to reveal the area of dysplasia for biopsy. If Monsel's solution is applied to the cervix instead of Lugol's solution, the biopsy area may be damaged by the cauterization effects of the acids. The scrub and circulator must verify both solutions during delivery to the back table, the containers must be labeled immediately, and the name of the agent called out as it is handed to the surgeon to avoid this dangerous medication error.

Systemic Coagulants

Systemic coagulants are agents that replenish deficiencies in the natural clotting mechanism. If needed, systemic coagulants are usually administered preoperatively. Occasionally, the anesthesia care provider may administer a systemic coagulant intraoperatively. Systemic coagulants may be used to replace calcium, vitamin K, or some of the coagulation factors in the blood. Such deficiencies in coagulation substances may be because of heredity, such as in hemophilia, or they may be acquired, such as a vitamin K deficiency. Systemic coagulants may be administered intravenously, intramuscularly, orally, or subcutaneously, depending on the medication used. See Box 9.2 for a summary of systemic coagulants.

CALCIUM SALTS

Calcium, which is the body's most common mineral, is critical for numerous body functions, including blood coagulation. If calcium levels fall during surgery, natural coagulation becomes less efficient, so calcium salts may be administered intravenously to assist the mechanism. For example, during transfusions, anesthesia care providers must monitor blood calcium levels very closely because the processing of donated blood tends to strip it of calcium. Typically, an injection of a 10% solution of calcium chloride ($CaCl_2$) is used to restore calcium levels intraoperatively. Calcium may also be given preoperatively. In the medical setting, calcium may be given by mouth in tablet form (Citracal) or injected intramuscularly.

> **! CAUTION**
>
> Calcium salts are not given to patients with a history of malignant hyperthermia (MH). Why? Because one aspect of MH is increased calcium release from muscle cells (see Chapter 15).

VITAMIN K

Vitamin K is a fat-soluble vitamin; it promotes blood clotting by increasing synthesis of coagulation factors. Recall that vitamin K is necessary to synthesize prothrombin (factor II), proconvertin (factor VII), PTC (factor IX), and the Stuart-Prower factor (X). In the surgical patient, a deficiency in vitamin K can lead to excessive bleeding. Decreased vitamin K levels are seen in patients on oral anticoagulants, such as coumarin derivatives. Some antibacterial therapies also cause vitamin K deficiency. If needed, vitamin K may be administered orally or by subcutaneous injection preoperatively, but it takes up to 24 hours to produce an acceptable effect. When surgery is needed urgently, vitamin K may be given intravenously, but there is an increased risk of anaphylaxis and it takes approximately 6 hours to produce an acceptable effect. When emergency surgery is necessary and cannot be delayed for vitamin K, 10 to 15 mL/kg of patient's weight of fresh frozen plasma may be administered for immediate hemostasis (4–6 units in a 70-kg adult).

Vitamin K is also used in the medical setting to counteract anticoagulant-induced prothrombin deficiency. It does not directly counteract oral anticoagulants but stimulates prothrombin formation by the liver. Vitamin K will not counteract the action of heparin. Administration of vitamin K intravenously has resulted in severe anaphylactic reactions; therefore, it is given intravenously only when other routes are not feasible and when the risks have been recognized and considered. Vitamin K is available as phytonadione (Mephyton Oral) for oral administration or as phytonadione (Vitamin K) for injection.

BLOOD COAGULATION FACTORS

Deficiency of any clotting factor interferes with effective coagulation. Two blood factors administered intravenously in the medical setting are AHF, known as *factor VIII*, and factor IX complex. Factor VIII, a plasma protein essential for conversion of prothrombin to thrombin, is prepared from human blood plasma. This factor is absent in patients with hemophilia A and must be administered intravenously, as needed, before an operative procedure. AHF is available as Hemofil-M, Koate-DVI, and many others. Factor IX complex is a concentrate of dried plasma fractions—mainly coagulation factors II, VII, IX, and X. Factor IX complex may be administered preoperatively, as needed, in patients with hemophilia B. It is also used in the medical setting to reverse coumarin-induced hemorrhage. Factor IX complex is available as Profilnine SD, Proplex T, AlpaNine SD, and many others.

BOX 9.2 Systemic Coagulants

Calcium Salt	Blood Coagulation Factors
Calcium chloride	*Antihemophilic Factor (VIII)*
Citracal	Hemofil-M
	Koate-DVI
Vitamin K	
Mephyton	*Factor IX Complex*
	AlpaNine SD
	Profilnine SD
	Proplex T

ANTICOAGULANTS

Anticoagulants are drugs that prevent or interfere with blood coagulation; they do not dissolve clots that are already formed. Anticoagulants are administered in the medical setting to prevent venous thrombosis, especially those in the lower extremities called DVT (refer to the section on advanced practices of this chapter for more information). Anticoagulants are also used to prevent PE, acute coronary occlusions after MI, and strokes caused by an embolus or cerebral blood clot. Anticoagulants do not dissolve existing clots; rather, they help to prevent new clots from forming. A surgical patient who has a history of arterial stasis or who must be immobilized for a prolonged period of time after surgery may be placed on prophylactic anticoagulant therapy. Anticoagulants are used in surgery to help prevent clot formation as a response to trauma or manipulation of blood vessels. Patients receiving anticoagulants are carefully monitored for signs of hemorrhage, a common side effect. Minor hemorrhage may be evident as bruising, nosebleed (epistaxis), blood in urine (hematuria), or bloody stools (melena).

Parenteral Anticoagulants

Parenteral anticoagulants are drugs administered intravenously, subcutaneously, or topically that interfere with blood clotting. Heparin sodium is the most common parenteral anticoagulant, and it is used in both medical and surgical settings. It is a highly negatively charged sugar molecule derived from porcine intestinal mucosa. Heparin acts by binding to antithrombin III (AT III, a protein), which greatly increases AT III's ability to inhibit the action of coagulation factors thrombin, Xa, and IXa. Binding with AT III enables heparin to work at several points in the clotting cascade by inhibiting factor X, interfering with the conversion of prothrombin to thrombin, and by inactivating thrombin, thus preventing conversion of fibrinogen to fibrin. Heparin also interferes with platelet aggregation and the formation of a stable fibrin clot. Heparin binds nonspecifically to plasma proteins, which may account for the variation of effects among patients. It is metabolized in the liver by heparinase. Heparin does not cross the placental barrier; however, there are no adequate studies on its use in pregnant women. Thus heparin used during pregnancy should be considered only if the potential benefit justifies the potential risk to the fetus.

Heparin is measured in units rather than milligrams and is available in doses of 10 to 40,000 units/mL for injection (see Caution), and in parenteral form only because it is poorly absorbed through the gastrointestinal tract. Heparin injection is available in 1-mL, single-dose vials and in premixed forms. See Table 9.5 for strengths. Hep-Lock catheter flush heparin is supplied in 10 and 100 units/mL. Onset of action is rapid, usually within 5 minutes, with duration of 2 to 4 hours. Adverse reactions include increased risk of hemorrhage and thrombocytopenia (decrease in platelets), so heparin is contraindicated in patients with existing severe thrombocytopenia. Coagulation studies (Insight 9.2) are used to monitor heparin's therapeutic action.

❓ QUICK QUESTION

Can you name two routes of administration for heparin as it is given in parenteral form only? Refer to Drug Administration Routes in Chapter 1 for the answer.

TABLE 9.5 Heparin Strengths

Strength	Volume (mL)
Single-Use Vials	
Heparin Injection	
1000 units/mL	1
5000 units/mL	1
10,000 units/mL	1
20,000 units/mL	1
Multidose Vials	
Heparin Injection	
10,000 units	10
30,000 units	30
50,000 units	10
40,000 units	4
Hep-Lock Flush	
10 units/mL	1
100 units/mL	1
Premixed Heparin Strengths	
1000 units	500
2000 units	1000
12,500 units	250
25,000 units	250
25,000 units	500

INSIGHT 9.2 Blood Coagulation Studies

Two laboratory tests are routinely used to assess blood coagulation. Prothrombin time (PT) is an evaluation of the extrinsic and common coagulation system. PT is used to monitor anticoagulant therapy by vitamin K antagonists, such as warfarin. PT screens for adequate amounts of factors I, II, VII, and X. Partial thromboplastin time (PTT) and activated partial thromboplastin time (aPTT) evaluate the intrinsic and common coagulation pathways. PTT is used to monitor heparin therapy. PTT screens for deficiencies of all coagulation factors except VII and XIII. Previously, results of PT varied by the method used and so were reported with the appropriate reference range. The reporting of PT results has been standardized with the use of the international normalized ratio (INR). The INR is the PT ratio obtained with the World Health Organization's reference preparation as the source of thromboplastin.

If a high risk of PE or DVT exists, heparin may be administered preoperatively by subcutaneous injection at least 1 hour before a surgical procedure. Interestingly, orthopedic procedures are known to be associated with a higher risk of DVT and PE than other categories of major surgical procedures.

Heparin is the primary anticoagulant used intraoperatively, most commonly in peripheral and cardiovascular procedures. For example, it is administered intravenously by the anesthesia care provider, 3 minutes before placement of an arterial occluding clamp. Three minutes is usually sufficient to allow systemic distribution of heparin, helping to prevent the formation of blood clots caused by arterial stasis and vessel manipulation. It may be of historical interest to note that some older types of vascular graft materials had to be preclotted before insertion to minimize blood loss. Preclotting a graft required saturation with the patient's blood, which had to be withdrawn *before* systemic heparinization to be effective.

According to the FDA, "Serious injuries and deaths have been associated with the use of heparin, a blood-thinning drug that contained active pharmaceutical ingredient from China. The adverse events have included allergic or hypersensitivity-type reactions, with symptoms, such as low blood pressure, angioedema, shortness of breath, nausea, vomiting, diarrhea, and abdominal pain. In February 2008 Baxter Healthcare Corporation recalled multidose and single-dose vials of heparin sodium for injection, as well as Hep-Lock heparin flush products. After launching a far-ranging investigation, FDA scientists identified a previously unknown contaminant in the heparin." This resulted in a change to the US Pharmacopeia (USP) monograph for heparin, effective October 1, 2009. This action now requires that all manufactured heparin undergo testing to detect impurities. It also reconciles the USP unit dose with the World Health Organization International Standard unit dose, which will result approximately in a 10% reduction in the potency of the heparin marketed in the United States. This change may affect the surgical use of heparin in vascular procedures because it is administered as a bolus intravenous dose, and an immediate anticoagulant effect is necessary. Dosage adjustments may be made to accommodate the change.

Heparin is also frequently used from the sterile back table during peripheral and cardiovascular procedures. A dilute solution, such as 5000 units of heparin in 1000 mL of normal saline, is commonly used in topical arterial irrigation.

! CAUTION

Careful attention must be paid to identifying the correct strength of heparin administered because 1 mL of heparin can contain 10, 100, 1000, 5000, or 10,000 units. Remember that the dose of drug administered is the strength *times* the volume. It is possible to administer the same volume of heparin yet give a dose 1000 times more than ordered. The circulator and scrub must always read aloud and verify the number of *units* of heparin placed in solution for irrigation, as well as the volume. The container must be carefully labeled, and the scrub must repeat the solution strength to the surgeon when passing it (Insight 9.3).

INSIGHT 9.3   **Heparin Tragedy**

In November 2007 at Cedars-Sinai Hospital in Los Angeles, infant twins were given doses of heparin that were 1000 times stronger than intended. Instead of the prescribed 10 units/mL dose of the Hep-Lock to flush out their IVs, they were given adult doses of 10,000 units/mL. They had internal and external bleeding until it was stopped with protamine sulfate. The twins survived, but similar incidents had occurred a year earlier at another hospital, which resulted in the deaths of three infants.

The twins were the babies of actor Dennis Quaid, who then led a campaign for safer medication practices and sued the drug company. Since that time, heparin labels have changed. They must now clearly state the strength of the entire container, as well as how much of the drug is in 1 mL. This is intended to eliminate the need for healthcare providers to calculate the total amount of heparin of more than 1 mL. Implementation date for the change was May 1, 2013. In addition, the labels are color coded to reflect the different strengths, key information on the label is enlarged, and the medication container caps are color coded to match the labels. Refer to the heparin bottle in Fig. 2.4.

✎ TECH TIP

If more than one strength of heparin is to be used from the sterile back table, use a different type/size container for the different strengths of heparin. This will assist you in differentiating the medications (Fig. 9.6).

Heparin may be used from the sterile back table in many types of vascular procedures. During a femoral embolectomy, heparin is administered directly into the affected artery (intraarterial) through an arterial irrigating catheter to clear the artery of remaining clot or embolic debris. In cardiovascular procedures requiring extracorporeal circulation, heparin is administered

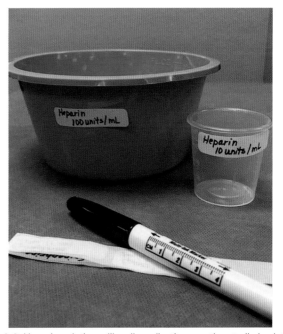

Fig. 9.6 Heparin solutions, like all medications on the sterile back table, must be labeled and their strengths clearly identified.

through the cardiopulmonary bypass pump to prevent coagulation of blood in the pump tubing. Heparin in various strengths is also used during placement of a venous access port or catheter. This is considered an intravenous administration of heparin because ports and catheters distribute medication directly into a vein. Again, proper identification—and careful labeling—of different strengths of heparin on the back table is mandatory. For example, a port or catheter may be flushed before insertion with a mild heparin solution, such as 10 units/mL; then when it is in position, it may be flushed with a solution of 100 units/mL. The scrubbed surgical technologist is responsible for passing the correct heparin solution at the correct time. It is imperative that the scrubbed surgical technologist call out the strength of heparin when passing it to the surgeon.

The antagonist (counteractive agent) for heparin is protamine sulfate, a parenteral anticoagulant that binds with and inactivates heparin. Protamine is a highly positively charged protein, isolated from salmon. Recall that heparin is a highly negatively charged molecule. By binding to heparin, protamine interferes with heparin's ability to bind to AT III and exert its effects to inhibit clotting. Protamine may be used to treat a heparin overdose or to reverse heparin-induced anticoagulation. Protamine is administered by slow intravenous injection. In surgery, protamine may be administered by the anesthesia care provider before wound closure if anticoagulation is still evident. If it is necessary to reverse heparin after cardiopulmonary bypass, 1 mg of protamine may be administered for every 100 units of heparin that was given, depending on the time interval when heparin was administered.

> **NOTE:** Protamine sulfate is also an anticoagulant when used alone. However, when given with heparin, protamine sulfate inhibits heparin's anticoagulant action.

LOW-MOLECULAR-WEIGHT HEPARINS

Unfractionated heparin was the first line of treatment for many years, but it has been replaced in many situations by low-molecular-weight heparins (LMWHs). These smaller molecules are used for the same purposes as regular heparin, such as preventing or treating DVT and PE. Like traditional heparin, LMWHs bind to AT III and increase its activity, but LMWHs have a lower affinity for plasma protein binding, so there is less variability among patients. LMWHs can be used outside the hospital setting because patients and their caregivers can be taught to administer the drug subcutaneously. Unlike unfractionated heparin, some LMWHs cannot be reversed reliably with protamine. LMWHs include dalteparin sodium (Fragmin) and enoxaparin sodium (Lovenox).

Enoxaparin is an LMWH used to prevent postoperative DVT after abdominal surgery and hip and knee replacement. Derived from porcine intestinal mucosa, enoxaparin is administered by subcutaneous injection. A preparation of the drug can be sent home with the patient, avoiding prolonged hospitalization for anticoagulant therapy. Enoxaparin is contraindicated in patients with active major bleeding or those with hypersensitivity to

heparin or pork products. It should not be given in combination with other anticoagulants, including aspirin. Side effects include local irritation, pain at the injection site, fever, and nausea. Rare adverse effects include hemorrhagic complications and thrombocytopenia. When necessary, enoxaparin may be *partially* reversed by protamine (1 mg protamine slowly intravenously for 1 mg of enoxaparin, depending on the time interval when enoxaparin was administered).

> **! CAUTION**
>
> LMWH and factor Xa inhibitor contain an FDA "boxed" warning regarding epidural or spinal hematomas: "Epidural or spinal hematomas may occur in patients who are anticoagulated with LMWH, heparinoids, or fondaparinux sodium and are receiving neuraxial anesthesia or undergoing spinal puncture. These hematomas may result in long-term or permanent paralysis."

FACTOR XA INHIBITOR

Fondaparinux sodium (Arixtra) is a factor Xa inhibitor used for postoperative and long-term prophylaxis of DVT and PE in orthopedic fracture, total joint, and abdominal surgery patients. It is a synthetic chemical, identical in structure to the part of the heparin molecule that binds with AT III. Fondaparinux sodium selectively affects only factor Xa, without directly affecting thrombin. It is administered subcutaneously *only*, no earlier than 6 to 8 hours after surgery once daily in a dose of 2.5 mg/day for 5 to 9 days. There is no reversal agent for fondaparinux. Factor Xa inhibitors that are taken orally include rivaroxaban (Xarelto) and apixaban (Eliquis).

> **! CAUTION**
>
> Do not confuse the medications Arista and Arixtra. The brand names are similar, yet they are very different agents. Arista is a topical hemostatic agent, and Arixtra is an anticoagulant.

Oral Anticoagulants

Oral anticoagulants have a delayed onset of action and should not be used in emergency situations. They are used for long-term medical management of thromboembolic disease, such as DVT or PE. Oral anticoagulant therapy is also used to prevent blood clots associated with cerebrovascular thromboembolic disease. Warfarin sodium, a coumarin derivative, is a widely prescribed oral anticoagulant. Coumarin derivatives act by inhibiting vitamin K activity in the liver, thereby preventing formation of coagulation factors II, VII, IX, and X. Warfarin, which is highly bound to plasma proteins (see Chapter 1), is metabolized in the liver and excreted in the urine. The onset of action of warfarin is prolonged, usually more than 2 days, and its duration is 2.5 to 5 days after discontinuation. The effectiveness of warfarin therapy is assessed by measuring prothrombin time, which should be approximately twice normal. (Refer to the section on advanced practices in this chapter for more information.) More food, drug, and herbal interactions are associated with warfarin than with any other drug, so all other medications must be closely monitored. Herbal supplements must be closely monitored as well. Some common side effects include hemorrhagic episodes, such as epistaxis, hematuria, and bleeding gums. The antidote for excessive warfarin anticoagulation is vitamin K, but it takes 48 to 72 hours to be effective.

Oral anticoagulant therapy poses a particular problem when a patient requires surgical intervention. In select cases warfarin may be temporarily discontinued approximately 1 week before an elective surgical procedure, but patients receiving oral anticoagulants who require emergency surgery exhibit prolonged bleeding times. As discussed previously, fresh frozen plasma may be administered to infuse coagulation factors in emergency situations. Meticulous hemostasis is also necessary to minimize blood loss in patients on oral anticoagulant therapy.

Aspirin, also called *acetylsalicylic acid* or *ASA*, is an antiplatelet drug that is considered an oral anticoagulant; it prevents clot formation by inhibiting platelet aggregation. Aspirin may be given after MI or recurrent transient ischemic attacks to reduce risk of further incidence. The administration of just 300 mg of aspirin can double normal bleeding time for up to 7 days. Thus if possible, patients receiving aspirin therapy should discontinue use at least 1 week before elective surgery. An example of aspirin is Bayer.

In addition to aspirin, there are many other antiplatelet drugs; among these are dipyridamole (Persantine) and clopidogrel (Plavix). These drugs have similar effects and uses as aspirin. It has been stated that clopidogrel, when taken with aspirin, is shown to be more effective in inhibiting platelet aggregation. Refer to the section on advanced practices in this chapter for more information.

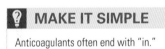

MAKE IT SIMPLE

Anticoagulants often end with "in."

Thrombolytics

Thrombolytics (Table 9.6) are agents given intravenously in the medical setting to help dissolve blood clots. These drugs activate plasminogen to form plasmin, which digests fibrin. When fibrin breaks down, the clot dissolves. Thrombolytics are used to treat acute MI when coronary artery thrombosis is present. Anticoagulant therapy may be used in conjunction with

thrombolytic agents because clot formation is an ongoing process. The major side effect of thrombolytics is significant hemorrhage, so patients are closely monitored. Mild side effects include skin rash, itching, nausea, and headache.

Two second-generation thrombolytics are alteplase tissue-type plasminogen activator (tPA) (Activase) and tenecteplase TNK-tPA (TNKase). Both are thrombolytic agents produced by recombinant deoxyribonucleic acid technology. These proteins are biosynthetic forms of a naturally occurring enzyme, human tPA, and are made by the ovarian cells of a Chinese hamster. The agents are administered intravenously in the medical setting to reduce patient mortality in acute MI. Tenecteplase is administered as a bolus. Alteplase is also administered as a bolus but is then infused over a 90-minute time frame. In specific cases, alteplase may also play a role in the treatment of strokes, pulmonary emboli, and peripheral vascular occlusions. Because tPA is a human enzyme, fewer allergic and hypersensitivity reactions occur with alteplase and tenecteplase than with first-generation thrombolytic agents. Another advantage of tPA is its ability to act specifically targeting clots rather than exerting systemic effects.

MAKE IT SIMPLE

Thrombolytic medications often end with "ase."

KEY CONCEPTS

- Blood naturally contains both coagulants and anticoagulants, but anticoagulants are normally dominant because they keep blood in its flowing, liquid form.
- Blood coagulation is a process that minimizes blood loss when small blood vessels are disrupted. The formation of a blood clot is the result of a three-stage cascade of events.
- Clot formation may be initiated via two different pathways: extrinsic or intrinsic.
- Thrombosis is the formation of a blood clot within an unbroken blood vessel. If natural coagulation or anticoagulation is inadequate, medical or surgical intervention may be necessary.
- Drugs that affect blood coagulation fall into two main categories: coagulants and anticoagulants.
- Coagulants assist the body's natural clotting mechanism. Coagulants applied topically during surgery to control minor bleeding and capillary oozing are called *hemostatics*.
- Anticoagulants work to prevent undesired clotting, to slow the normal clotting mechanism, or to help break up existing clots.
- Anticoagulants fall into three basic categories: parenteral anticoagulants, oral anticoagulants, and thrombolytics.
- Heparin is the most common parenteral anticoagulant used in surgery, usually during peripheral and cardiovascular procedures.
- Thrombolytics are administered intravenously to break up existing blood clots.

TABLE 9.6 Thrombolytics	
Generic Name	**Trade Name**
alteplase tissue-type plasminogen activator (tPA)	Activase
tenecteplase TNK-tPA	TNKase

LEARNING THE LANGUAGE (KEY TERMS)

Using your textbook or a standard medical dictionary, look up and write the definition of each term.

antagonist

anticoagulants

antiplatelet drugs

coagulants

DVT

hemostatics

platelet aggregation

PE

thrombolytics

REVIEW QUESTIONS

1. Why are hemostatics used? Can you name some?
2. For what purpose are systemic coagulants used? Can you name some?
3. Name three surgical procedures that usually require heparin ready on the back table. In what strengths?
4. How does oral anticoagulant therapy affect the patient about to undergo a surgical procedure?
5. Why are thrombolytics administered?

CRITICAL THINKING

Scenario 1

You are scrubbed for a repair of an abdominal aortic aneurysm. The preference card indicates that Dr. Fromm wants 5000 units of heparin in 500 mL of saline for topical irrigation. The circulator can find only carpules containing 10,000 units/mL of heparin.

1. What is one solution to this problem?
2. What is another solution to this problem?

Scenario 2

Mr. Davis is a 67-year-old man admitted to surgery for an immediate laparoscopic cholecystectomy for acute cholecystitis. Review of his medical chart reveals that he is on warfarin.

1. What complications do you expect to see during this procedure?
2. What additional supplies should you bring in the room in preparation for these complications?
3. What actions may be taken during surgery to treat these complications?

BIBLIOGRAPHY

Fulcher EM, Fulcher RM, Soto CD: *Pharmacology: principles and applications*, ed 3, St Louis, 2012, Saunders/Elsevier.

Kee JL, Hayes ER, McCuistion LE: *Pharmacology: a patient-centered nursing approach*, ed 8, St Louis, 2015, Saunders/Elsevier.

Skidmore-Roth L: *Mosby's drug guide for nursing students*, ed 11, St Louis, 2015, Mosby/Elsevier.

INTERNET RESOURCES

Arixtra: http://www.drugs.com/pro/arixtra.html.

Baxter BioSurgery, COSEAL (Surgical Sealant): https://advanced surgery.baxter.com/coseal.

Baxter BioSurgery, FLOSEAL (Hemostatic Matrix): https://advancedsurgery.baxter.com/floseal.

Baxter BioSurgery, TISSEEL (Fibrin Sealant): https://advancedsurgery.baxter.com/tisseel.

Cascade Autologous Platelet System: www.ncbi.nlm.nih.gov/pmc/articles/PMC3839008.

C.B.S. News, *Dennis Quaid recounts twins' drug ordeal*: www.cbsnews.com/news/dennis-quaid-recounts-twins-drug-ordeal/.

Integra, DuraSeal Dural Sealant System: https://www.integralife.com/duraseal-dural-sealant-system-5-ml/product/dural-repair-sealants-duraseal-dural-sealant-system-5-ml.

CryoLife, BioGlue Surgical Adhesive: www.cryolife.com/products/bioglue-surgical-adhesive.

DailyMed, Calcium Chloride Injection, USP 10%: https://dailymed.nlm.nih.gov/dailymed/drugInfo.cfm?setid=90b8936e-61f2-5318-e053-2995a90aac44.

Drugs.com, Calcium Salts Monograph for Professionals: https://www.drugs.com/monograph/calcium-salts.html.

Drugs.com, Professionals, Arixtra: www.drugs.com/pro/arixtra.html.

Drugs.com, Professionals, FDA PI, Heparin, FDA prescribing information, side effects and uses: www.drugs.com/pro/heparin.html.

Drugs.com, Professionals, FDA PI, Hep-Lock, FDA prescribing information, side effects and uses: www.drugs.com/pro/hep-lock.html.

Drugs.com, Professionals, FDA PI, Lovenox, FDA prescribing information, side effects and uses: www.drugs.com/pro/lovenox.html.

Ethicon, EVICEL Solutions for Sealant: https://www.ethicon.com/na/epc/code/3905?lang=en-default.

Ethicon, Adjunctive Hemostats: https://www.jnjmedtech.com/en-US/platform/adjunctive-hemostats.

FloSeal (Hemostatic Matrix): www.floseal.com/us.

Gynex Corporation, Monsel's (ferric subsulfate paste): https://www.gynexcorporation.com/product/monsels-ferric-subsulfate-solution/.

Mayo Clinic, Antihemophilic Factor (Intravenous Route) Description and Brand: www.mayoclinic.org/drugs-supplements/antihemophilic-factor-viii-and-von-willebrand-factor-complex-intravenous-route/description/drg-20073496.

Mayo Clinic, Drugs and Supplements, Streptokinase (intravenous route, intracoronary route) Description and Brand Names: www.mayoclinic.org/drugs-supplements/streptokinase-intravenous-route-intracoronary-route/description/DRG-20070834.

MedicineNet.com, Alteplase: www.medicinenet.com/alteplase/article.htm.

MedicineNet.com, Vitamin K-1, phytonadione (Mephyton): www.medicinenet.com/vitamin_k-injection/article.htm.

Medline Plus, Medical Encyclopedia, Thrombolytic therapy: www.nlm.nih.gov/medlineplus/ency/article/007089.htm.

Medscape, Drugs & Diseases, Silver Nitrate: http://reference.medscape.com/drug/silver-nitrate-343589.

Medtronic, Healthcare Professionals: https://www.medtronic.com/us-en/healthcare-professionals/products/spinal-orthopaedic/bone-grafting.html.

Merriam-Webster, Hemostasis: www.merriam-webster.com/medical/hemostasis.

Pfizer, Gelfoam: https://www.pfizermedicalinformation.com/en-us/gelfoam-absorbable-gelatin-powder.

Quikclot: www.quikclot.com.

R.E.C.O.T.H.R.O.M. Thrombin, Topical (Recombinant): https://advancedsurgery.baxter.com/recothrom.

RxList, Rx.List, Heparin: www.rxlist.com/heparin-drug.htm.

RxList, Innohep: www.rxlist.com/innohep-drug.htm.

RxList, Kinlytic: www.rxlist.com/kinlytic-drug.htm.

RxList, Lovenox: https://www.rxlist.com/lovenox-drug.htm.

RxList, Thrombin, Indications & Dosages: www.rxlist.com/thrombin-drug/indications-dosage.htm.

Smiths Medical: www.smiths-medical.com/products/vascular-access/implantable-ports/portacath-implantable-venous-access-systems.

Surgiflo: https://www.jnjmedtech.com/en-US/product/surgiflo-hemostatic-matrix.

The Medical Biochemistry Page, Blood Coagulation: Hemostasis: http://themedicalbiochemistrypage.org/blood-coagulation.php.

Tisseel [Fibrin Sealant], Preparation & Use: www.tisseel.com/us/preparation_use.html.

US Food and Drug Administration, FDA Public Health Alert: Change in Heparin USP Monograph: www.fda.gov/Drugs/DrugSafety/PostmarketDrugSafetyInformationforPatientsandProviders/ucm207506.htm.

US Food and Drug Administration, Information on Heparin: www.fda.gov/Drugs/DrugSafety/PostmarketDrugSafetyInformationforPatientsandProviders/ucm112597.htm.

Weber State University Health Sciences, Mechanisms of Blood Coagulation: http://departments.weber.edu/chpweb/hemophilia/mechanisms_of_blood_coagulation.htm.

KEY TERMS

activated partial thromboplastin time (aPTT)
anticoagulation therapy
INR

partial thromboplastin time (PTT)
thrombocytopenia

ANTICOAGULATION THERAPY

A common medication protocol that affects the vascular system is anticoagulation therapy. It is crucial that the surgical first assistant be familiar with medications and how anticoagulation therapy is used in the preoperative, intraoperative, and postoperative settings. In anticoagulation therapy, the blood-clotting action is diminished or eliminated. It can be implemented as short- or long-term therapy. A higher degree of anticoagulation carries a higher risk of bleeding. These patients must be thoroughly educated on the effects of anticoagulation medications, and they are closely monitored while the therapy is in progress. There are various medications used for anticoagulation depending upon the conditions being treated and the length of time the treatment is required (Table 9.A).

SHORT-TERM THERAPY

Short-term anticoagulation therapy is used intraoperatively on vascular procedures and for the postoperative prevention of deep vein thrombosis (DVT) or pulmonary embolism (PE) in the surgical patient. The most common medication used for short-term therapy is heparin sodium. It is the medicine of choice for intraoperative anticoagulation because of its relatively short half-life of 1 hour (dependent on the dose given). For example, in cardiac surgery using cardiopulmonary bypass, the usual dosage with heparin administered intravenously is not less than 150 and up to 400 units/kg (units per kilogram of patient weight). This is to obtain total anticoagulation of the patient's blood; however, heparin dosage may vary between individuals. The surgeon should be notified after 1 hour has lapsed since the last dosage. Additional doses may be required to maintain anticoagulation for the remainder of the procedure. As stated, heparin is used as the first line of treatment for DVT and PE. In addition, it is used for treatment of chronic disseminated intravascular coagulation. partial thromboplastin time (PTT) and activated partial thromboplastin time (aPTT) are laboratory tests used to monitor the patient and verify the correct dosage of heparin. Heparin can cause thrombocytopenia,

a decrease in platelet count. Protamine sulfate is administered to reverse the effects of heparin. Protamine sulfate should be administered very slowly to prevent hypotension.

> **! CAUTION**
> Heparin sodium comes in many strengths, as discussed in this chapter. Always check the strength before mixing or allowing administration of this medication.

LONG-TERM THERAPY

Long-term anticoagulation therapy is usually necessary for patients with vascular disease or vascular implants, such as stents or heart valves. It carries the high risk of bleeding, which can be a major or life-threatening complication. The risk of thrombus or embolus formation must outweigh the risk of bleeding. Warfarin sodium is used for long-term anticoagulation to treat any thromboembolic condition, such as DVT and PE. It is also used to prevent thrombus formation for patients with atrial fibrillation and/or cardiac valve replacement. Warfarin is an oral anticoagulant that suppresses the amount of vitamin K produced in the liver. When the amount of vitamin K is reduced, clotting factors II, VII, IX, and X are suppressed. Warfarin's medication levels peak a few days after its administration, and it remains in the body for 2 to 5 days after it has been discontinued.

Warfarin prolongs the clotting time that is assessed by the prothrombin time (PT) laboratory test and must be closely monitored. Laboratory values of PT may be different between specific laboratories depending on the type of reagent used. For this variability to be controlled, the international normalized ratio (INR) laboratory test was introduced (see Insight 9.2). This has been widely accepted as the test of choice to monitor and adjust the effects of warfarin to maintain the appropriate level of anticoagulant in the patient. The effects of warfarin can be different among the patient population, making dosage difficult to control, especially at the beginning of the therapy. Initial and maintenance dosages are individualized according to the INR results. The INR is mathematically calculated from a PT

TABLE 9.A Anticoagulant and Antiplatelet Medications[a]

Drug	Route	Indications	Dosage	Side Effects	Adverse Reactions
Anticoagulants					
heparin sodium[b]	SC, IV bolus, IV drip	Treat thromboembolism, DVT, PE, prevent blood clotting	SC: 5000–10,000 units every 4–12 h IV: bolus 5000 units 20,000–40,000 daily IV drip based on aPTT	Bleeding, itching, burning	Bleeding, hematuria, thrombocytopenia
enoxaparin sodium (Lovenox)	SC, IV	Prophylactic treatment and acute treatment of DVT and MI	30–40 mg SC daily or bid postoperatively[c]	Anemia, diarrhea, nausea, bruising	Bleeding, thrombocytopenia, dyspnea
warfarin sodium	PO	Long-term prophylaxis for thromboembolism	5–10 mg/day × 2–5 days then 2–10 mg/day maintenance or dependent on the INR results	Rash, fever, nausea, mild abdominal cramps, anorexia, diarrhea	Bleeding, petechiae, hematemesis
dabigatran (Pradaxa)	PO	Prophylactic treatment of DVT and PE	75–150 mg bid	Abdominal pain and discomfort, nausea, bruising	GI bleeding, hematuria, hemoptysis
Antiplatelets					
aspirin (Bayer)	PO, rectal suppository	Prophylaxis for MI, stroke, TIA	81–650 mg/day	Bleeding, bruising, GI symptoms	GI distress, peptic ulcers, perforation
clopidogrel (Plavix)	PO	Prophylaxis for MI, stroke, TIA, and thromboembolism	Loading dose: 300 mg, then 75 mg/day May be combined with aspirin	Heartburn, dizziness, aching muscles, GI discomfort, headache	Thrombocytopenia, hypotension, bronchiospasm
dipyridamole (Persantine)	PO	Prophylaxis for thromboembolism post-MI, to prevent clots postop prosthetic device surgery (heart valves, hip replacement)	75–100 qid	Abdominal distress, dizziness, headache, muscle or joint pain	Weakness, fainting, unusual bleeding, tachycardia

aPTT, Activated partial thromboplastin time; *bid*, twice per day; *DVT*, deep venous thrombosis; *GI*, gastrointestinal; *INR*, international normalized ratio; *IV*, intravenous; *MI*, myocardial infarction; *PE*, pulmonary embolism; *PO*, per os (by mouth); *qid*, 4 times per day; *SC*, subcutaneous; *TIA*, transient ischemic attack.

[a]All doses are individualized for each patient according to the patient's INR response to the medication.
[b]Heparin sodium is also used topically from the sterile back table, as discussed in this chapter.
[c]One dose of enoxaparin sodium can also be given 12 hours preoperatively when used prophylactically.

(clotting time). Therapeutic ranges of anticoagulants are controversial within the medical community. It is commonly accepted that an INR range of 2.0 to 3.0 is sufficient to maintain a level of anticoagulation that is beneficial for the treatment of most thromboembolus conditions. Patients should be monitored for bruising, bloody stools, bleeding gums, and hematuria.

Enoxaparin sodium (Lovenox), a sterile aqueous solution, is a low-molecular-weight heparin (LMWH). It comes in prefilled syringes and multiple-dose vials for subcutaneous and intravenous use. Unlike heparin, the medication may be administered by patients at home using a prefilled syringe (with physician-prescribed dosage) and injecting it (subcutaneously) into the fatty tissues of the abdomen. Enoxaparin sodium is indicated in the prophylactic treatment of DVT in abdominal surgery, hip and knee replacement, and for treatment of DVT with or without PE. Thrombocytopenia can occur with enoxaparin

sodium use. Therefore, blood tests for platelet monitoring are performed.

Dabigatran etexilate (Pradaxa) is a direct thrombin inhibitor that keeps platelets from coagulating and so prevents clots from forming in blood vessels. It is used to prevent blood clots in DVT and PE, to decrease the risk of stroke, and in certain types of heart rhythm disorders. Dabigatran is indicated to reduce the risk of recurrence of DVT and PE in patients who have been previously treated with parenteral anticoagulants for 5 to 10 days. It comes in 75- and 150-mg capsules for oral administration, and unlike other anticoagulants, it does not require routine coagulation monitoring.

Other oral medications that affect the clotting factor of blood are antiplatelet medicines. As discussed in the chapter, these drugs suppress aggregation (clumping) of platelets. The most common is aspirin, which is often discounted by healthcare workers as a drug therapy. Aspirin is used mainly for prophylactic coverage to prevent the formation of a thrombus in arteries. Patients at risk of myocardial infarction (MI), stroke, or transient ischemic attack (TIA) will benefit from aspirin therapy. Tablets come in strengths of 81, 162, 325, 500, or 650 mg and are taken orally or by rectal suppository. Aspirin reaches its maximum effect on platelets within 30 minutes after administration. Because of its long-acting effects, patients requiring surgery of any kind should discontinue the use of aspirin at least 7 days before their procedures. Adverse effects include heartburn, gastrointestinal symptoms, and nausea.

> **NOTE:** Reye syndrome has been reported in children and teens who took aspirin for chickenpox or flu-like symptoms. A physician should always be consulted.

Other antiplatelet medications include clopidogrel (Plavix) and dipyridamole (Persantine). These medicines may be prescribed individually or be used in combination with an anticoagulation medication. Indications for use as a stand-alone therapy are usually in patients with high risk of or a history of a thromboembolic event. These include prevention of MI, stroke, and TIA. These medications have relatively long half-lives and should be discontinued several days in advance of any surgical procedures.

Clopidogrel (Plavix) is prescribed to prevent formation of thrombus in arteries. Like aspirin, clopidogrel is used as a prophylactic therapy for patients with history or high risk for arterial thromboembolic event, MI, stroke, or TIA. Recommended dosage is 75 mg/day orally. Its peak effect may take up to 4 days to be reached. Common side effects may include gastrointestinal discomfort, headache, dizziness, aching muscles, and heartburn. Excessive bruising may also occur while taking this medication.

Dipyridamole (Persantine) is used to prevent thrombus in patients who have had heart valve surgery. As stated, it may also be used in combination with other medications (such as aspirin) to reduce the damage from an MI, to prevent a recurrence, and to prevent complications during heart bypass surgery. Usual dosage is 75 to 100 mg orally 4 times a day. Common side effects may include abdominal distress, dizziness, headache, and itching.

> **! CAUTION**
>
> When epidural and spinal anesthesia or spinal puncture is performed, patients anticoagulated or scheduled to be anticoagulated with LMWHs, heparinoids, and/or some oral anticoagulants are at risk of developing an epidural or spinal hematoma. This can result in long-term or permanent paralysis. The risk increases with the use of an indwelling epidural catheter and by traumatic or repeated epidural and spinal punctures.

> **NOTE:** Antiplatelet drugs are best for preventing arterial thrombi, and anticoagulants are best for preventing venous thrombi.

ADVANCED PRACTICES: REVIEW QUESTIONS

1. Why is it necessary for patients on anticoagulation therapy to be closely monitored?
2. What type of procedures may require short-term anticoagulation therapy?
3. What condition is treated with short-term anticoagulation therapy postoperatively?
4. The most common medication used for short-term anticoagulation is _____ and its normal dosage is _____ units/kg of patient weight.
5. One indication for long-term anticoagulation therapy is _____.
6. How does warfarin produce its anticoagulation effect?
7. List three oral anticoagulant medications and an indication for each.

ADVANCED PRACTICES: BIBLIOGRAPHY

Fulcher EM, Fulcher RM, Soto CD: *Pharmacology: principles and applications,*, ed 3, St Louis, 2012, Saunders/Elsevier.

Kee JL, Hayes ER, McCuistion LE: *Pharmacology: a patient-centered nursing process approach*, ed 8, St Louis, 2015, Saunders/Elsevier.

Martini R, Ober B, Nath J: *Visual anatomy & physiology*, San Francisco, 2011, Benjamin Cummings/Pearson.

Skidmore-Roth L: *Mosby's drug guide for nursing students*, ed 11, St Louis, 2015, Mosby/Elsevier.

ADVANCED PRACTICES: INTERNET RESOURCES

Bayer HealthCare, Bayer Aspirin, Frequently Asked Questions: www.wonderdrug.com/faqs.

Drugs.com, Aspirin: www.drugs.com/aspirin.html.

Drugs.com, Dabigatran Dosage: www.drugs.com/dosage/dabigatran.html.

Drugs.com, Persantine, Side effects: www.drugs.com/cdi/persantine.html.

O'Carroll-Kuehn BU, Meeran H: Management of coagulation during cardiopulmonary bypass, *Contin Educ Anaesth Crit Care Pain* 7(6):195–198, 2007. http://ceaccp.oxfordjournals.org/content/7/6/195.full

MedlinePlus, Drugs, Herbs and Supplements, Dipyridamole: www.nlm.nih.gov/medlineplus/druginfo/medmaster/a682830.html.

Medline Plus, Medical Encyclopedia, Partial Thromboplastin Time (PTT): www.nlm.nih.gov/medlineplus/ency/article/003653.htm.

Medscape, Disseminated Intravascular Coagulation, Treatment and Management: http://emedicine.medscape.com/article/199627-treatment.

Medscape, Plavix: https://reference.medscape.com/drug/plavix-clopidogrel-342141.

Pradaxa (dabigatran etexilate), U.S. Healthcare Professionals: www.pradaxa.com/.

RxList, Heparin: www.rxlist.com/heparin-drug.htm.

RxList, Lovenox (enoxaparin sodium injection): www.rxlist.com/lovenox-drug.htm.

RxList, Persantine (dipyridamole USP): www.rxlist.com/persantine-drug.htm.

RxList, Plavix: www.rxlist.com/plavix-drug.htm.

RxList, Pradaxa (dabigatran etexilate mesylate): https://www.rxlist.com/pradaxa-drug.htm.

U.C. San Diego Health, LMWH Reversal Anticoagulation Clinic: https://health.ucsd.edu/specialties/anticoagulation/providers/lmwh/Pages/reversal.aspx.

WebMD, Partial Thromboplastin Time: www.webmd.com/a-to-z-guides/partial-thromboplastin-time.

10

Ophthalmic Agents

Ophthalmic surgical procedures often require the use of several categories of medications (Box 10.1) from the sterile back table. Initially, the scrubbed surgical technologist must properly identify and label all medications received into the sterile field. In addition, the surgical technologist must understand the purpose of each drug to pass it to the surgeon at the appropriate time. This is especially important during procedures in which the operative microscope is used. The surgeon must focus attention and vision through the microscope lens and should not have to continually refocus away from the operative field. In this chapter we discuss definitions, purposes, routes, and agents in each ophthalmic drug category used in surgery. A review of basic anatomy is included for reference.

BOX 10.1 Categories of Agents Used in Ophthalmic Surgery

Ophthalmic prep solutions
Irrigation solutions and lubricants
Ophthalmic viscosurgical devices (OVD)
Miotics
Mydriatics and cycloplegics
Ophthalmic antiinfectives
Anesthetics
Antiglaucoma agents
Antiinflammatory agents
Diagnostic agents

ANATOMY REVIEW

The eye (Fig. 10.1) is a complex sensory organ that receives visual stimuli and transmits signals via the optic nerve (cranial nerve II) to the brain for interpretation. Each eyeball is controlled by cranial nerves III, IV, and VI and attached to six extraocular muscles for movement. These are the medial, lateral, superior, and inferior rectus muscles and the inferior and superior oblique muscles. Accessory structures include eyebrows, eyelids, eyelashes, and the lacrimal system. The lacrimal system produces, distributes, and removes tears, which keep eye surfaces moist and clean. A thin, transparent mucous membrane called the *conjunctiva* lines the inside of the eyelids and the anterior surface of the eyeball (globe). Only about 17% of the globe is visible; the remainder is protected within the bony orbit, where it is supported on a cushion of fat and fascia. The globe consists of three layers of tissue: fibrous, vascular, and nervous. The fibrous outer coat of the eye is composed of a dense, white connective tissue called *sclera*. Sclera gives the globe its shape, provides protection, and can be seen through the conjunctiva as the "white" of the eye. The anterior covering of the eye is made of clear, nonvascular fibrous tissue called the *cornea*. The cornea does not contain blood vessels to provide its nourishment; rather, it is nourished by being bathed in a solution called *aqueous humor* and from oxygen in the air. It serves as the "window" of the eye. The area where the cornea and sclera meet is called the *limbus*. Deep to the limbus is a venous sinus called *Schlemm's canal*.

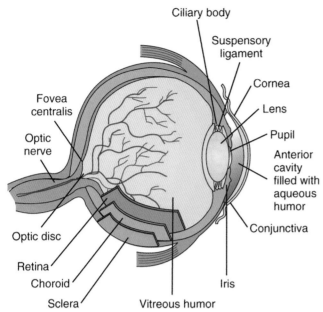

Fig. 10.1 Anatomy of the eye. (From Young AP, Proctor DB: *Kinn's the medical assistant: an applied learning approach*, ed 11, St Louis, 2011, Saunders.)

? QUICK QUESTION

Which structure of your eye defines its color? For the answer, review your eye anatomy.

The vascular layer of the eye is called *choroid*. The anterior and thickest portion of choroid is the ciliary body. The ciliary body secretes aqueous humor from structures called *ciliary processes*. Ciliary muscle arises in the ciliary body and attaches to the lens, altering its shape to accommodate near or distant vision. The iris is attached to the ciliary process and is positioned between the cornea and lens. The pigmented iris consists of radial and circular muscle fibers whose function is to change the size of its opening, called the *pupil*. The pupil regulates the amount of light entering the eye by constricting (making an opening smaller) or dilating (making an opening larger). The nervous layer of the eye, called the *retina*, is present only posteriorly and covers the choroid. Images focused onto the retina trigger sensory receptors characterized as rods and cones. Signals are then transmitted via the optic nerve to the occipital lobe of the brain for recognition.

The lens is positioned just behind the iris and serves to focus images onto the retina. The lens consists of protein fibers arranged in onion-like layers. The lens, which is normally transparent, is covered by a clear fibrous capsule and held in place by suspensory ligaments called *zonula*.

? MAKE IT SIMPLE

The parts of the ocular lens may be compared with a pitted fruit, such as a peach. The nucleus of the lens is like the pit of the fruit, the cortex of the lens is like the flesh of the fruit, and the lens capsule is like the skin of the fruit.

The interior portion of the globe contains two cavities, anterior and posterior, separated by the lens. The anterior cavity is further separated into anterior and posterior chambers. The anterior chamber is posterior to the cornea and anterior to the iris. The posterior chamber is behind the iris and anterior to the lens. The entire anterior cavity is filled with aqueous humor (fluid) secreted by the ciliary processes. Aqueous humor flows forward in the anterior cavity and drains through the trabecular meshwork into Schlemm's canal. If a blockage occurs in the trabecular meshwork, intraocular pressure (IOP) builds, causing glaucoma. *Glaucoma* is the term used to describe a group of ocular conditions characterized by increased IOP. The posterior cavity, which is between the lens and retina, is filled with a thick substance called *vitreous humor*. Vitreous humor gives the globe its shape, keeps the retina in position, and contributes to IOP. Unlike aqueous humor, vitreous humor is not naturally replaced by the body.

The eye contains a barrier similar to the blood-brain barrier. The blood-eye barrier prevents effective absorption of most systemically administered medications. For this reason, the most common administration route for ophthalmic medications is topical application: as drops, suspensions, ointments, and on medicated disks or pledgets inserted onto the eye. A few agents may be given orally or parenterally. Ophthalmic agents administered topically enter systemic circulation through the conjunctival vessels and the nasolacrimal system. Approximately 80% of eye drops enter the nasolacrimal system, then drain from nose to mouth and enter the stomach, where absorption takes place. Fig. 10.2 illustrates the proper administration of topical ophthalmic solutions and ointments. After administration of the medications, compression of the lacrimal sac prevents rapid drainage of medication into the lacrimal system, where it is carried away from the eye.

? QUICK QUESTION

A few ophthalmic agents may be administered *parenterally*. Do you remember what this term means? Refer to Drug Administration Routes in Chapter 1 for the answer.

NOTE: It is important to follow aseptic technique when applying ophthalmic medications. The tip of the medication applicator should not touch the patient's tissue or the bottle is considered to be contaminated and must be discarded immediately after use. Such contact could also result in a corneal abrasion. When ointments are used for the first time, the first quarter inch should be squeezed from the container and discarded.

Topical administration may limit a drug's effectiveness because of dilution by lacrimal fluid and drainage, as well as systemic absorption. Sustained-release delivery systems, such as pilocarpine ophthalmic, a wafer-thin disk used to produce miosis and decrease IOP for the treatment of glaucoma, have been developed to overcome lacrimal medication dilution. The disk is placed into the lower conjunctival sac, where it delivers the appropriate amount of medication every hour for 7 days.

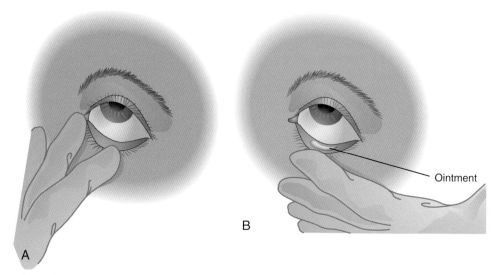

Fig. 10.2 Administration of eye medications. Step 1: Gentle retraction of the lower lid to expose conjunctival sac (A). Step 2: Place drops or ointment onto the lower cul-de-sac (B). Step 3: Hold light finger pressure over lacrimal sac for approximately 1 minute; then, with eye closed, remove excess medication from the inner corner of the eyelid with a cotton ball. (From Kee JL, Hayes ER, McCuistion LE: *Pharmacology: a patient-centered nursing process approach*, ed 8, St Louis, 2015, Elsevier.)

The patient must remove and replace the wafer as directed. Other innovative medication delivery systems are being continually introduced. DuraSite is a drug delivery vehicle that binds drug molecules in matrix that enables release of the medication in a gel-like drop. Added to the antibiotic azithromycin, DuraSite extends the length of time the antibiotic is in contact with the ocular surface. This method is used in the treatment of blepharitis.

Another method for instilling ophthalmic medications preoperatively is with the use of pledgets. Medication-soaked pledgets are placed in the conjunctival cul-de-sac after the eye has been anesthetized with local anesthetic drops. An example of this method is instilling mydriatic or cycloplegic medication preoperatively. Antibiotic and local anesthetic medications can also be added to the pledget mixture (placing all medications into a sterile medicine cup), and then the pledget inserted with sterile tissue forceps. It should be noted that corneal abrasion and patient discomfort have been reported with the use of some pledgets. Intraoperatively, medications, such as antibiotics, may also be administered directly into the anterior chamber of the eye. This is referred to as *intracameral administration* and would have a systemic effect. Intracameral injections require methylparaben-free (MPF) medication.

A 21st-century method for medicine delivery is the use of nanoparticles. A nanoparticle is a microscopic particle so small that it is measured in nanometers (one nanometer equals one billionth of a meter). It acts as a whole unit in terms of its properties and measures 100 nm or less. Nanoparticles are an area of intense scientific and medical research. Polymeric nanoparticles with a size of 10 to 1000 nm are being used in ophthalmic drug delivery because they can be easily manipulated for both passive and active drug targeting and made to control and sustain the release of the drug to the target tissue. More on the use of nanoparticles is discussed in Chapter 6.

> **! CAUTION**
>
> It is important to remember how easily the cornea can be scratched (abraded) or damaged. Never use a regular sponge to wipe across the eye and remember that corneal damage can result even when the eyelid is closed.

CATEGORIES OF OPHTHALMIC AGENTS

Ophthalmic Prep Solution

Delicate tissues of the eye require special prep solutions. Betadine Ophthalmic 5% Prep Solution is a sterile, dark-brown liquid stabilized by glycerin that contains 5% povidone-iodine. It is used to prep the ocular region that also includes the eyelids, brows, and cheeks. It can be used to irrigate and is a broad-spectrum microbicide. Betadine Ophthalmic should be left in contact with the prepped areas for 2 minutes, then the eyes should be flushed with sterile saline to remove any residual solution.

Irrigating Solutions and Lubricants

Irrigating solutions are used during ophthalmic procedures to cleanse the operative site and keep the cornea moist. The most common ophthalmic irrigating solution is balanced salt solution (BSS) (Fig. 10.3). BSS is a sterile, physiologically balanced irrigant. It is packaged in sterile containers of 15 and 30 mL for topical use from the sterile field; it also comes in bottles of 250 and 500 mL for infusion with administration tubing sets during procedures, such as phacoemulsification (a type of cataract surgery). BSS PLUS solution is enriched with bicarbonate, dextrose, and glutathione. It comes in a two-part system that is combined before use. It has no preservatives and must be used within 6 hours of mixing. As with regular BSS, it is not for intravenous use or injection. During most ophthalmic procedures (and any other procedures that involve blood in the eye area), the scrubbed surgical technologist will periodically irrigate the

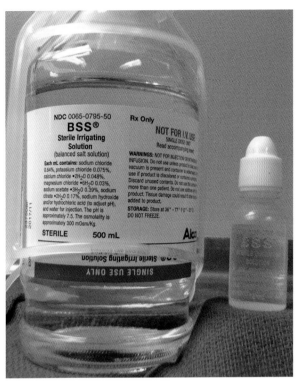

Fig. 10.3 Balanced salt solutions.

cornea with BSS beginning at the inner canthus and allowing the solution to flow out the corner of the eye. Other ophthalmic irrigating solutions are available for over-the-counter (OTC) purchase.

Lubricants are agents in ointment form that are used to moisten and protect the eye. Ophthalmic lubricants may be used when a general anesthetic is administered for any surgical procedure. With patients under general anesthesia, eyelids are relaxed, and the corneal reflex is absent. To prevent corneal drying or damage and maintain integrity of the epithelial surface, a nonionic ointment or lubricant, such as lanolin alcohol (Refresh Lacri- Lube) or polyvinyl alcohol (Liquifilm, LubriFresh PM), is applied to each eye. Then the eyelids are taped closed or special foam eye masks with plastic shields are used. On emergence from anesthesia, patients may exhibit blurred vision; although this blurring is caused by the ointment, they should be prevented from rubbing their eyes. Be alert to any patient allergic reactions to preservatives found in these medications.

> **! CAUTION**
>
> It is possible for the semi-awake patients to injure their cornea, even through closed eyelids. All members of the surgical team are responsible for observing and ensuring the safety of their patients.

Viscoelastic Agents

Viscoelastic agents are thick, jelly-like substances injected into the eye during certain ophthalmic procedures. These agents are often injected into the anterior chamber during cataract extraction (phacoemulsification) to keep the chamber expanded,

prevent injury to surrounding tissue, and protect the cornea. Viscoelastic agents may also be used as a vitreous substitute or tamponade (compression). An example of a viscoelastic agent is sodium hyaluronate (Vitrax). Viscoelastic agents are supplied in premeasured sterile syringes with blunt-tipped cannulas. Most should be kept refrigerated until use. Side effects include a transient rise in IOP, iritis, corneal edema, and corneal decompensation. Note that the term *ophthalmic viscosurgical device* (OVD) is being used for viscoelastic agents because they are no longer considered as the only medications used to maintain space and coat ocular tissues. Rather, they are an integral part of cataract surgery and are being used in combinations as newer techniques for ophthalmic surgery are being developed.

Miotics

Miotics are medications that constrict the pupil by stimulating the sphincter muscle of the iris. Because constriction of the pupil (miosis) reduces IOP, miotics are frequently used in short-term treatment of glaucoma. Miotics may be used intraoperatively when pupillary constriction is indicated, as in laser iridectomy. Occasionally, miotics are used to maintain the position of an implanted lens after cataract extraction (Fig. 10.4). Miotics may be administered by injection or topical application. Side effects include eye, eyebrow, or eyelid pain; blurred vision; abdominal cramps; and diarrhea.

Acetylcholine chloride is a miotic agent available in a solution of mannitol marketed as Miochol-E. It may be used for the initial treatment of chronic open-angle glaucoma and acute glaucoma; this is because miosis facilitates drainage of aqueous humor. Miochol-E may be injected during surgery to decrease IOP and to cause miosis if needed. Miosis lasts approximately 10 minutes. Miochol-E should be reconstituted immediately before use. Carbachol (Isopto Carbachol) is used topically to reduce IOP in glaucoma and by injection (Miostat) into the anterior chamber, as needed, intraoperatively.

Mydriatics and Cycloplegics

Both mydriatics and cycloplegics are paralytic agents used to dilate the pupil before ophthalmoscopy. Both kinds of agents cause *mydriasis*—dilation of the pupil—by paralyzing the sphincter muscle of the iris. Cycloplegics also paralyze the accommodation mechanism. (This means that patients may be unable to see near objects clearly.) After topical instillation of mydriatics or cycloplegics, the lacrimal sac should be compressed for 2 to 3 minutes to avoid rapid systemic absorption of the medication. Common mydriatic agents are atropine sulfate and phenylephrine. Atropine sulfate (Atropisol, Isopto Atropine Ophthalmic), an anticholinergic agent and a belladonna alkaloid, is available for ophthalmic use in solutions of 0.25% and 2% and in ointment of 0.5% and 1% for topical application. Atropine may be used to dilate the pupil for a few weeks after surgery, if needed. Atropine's onset is approximately 30 minutes, whereas peak effect is seen in 30 to 40 minutes; duration is 7 to 10 days. Atropine is also a potent cycloplegic. Homatropine hydrobromide (Isopto Homatropine) is similar to atropine but has a faster onset of approximately 10 to 30 minutes and a shorter duration of up to 3 days. Some medications that dilate

Cataract Extraction

Preoperative Orders:
1. Have consent signed for Extracapsular Cataract Removal with Insertion of Intraocular Lens Prosthesis, Right or Left Eye
2. Lab reports as indicated on the surgery order form. Send abnormal lab results to family physician.
3. NPO 6-8 hours pre-anesthesia. May take heart and blood pressure medication with a sip of water early morning.
4. Site/side verification per surgeon as per policy. (Surgeon places "yes" above correct eye).
5. Phenylephrine HCl 2.5% and cyclopentolate HCl 1% 1 gtt of each in operative eye every 10 minutes × 3. If difficult to dilate, substitute phenylephrine HCl 10% for the phenylephrine 2.5%, continue to instill 1 gtt every 10 minutes along with the cyclopentolate HCl 1% until pupil is dilated.
   Time given: _____, _____, _____.
6. Flurbiprofen sodium 0.03% 1 gtt in operative eye every 10 minutes × 3 following prior series of eye drops.
   Time given: _____, _____, _____.
7. Start IV lactated Ringer's 1000 mL at KVO.
8. Have patient void prior to going to surgery.

   _____

Intraoperative Orders:
1. Instill 1 gtt tetracaine 0.5% in the operative eye immediately prior to the eye prep.
2. Add 0.3 mL epinephrine (1 mg/mL) to 500 mL BSS or BSS PLUS
3. Open Duovisc and 15 mL BSS onto sterile table for use by doctor.
4. Instill 1 gtt Betadine 5% in operative eye. Leave in eye for 3 minutes. Meanwhile prep around eye with Betadine 5%.
5. Irrigate eye with 15 mL BSS.
6. Instill Zymaxid 2 gtts, Pred Forte 2 gtts, and Bromday 1 gtt in operative eye immediately following procedure.

   _____

Postoperative Orders:
1. Admit to PACU.
2. O_2 via nasal cannula at 2 L/min for O_2 Sat less than 95%.
3. Vital signs every 10 minutes until discharge criteria are met.
4. Diamox Sequel 500 mg PO before discharge if not allergic to sulfa.
5. Zofran 4 mg IV PRN for nausea or vomiting.
6. Contact surgeon for blood pressure less than 80/50, O_2 Sat less than 90%, and/or respirations less than 12 breaths per minute.
7. Discontinue IV and discharge when discharge criteria are met.
8. Give patient card with appointment time for follow-up.
9. Give patient medication prescription per doctor.
10. Patient to follow discharge instruction sheet for post-op cataract.
11. Medications to be used in operative eye at home:
    a. Zymaxid 1 gtt every 2 hours day of surgery and the next day, then 4 times a day in operative eye.
    b. Pred Forte 1 gtt 4 times a day in operative eye.
    c. Bromfenac 1 gtt to operative eye 1 time daily.

   _____

(Patient Label)

Fig. 10.4 Surgeon's routine order sheet for cataract surgery using phacoemulsification.

the pupil are actually decongestants. They are also vasoconstrictors that act by narrowing blood vessels. An example is phenylephrine (Neo-Synephrine Ophthalmic, AK-Dilate) that is available in solutions of 2.5% and 10% for topical ophthalmic use. Its onset is approximately 30 minutes, with effects lasting 2 to 3 hours. Cycloplegic agents include cyclopentolate HCl (Cyclogyl, AK-Pentolate) available in 0.5% to 2% solutions and

tropicamide (Mydral, Mydriacyl) available in 0.5% and 1% solutions. Side effects include tachycardia, photophobia, dry mouth, edema, conjunctivitis, and dermatitis.

Another agent used to dilate the pupil, used especially for phacoemulsification procedures, is lidocaine 1% MPF administered by intracameral injection. In this case the lidocaine acts as an anesthetic and a mydriatic.

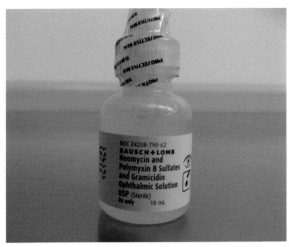

Fig. 10.5 Neomycin, polymyxin B sulfates, and gramicidin ophthalmic solution.

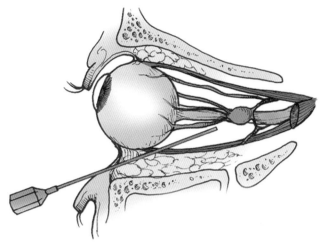

Fig. 10.6 Retrobulbar block. (From Rothrock J: *Alexander's care of the patient in surgery*, ed 15, St Louis, 2014, Elsevier.)

Ophthalmic Antiinfectives

Antiinfectives are frequently used in ophthalmology to treat external ocular infections and as prophylaxis against postoperative infections. Ophthalmic antibiotic preparations include aminoglycosides, such as gentamicin, neomycin, and tobramycin. Interestingly, no nephrotoxicity or ototoxicity has been noted with ophthalmic use of aminoglycosides (see Chapter 5). Gentamicin (Garamycin, Genoptic) is available in 0.3% solution or ointment, tobramycin (Tobrex) in 0.3% solution or ointment, and neomycin in a solution of 2.5 mg/mL or an ointment of 5 mg/g. Tobramycin may be combined with the antiinflammatory agent dexamethasone in Tobradex solution or ointment. Neomycin is also available as Neosporin combined with polymyxin B sulfates and bacitracin zinc (commonly referred to as *triple antibiotic ophthalmic ointment*). Neomycin combined with polymyxin B sulfates and gramicidin as another trio of topical antibiotics that work together to stop bacterial growth (Fig. 10.5). This combination can also be used to treat eye infections, such as conjunctivitis and keratitis. Other common ophthalmic antiinfectives include bacitracin ointment (Baciguent) in 500 units/g, erythromycin (Ilotycin) 0.5% ointment, and sulfacetamide (Bleph-10, Sodium Sulamyd) in 10% and 30% solution and 10% ointment. Moxifloxacin (Vigamox) 0.5% solution, gatifloxacin (Zymaxid) 0.5% solution, ciprofloxacin (Ciloxan) 0.3% solution and 0.3% ointment, and ofloxacin 0.3% solution (Ocuflox) are more examples of antiinfectives.

❓ QUICK QUESTION

Look at the medication label in Fig. 10.5. Can you answer the following questions: How do you know this medication is used on eyes?

How much medicine is in this container? Can it be purchased OTC? Refer to Chapter 2 under Medication Labeling if you need help.

ANESTHETICS

Anesthetics are medications that interfere with normal transmission of pain impulses to the brain. Most ophthalmic surgical procedures require the use of a topical or an injected anesthetic agent. Cocaine solution (1% and 4%) was the initial topical anesthetic agent used in ophthalmology; however, it is currently used predominantly in otolaryngology. Two common topical ophthalmic anesthetics are tetracaine hydrochloride (Pontocaine) and proparacaine hydrochloride (Alcaine, Ophthaine). Both medications are available in a 0.5% ophthalmic solution. Their onset is under 1 minute, and duration is 10 to 20 minutes. With these medications, the patient's blink reflex is temporarily lost. Tetracaine is also available in gel form (TetraVisc, TetraVisc FORTE) for sustained contact time and increased anesthetic effect. Many ophthalmic procedures are scheduled with an anesthesia care provider present to administer sedation and monitor the patient. This is called *monitored anesthesia care* (see Chapter 13).

Ophthalmic procedures requiring an extensive area of anesthesia are performed under a regional, retrobulbar (see Chapter 13) or peribulbar block. This type of anesthesia, which provides both sensory and motor (movement) block, is performed with a local anesthetic, such as lidocaine (Xylocaine 4% MPF) or bupivacaine (0.75%). In retrobulbar block, the agents are injected near the optic nerve (Fig. 10.6). In peribulbar block, the injections are made in the soft tissue superior (above) and inferior (below) to the eyeball. Other agents may be added to the anesthetic, such as hyaluronidase (Vitrase). Hyaluronidase is an enzyme mixed with anesthetics to increase diffusion of the anesthetic through the tissue and to improve the effectiveness of the block. This is contraindicated if a malignancy is present. Another agent added to an anesthetic is epinephrine. Epinephrine is a powerful vasoconstrictor; it is used to prevent rapid absorption of the anesthetic, thereby prolonging the block.

ANTIGLAUCOMA AGENTS

The word *glaucoma* is a general term that refers to a group of conditions characterized by increased IOP. There are two main causes for this condition: either aqueous humor is overproduced or the drainage mechanism is blocked. Normal IOP is between 10 and 22 mm Hg, and pressure greater than 25 mm Hg is considered abnormal. This pressure damages the optic nerve and may cause blindness. Although glaucoma is easily treated in the medical setting, untreated it can lead to blindness.

> **NOTE:** Most antiglaucoma agents discussed in this section are administered in the medical setting rather than in the surgical setting.

The most common form of glaucoma is chronic open-angle glaucoma. In open-angle glaucoma, the trabecular meshwork cannot drain aqueous fluid effectively. A far rarer form is narrow-angle glaucoma (also called *angle-closure glaucoma*), which may be acute or chronic and is found in only approximately 5% of all glaucoma patients. Angle-closure glaucoma is caused by an abnormally narrow junction between the cornea and iris, blocking the flow of aqueous humor into the trabecular meshwork. Surgical treatments for angle-closure glaucoma include iridectomy and trabeculectomy.

Because pupillary constriction (miosis) may open the trabecular meshwork and facilitate drainage of excess fluid, short-term treatment often involves the use of miotic agents (as discussed previously). However, long-term management of increased IOP may be accomplished with several different types of agents, including prostaglandin analogues (PGAs), miotics, β-adrenergic blockers, α-adrenergic agonists, and diuretics (see Chapter 7), particularly carbonic anhydrase inhibitors (Box 10.2).

Carbonic anhydrase is an enzyme present in the ciliary body; it catalyzes secretion of aqueous humor. A carbonic anhydrase inhibitor, such as acetazolamide (Diamox Sequel), interferes with production of carbonic anhydrase; thus it reduces production of aqueous humor and decreases IOP. Acetazolamide, which reduces aqueous humor production by 50% to 60%, is administered orally to manage chronic open-angle glaucoma or given intravenously to treat acute angle-closure glaucoma. With oral administration, ocular effects are seen in 1 to 2 hours, with a duration of 3 to 5 hours. Other carbonic anhydrase inhibitors include brinzolamide (Azopt) and dorzolamide (Trusopt). Side effects may include lethargy, anorexia, drowsiness, nausea, vomiting, and hypokalemia.

Osmotic diuretics may also be used for short-term treatment of glaucoma. By raising the osmotic pressure of blood, osmotic diuretics cause fluid to be drawn out of the eye, lowering IOP. Ocular effects of osmotic diuretics last approximately 4 hours.

Osmotic diuretics may be used immediately before surgery to reduce IOP, or they may be given during procedures to treat retinal detachment to aid in scleral closure. Osmotic diuretics are also used in cases of acute angle-closure glaucoma to facilitate the response of the iris muscle to miotics. The most common osmotic diuretic used in ophthalmic surgery is mannitol (Osmitrol). Mannitol in a 5% to 20% solution is given intravenously in a dose of 0.25 to 2 g/kg of patient weight. For example, 500 mL of a 20% mannitol solution may be administered over a period of 30 to 60 minutes. When mannitol is administered preoperatively, an indwelling urinary catheter is usually inserted into the patient's bladder to accommodate resulting diuresis (increased excretion of urine). Maximum effect is noted approximately an hour after administration. Another osmotic diuretic used in ophthalmology is glycerin 50% solution (Osmoglyn, Ophthalgan) administered orally. Side effects from osmotics are commonly headache, nausea, vomiting, and diarrhea.

Another category of medications used to treat glaucoma is the α-adrenergic agonists (also called *sympathomimetics*), administered as eye drops. These agents are considered the third line of treatment for glaucoma, reducing production of aqueous humor and increasing outflow. Examples of these agents include apraclonidine (Iopidine), brimonidine (Alphagan), epinephrine, and dipivefrin (Propine), a prodrug that is converted to epinephrine in the eye.

A group of medications known as *β-adrenergic blockers* are also used to treat glaucoma. By blocking β-adrenergic receptor sites, these drugs reduce aqueous fluid production. Systemic side effects of β-adrenergic blockers include decreased heart rate and blood pressure. Timolol maleate (Timoptic) is used to treat chronic open-angle glaucoma. Although its exact mechanism is not yet known, it has been reported to decrease production of aqueous humor and increase outflow. Timolol, in 0.25% or 0.5% ophthalmic solution, is administered in a dosage of one drop in the affected eye twice a day. One dose of timolol may reduce IOP for up to 24 hours. Unlike miotics, no accommodation problems are noted with use. Other β-adrenergic blockers include betaxolol (Betoptic S) 0.25% to 0.5% solution, metipranolol (OptiPranolol) 0.3% solution, and levobunolol (Betagan) 0.25% and 0.5% solution. Side effects include mild ocular irritation, eye pain, headache, decreased corneal sensitivity, transient dry eye syndrome, and blurring of central vision.

? MAKE IT SIMPLE

The names of β-adrenergic blockers usually end in "-olol."

Currently, the first line of glaucoma treatment is a group of drugs known as *PGAs*. These agents significantly reduce IOP by increasing uveoscleral outflow, a different route than the trabecular meshwork. PGAs may be used alone or in combination with other categories of agents, such as carbonic anhydrase inhibitors or β-adrenergic blockers. Bimatoprost (Lumigan 0.03%), latanoprost (Xalatan 0.005%), and travoprost (Travatan 0.005%) are all PGAs.

BOX 10.2 Categories of Medications Used to Treat Glaucoma

Carbonic anhydrase inhibitors
Osmotic diuretics
α-Adrenergic agonists
β-Adrenergic blockers
Cholinergics (miotics)
Prostaglandin analogues

Antiinflammatory Agents

Two categories of antiinflammatory agents are used in ophthalmology: steroids and nonsteroidal antiinflammatory drugs (NSAIDs). Steroids are hormones (see Chapter 8) with a wide range of effects; they are used in ophthalmology to decrease ocular inflammatory response to trauma, to decrease corneal inflammation, to protect the eye from scarring, and postoperatively to decrease swelling. They are contraindicated in the presence of infection because steroids are not bactericidal and tend to hide the symptoms of infection. Steroid preparations are also available in combination with antimicrobial agents. Examples are Tobradex, which combines the antiinflammatory action of dexamethasone 0.1% with the antibiotic tobramycin 0.3%; PRED-G, which is prednisolone in combination with the antibiotic gentamicin; and Maxitrol ointment, which combines the antibiotics neomycin and polymyxin B with dexamethasone. Steroids may be administered through four routes: topical, systemic, periocular, or intravitreal. Common steroids used are betamethasone (Celestone Soluspan), dexamethasone (Maxidex suspension, Decadron ointment and solution), and prednisolone (Inflamase Forte and Inflamase Mild, Pred Forte suspension and solution).

Ocular NSAIDs are used to prevent or treat cystoid macular edema, iritis, and conjunctivitis. They are also used to reduce postoperative inflammation following cataract surgery. Ophthalmic solutions of ketorolac 0.5% (Acular), diclofenac sodium 0.1%, nepafenac 0.1% (Nevanac), and bromfenac 0.09% (Xibrom, Bromday) are available. NSAIDs may also be used to inhibit intraoperative miosis, particularly flurbiprofen 0.03% (Ocufen). Side effects include eye redness, burning, and stinging when administered.

Diagnostic Stains

Staining agents (also referred to as *dyes*) color or mark tissue and are used as diagnostic tools in ophthalmology. These agents are instilled topically to diagnose abnormalities of the cornea and conjunctival epithelium or to locate foreign bodies. Diagnostic stains may also be used to observe the flow of aqueous humor or to demonstrate lacrimal system function. Examples are fluorescein sodium, rose bengal, and lissamine green. They are available as individually wrapped sterile paper strips, which are moistened with a sterile solution and applied to the anterior surface of the eye. Fluorescein sodium (Fluor-I-Strip, Ful-Glo, Fluorescite) is a nontoxic, water-soluble dye that is applied to the cornea or conjunctiva to identify denuded areas of epithelium or foreign bodies. It diagnoses corneal abrasions by staining damaged or diseased corneal tissue bright green, which is best illuminated with the aid of ultraviolet or cobalt light. A foreign body will be surrounded by a green ring.

Fluorescein sodium should not be used with soft contact lenses because they may absorb the dye. Rose bengal and lissamine green in 1% solutions stain devitalized cells better than fluorescein sodium. These agents are primarily used for demarcation of devitalized conjunctival epithelium seen in "dry eye" syndrome (keratoconjunctivitis sicca, or KCS).

Indocyanine green (IC-Green) is a diagnostic dye used for ophthalmic angiography. It is given intravenously outside the surgical setting to visualize the choroidal vascular network. The dye leaks slowly from these choroidal capillaries, which allows vessels in the deeper tissues to be seen (because they are not masked by the dye). As these deeper layers are visualized, tumors and other problems that may not be detectable with regular angiography at this point can be located and treated. Indocyanine green is a fluorescent, sterile, water-soluble dye that comes in powder form and must be reconstituted with sterile water. Once prepared, it must be used within 10 hours. It contains sodium iodide, so caution must be used for patients with iodide allergies.

KEY CONCEPTS

- The eye is a complex sense organ comprising many anatomic structures.
- The blood-eye barrier prevents effective absorption of most systemically administered medications; thus the most common method of administration for ophthalmic medications is topical.
- Enzymes are used to increase anesthetic diffusion through tissue for nerve blocks.
- Irrigating solutions cleanse the operative site and keep the cornea moist, and lubricants are used to protect the cornea for patients undergoing general anesthesia for any category of surgical procedures.
- Viscoelastic agents are used to keep the anterior chamber expanded and to prevent injury to surrounding tissue.
- Miotics constrict the pupil and can be used for short-term treatment of glaucoma and to maintain position of the lens after cataract surgery.
- Mydriatics and cycloplegics dilate the pupil by paralyzing the sphincter muscle of the iris.
- Ophthalmic formulations of antibiotics are used to prevent and treat ocular infections.
- Ophthalmic anesthesia is achieved with topical agents, and when a more extensive area is involved, a retrobulbar or peribulbar block can be administered.
- Glaucoma is a general term referring to a group of conditions characterized by increased IOP.
- There are several categories of medications that are used to treat glaucoma: carbonic anhydrase inhibitors, osmotic diuretics, α-adrenergic agonists, β-adrenergic blockers, cholinergics, and PGAs.
- Steroids and NSAIDs are used as antiinflammatory agents in ophthalmology.
- Steroid preparations are available in combination with antimicrobials.
- Diagnostic agents are used in ophthalmology to observe the flow and amount of fluids and identify lesions or foreign objects.

▌LEARNING THE LANGUAGE (KEY TERMS)

Using your textbook or a standard medical dictionary, look up and write the definitions of each item.

constrict
cycloplegic
dilate
glaucoma
intracameral
IOP
miotic
mydriatic
phacoemulsification

■ REVIEW QUESTIONS

1. Why are enzymes used in ophthalmology?
2. What is the difference between a miotic and a mydriatic?
3. What types of ophthalmic medications are available in ointment form?
4. Which routes are used to administer ophthalmic medications?
5. How do various antiglaucoma agents work?
6. Can you name two ophthalmic antiinflammatory agents?
7. Why are dyes used in ophthalmology?

■ CRITICAL THINKING

1. Obtain a list of ophthalmic medications used at your facility or refer to Fig. 10.4 to answer the following questions.
   a. What local anesthetic medications are used?
   b. What viscoelastic agents are used?
   c. What miotics are used?
   d. What mydriatics and cycloplegics are used?

2. If you are in the clinical portion of your program, do the anesthesia care providers at your facility use ointments to help protect patients' eyes? If yes, what ointments are used?
3. List two ways in which aseptic technique is used to help to prevent infections during ophthalmic surgery.

BIBLIOGRAPHY

Bartlett JD, Jaanus SD: *Clinical ocular pharmacology*, ed 5, St Louis, 2008, Saunders/Elsevier.

Fulcher EM, Fulcher RM, Soto CD: *Pharmacology: principles and applications*, ed 3, St Louis, 2012, Saunders/Elsevier.

Kee JL, Hayes ER, McCuistion LE: *Pharmacology: a patient-centered nursing process approach*, ed 8, St Louis, 2015, Saunders/Elsevier.

Kumar A, Mansour H, Friedman A, et al: *Nanomedicine in drug delivery*, Boca Raton, 2013, CRC Press.

Nikeghbali A, Falavarjani KG, Kheirkhah A, et al: Pupil dilation with intracameral lidocaine during phacoemulsification, *J Cataract Refract Surg* 33(1):101–103, 2007.

Skidmore-Roth L: *Mosby's drug guide for nursing students*, ed 11, St Louis, 2015, Mosby/Elsevier.

INTERNET RESOURCES

Alcaine (Proparacaine Hydrochloride) – Drug Summary: www.pdr.net/drug-summary/alcaine?druglabelid=2828.

American Academy of Ophthalmology, Rapid clinical report: http://eyeanesthesia.org/resources/Documents/Wydase_Study_%2821301%29.pdf.

DailyMed, Tobramycin and dexamethasone: https://dailymed.nlm.nih.gov/dailymed/drugInfo.cfm?setid=d1d48422-8cfc-4e9e-a7f8-56c274d8eb83.

DailyMed, 4% Xylocaine: dailymed.nlm.nih.gov/dailymed/archives/fdaDrugInfo.cfm?archiveid=1647.

Drugs.com, Professionals, FDA PI, Bupivacaine: www.drugs.com/pro/bupivacaine.html.

Drugs.com, Professionals, FDA PI, Neomycin, polymyxin B, gramicidin: www.drugs.com/pro/neomycin-polymyxin-b-gramicidin.html.

Drugs.com, Professionals, FDA PI, Ofloxacin ophthalmic solution: www.drugs.com/pro/ofloxacin-ophthalmic-solution.html.

Drugs.com, Tobradex: www.drugs.com/tobradex.html.

Drugs.com, Zymaxid: www.drugs.com/zymaxid.html; www.allergan.com/assets/pdf/zymaxid_pi.pdf.

Glaucoma Research Foundation, Medications Guide: www.glaucoma.org/treatment/medication-guide.php.

Medline Plus, Drugs, Herbs and Supplements, Diclofenac Ophthalmic: www.nlm.nih.gov/medlineplus/druginfo/meds/a606003.html.

myalcon, B.S.S. PLUS Irrigating Solution: https://professional.myalcon.com/cataract-surgery/cataract-disposables/bss-sterile-irrigation-solution/.

myalcon, OVDS, DuoVisc: https://professional.myalcon.com/cataract-surgery/cataract-disposables/bss-sterile-irrigation-solution/.

National Center for Biotechnology Information, PMC: www.ncbi.nlm.nih.gov/pmc/.

Outpatient Surgery, Surgical Topics, Cataract Pledgets for Pre-Op Eye Dilation: https://www.aorn.org/outpatient-surgery/article/2003-October-mix-own-dilating-cocktail.

Phenylephrine Hydrochloride Ophthalmic: http://dailymed.nlm.nih.gov/dailymed/drugInfo.cfm?setid=21525f9e-f3a2-4871-81bf-90a0686968f0.

Pilocarpaine Hydrochloride Ophthalmic Solution USP. https://dailymed.nlm.nih.gov/dailymed/drugInfo.cfm?setid=84428e9a-f486-44d9-ad93-4ea9069a6787.

RxList, Genoptic: www.rxlist.com/genoptic-drug.htm.

RxList, Gentak: www.rxlist.com/gentak-drug.htm.

RxList, Isopto Carpine Side Effects Center: www.rxlist.com/isopto-carpine-side-effects-drug-center.htm.

RxList, Miochol-E.: www.rxlist.com/miochol-e-drug.htm.

RxList, Neo-Synephrine, Neo-synephrine patient information including side effects: www.rxlist.com/neo-synephrine-drug/patient-images-side-effects.htm.

RxList, VisionBlue, www.rxlist.com/visionblue-drug.htm.

RxList, Xibrom: www.rxlist.com/xibrom-drug.htm.

RxList, Zymar: www.rxlist.com/zymar-drug.htm.

WebMD, Lubrifresh P.M.: Ophthalmic: www.webmd.com/drugs/2/drug-60569/lubrifresh-pm-ophthalmic/details.

WebMD, Prostaglandin analogs for glaucoma: www.webmd.com/eye-health/prostaglandin-analogs-for-glaucoma.

What are nanoparticles? News Medical: www.news-medical.net/health/Nanoparticles-What-are-Nanoparticles.aspx.

KEY TERMS

extracapsular

intracapsular

CATARACT EXTRACTION

The surgical first assistant practicing in ophthalmology must combine the science of pathophysiology and anatomy of the eyes with a current knowledge of the pharmaceutical agents used in the treatment of eye disorders and surgical procedures. Statistics reveal one of the most common eye disorders is cataracts. Cataracts are the leading cause of decreased vision in the United States and, globally, are the leading cause of blindness. Approximately 20.5 million Americans have a cataract interfering with their vision. By the age of 80 years, more than half of all Americans have cataracts. The National Eye Institute (NEI), part of the National Institutes of Health, is the leading federal agency for vision research. The NEI's research into the cause of cataracts includes the effect of sunlight exposure associated with increased risk of developing cataracts, vitamin supplements and their ability to delay the progression of cataracts, and genetic studies for a better understanding of cataract development. With surgical removal being the only treatment, cataract surgery represents the most common and successful of all surgical procedures today. More than 3 million cataracts are removed each year. A cataract is defined as an opacity or clouding of the crystalline lens of the eye. Although most cataracts are age related (senile cataract), they may be associated with other factors. These include trauma, metabolic diseases, congenital factors, prolonged corticosteroid usage, and exposure to radiation or ultraviolet (UV) light. Cataracts may develop in one or both eyes. Each cataract tends to "mature" or develop at a different rate. Therefore, the patient's vision may be affected in one eye more than the other. Because of this differential, only one cataract is removed at a time. Cataract extraction is an intraocular procedure. Cataracts can be extracted by one of two methods: intracapsular or extracapsular. The most commonly performed surgical intervention for cataracts in the United States is extracapsular extraction with phacoemulsification and intraocular lens implant. It is not uncommon for the patient to be referred for surgery before the cataract has fully matured (i.e., produces swelling and opacity of the entire lens). It is safer with less risk of complications and easier removal of the cataract before this stage.

Today's patient undergoing an ophthalmic procedure, such as cataract extraction, is most likely to have surgery performed on an ambulatory (same-day surgery) basis. This means the perioperative team must coordinate patient preparations in a very short period. The success of surgical intervention depends on the skills and knowledge of the team.

> **! CAUTION**
>
> Medications that are intended for use in the eyes are potent, and one medication error can result in permanent blindness. Therefore, all medications and irrigating solutions should be confirmed and labeled immediately.

PREOPERATIVE MEDICATIONS

Refer to Fig. 10.4 for a discussion of the following.

Preoperative medications are extremely important to the outcome of the procedure and to the patient's safety. Conventionally, preoperative preparation for cataract extraction involved the installation of multiple drops. These may include, but are not limited to, a mydriatic for maximum pupil dilation that is essential for lens extraction. A short-acting mydriatic, such as phenylephrine hydrochloride (Neo-Synephrine Ophthalmic) 2.5% or 10%, is preferred. This can be used alone or in combination with a cycloplegic. Tropicamide (Mydriacyl) 1% is a commonly used agent that causes cycloplegia (paralysis of accommodation, inhibits focusing), and it also has a mydriatic effect. Another mydriatic cycloplegic is cyclopentolate hydrochloride 1% (Cyclogyl). A nonsteroidal antiinflammatory agent, such as flurbiprofen sodium (Ocufen) 0.03%, may be used to decrease the inflammatory process and to help to maintain pupil dilation. Then an intravenous (IV) of lactated Ringer's solution is started, and the patient is taken to the surgical room. A topical, broad-spectrum antiinfective agent, such as gatifloxacin (Zymaxid) 0.5% ophthalmic solution, may be used to sterilize the eye to prevent the intraocular introduction of bacteria and is prescribed for the patient postoperatively as well.

> **NOTE:** Ophthalmic medications are sterile when opened. Take care to prevent contamination when handling the container.

When prepping the site, povidone-iodine ophthalmic solution (Betadine Ophthalmic) 5% is used. Usually, one drop is inserted into the operative eye, and it should be left for a minimum of 2 minutes (the doctor's order sheet states, "Leave in eye for 3 minutes"). The eye is closed, and then the area around the site is prepped with regular povidone-iodine prep solution. The eye is then irrigated with balanced salt solution (BSS).

TOPICAL METHOD OF LOCAL ANESTHESIA

The topical method of local anesthesia for cataract extraction has increased in popularity. A combination of anesthetic eye drops, such as tetracaine hydrochloride (Pontocaine) 0.5%, is instilled into the eye and may be enhanced with infiltration anesthetic, such as methylparaben-free (MPF) lidocaine (Xylocaine) 1% or 2%, which is placed into the anterior chamber through the incision. Lidocaine (MPF) 4% ophthalmic drops may also be used before and during the procedure. Another topical anesthetic agent used is proparacaine (Alcaine) 0.5%, which can be instilled into the operative eye 1 hour preoperatively, then every so many minutes (such as 5–10) for a total of three doses, as per surgeon's preference. Notice the doctor's routine order sheet includes tetracaine 0.5% as the local anesthetic, and it is given immediately before the eye prep to decrease the patient's discomfort.

> **NOTE:** The patient may be given only topical local anesthesia to the eye and valium orally to calm nervousness. Therefore, it may not be necessary for the patient to be NPO (*nil per os* [nothing by mouth]); however, most surgeons and anesthesia care providers prefer to have an IV solution started before the procedure.

INTRAOPERATIVE MEDICATIONS

As discussed in the chapter, intraoperative medications may include BSS or BSS PLUS used for intraocular irrigation and to moisten the cornea during procedures. On the doctor's routine orders, 0.3 mL of adrenalin 1:1000 is added to the BSS 500-mL bottle for control of bleeding. Some doctors may add an antibiotic to the solution, such as vancomycin or gentamicin. A viscoelastic agent is injected into the anterior chamber to deepen and maintain the chamber and widen the pupil to facilitate the use of the phacoemulsification. These agents, now known as *ophthalmic viscosurgical devices* (OVDs), include Duovisc. After the placement of the intraocular lens implant, timolol maleate (Timoptic) 0.5% drops may be used to decrease intraocular pressure (IOP). A miotic, such as acetylcholine chloride (Miochol-E), may be used immediately after delivery of the lens to achieve constriction of the iris. Note that gatifloxacin (Zymaxid), which is mentioned in the section on preoperative medications, may be used again. An alternative to this is a subconjunctival injection of a corticosteroid and antibiotic, such as gentamicin sulfate (Garamycin). Some commonly used steroids (antiinflammatory agents) may include prednisone (Pred Forte) and a nonsteroidal antiinflammatory drug (NSAID), such as bromfenac (Bromday). Some surgeons prefer to patch and shield the eye after the procedure.

POSTOPERATIVE MEDICATIONS

The patient is usually released within a few hours postoperatively (unless there are complications). If the patient experiences nausea or vomiting, IV Zofran may be ordered before discharge. Medications sent home with the patient will usually include the same topical antiinflammatory agent (to reduce pain and swelling) and antibiotic agents used during the surgical procedure. The patient is instructed to avoid activities that could increase pressure in the eye and may also be sent home with a medication, such as acetazolamide (Diamox Sequel) 500 mg, taken orally with food, to decrease IOP. Normally the patient is seen the next day for postoperative evaluation.

ADVANCED PRACTICES: REVIEW QUESTIONS

1. Eye medications are considered
   a. Potent
   b. Weak
   c. Short acting
   d. Long acting

2. Multiple dosages of mydriatic drops may be needed to achieve pupil dilation on a patient with
   a. Blue eyes
   b. Brown eyes
   c. Glaucoma
   d. Diabetes

3. Which of the following agents would be used to achieve maximum pupil dilation?
   a. Neo-Synephrine
   b. Miostat
   c. Carbachol
   d. Timoptic
4. Betamethasone is what type of pharmacologic agent?
   a. Antiinflammatory
   b. Antibiotic
   c. Diuretic
   d. Vasoconstrictor

5. A substance used to lubricate and support the shape of the eye during lens extraction, now known as an OVD, is
   a. Healon
   b. Zymar
   c. Diamox Sequel
   d. Neo-Synephrine
6. The ophthalmic condition commonly treated with a miotic drug is
   a. Cataract
   b. Retinal detachment
   c. Pterygium
   d. Glaucoma

ADVANCED PRACTICES: BIBLIOGRAPHY

Fulcher EM, Fulcher RM, Soto CD: *Pharmacology: principles and applications*, ed 3, St Louis, 2012, Saunders/Elsevier.

Kee JL, Hayes ER, McCuistion LE: *Pharmacology: a patient-centered nursing process approach*, ed 8, St Louis, 2015, Saunders/Elsevier.

Skidmore-Roth L: *Mosby's drug guide for nursing students*, ed 11, St Louis, 2015, Mosby/Elsevier.

ADVANCED PRACTICES: INTERNET RESOURCES

National Eye Institute, Health Information, *At a glance: Cataracts*: https://www.nei.nih.gov/learn-about-eye-health/eye-conditions-and-diseases/cataracts.

Senile cataract, Medscape: http://emedicine.medscape.com/article/1210914-overview.

The Free Dictionary, Mature Cataract. http://medical-dictionary.thefreedictionary.com/mature+cataract.

11

Fluids and Irrigation Solutions

OBJECTIVES

After completing this chapter, you should be able to do the following:

1. Define terms and abbreviations related to fluids and irrigation solutions.
2. Briefly describe the physiology of fluid loss in the surgical patient.
3. List fluid electrolytes and their functions crucial to homeostasis.
4. State objectives of parenteral fluid therapy in surgery.
5. List common intravenous (IV) solutions and their purposes in surgery.
6. List and discuss supplies needed for an IV line.
7. Briefly describe the physiology of blood replacement in the surgical patient.
8. List basic functions and types of blood.
9. State average adult circulating volume of blood, hemoglobin, and hematocrit values.
10. List the formed elements present in blood.
11. Briefly describe antigen-antibody interactions in blood types.
12. List and describe indications for blood replacement in the surgical patient.
13. List available options for blood replacement and discuss autologous and homologous blood donation.
14. Describe components of whole blood used for replacement.
15. Describe the process of intraoperative autotransfusion.
16. List and describe volume expander solutions used in surgery.
17. Discuss hetastarch and hematopoietic growth factors.
18. List and describe oxygen therapeutics used in clinical trials.
19. Describe the procedure for blood replacement in surgery using donor blood from the blood bank.
20. List and describe fluids used as irrigation solutions in surgery.
21. List and describe supplies and equipment used for irrigation.

OUTLINE

One of the primary goals of the surgical team is to maintain the patient in as stable a physiologic state as possible. Because fluids are essential to survival, blood and fluid replacement are two of the most common means used in surgery to assist in maintaining homeostasis. Blood loss may be caused by trauma or by the surgical procedure itself. The volume of blood lost must be carefully assessed and replaced if significant. The surgical patient's fluid and electrolyte balance must also be assessed and monitored. Most surgical patients will have preoperative fluid and food restrictions before surgery, so fluid replacement is usually indicated. This is accomplished by administering intravenous (IV) fluids and medications. IV means administration of fluids or medications through a vein. There are three basic classifications of IV fluids: crystalloids (with or without added electrolytes) as IV solutions and some as volume expanders, colloids as volume expanders, and blood/blood products. IV fluids may be ordered for replacement of lost fluids, to maintain fluid and electrolyte balance, or to administer IV medications. *Replacement fluids* are often ordered to replenish losses caused by hemorrhage (in surgery) or vomiting and diarrhea (in the medical setting). *Maintenance fluids* sustain normal fluid and electrolyte balance. In addition, fluids are administered topically to irrigate body tissues during surgical procedures. These irrigation solutions must be physiologically acceptable to tissues, while providing visualization, removing blood and debris, and adding medications to the surgical site. The surgical technologist will observe blood or fluid loss and replacement and assist with irrigation during surgical procedures.

FLUID AND ELECTROLYTE MANAGEMENT

Physiology Review

In a healthy adult, approximately 60% of the total body weight is made up of fluids, electrolytes, and nonelectrolytes. Fluids are distributed into two distinct compartments: intracellular fluid (ICF) and extracellular fluid (ECF).

The major electrolytes break down into sodium (Na^+), chloride (Cl^-), potassium (K^+), calcium (Ca^{2+}), phosphate (HPO_4^{2-}), and magnesium (Mg^{2+}) ions. Other electrolytes are bicarbonate (HCO_3^-), sulfate (SO_4^{2-}), and carbonic acid (H_2CO_3). The nonelectrolytes present in normal body fluid are glucose, urea, and creatinine. Electrolytes have three main purposes in homeostasis: controlling the volume of body water by osmotic pressure, maintaining the acid-base balance, and serving as essential minerals. See Table 11.1 for a list of major electrolytes and functions. Alteration of normal concentrations of these elements can result in serious and possibly life-threatening complications.

Chloride is the most abundant anion in ECF and helps to regulate osmotic pressure between intracellular and extracellular spaces. Magnesium plays an important part in the sodium-potassium pump and also activates enzymes required to break down adenosine triphosphate (ATP). Phosphate is stored in teeth and bone and is released when needed. Phosphate is a necessary element in the formation of deoxyribonucleic acid and ribonucleic acid, in synthesis of ATP, and in buffering of acid-base reactions.

Two electrolytes with particular importance to surgery are calcium and potassium. Calcium is the most abundant mineral in the body and necessary for the formation and function of bones and teeth. Calcium is also involved in the blood-clotting process, neurotransmitter release, muscle contraction, and cardiac function. Too much calcium (hypercalcemia) or too little calcium (hypocalcemia) can cause the heart to beat irregularly (cardiac arrhythmias), muscle spasms, and weak heartbeats. Normal calcium levels are 8.9 to 10.2 mg/dL. Potassium is the major intracellular cation and serves several critical functions in homeostasis. Potassium helps to maintain fluid volume in cells, controls pH, and is vital in the transmission of nerve impulses. Either too much potassium (hyperkalemia) or too little potassium (hypokalemia) causes serious metabolic problems. Because potassium is critical to neuromuscular function, which includes the heart, cardiac arrhythmias are often seen in patients with potassium imbalances. Many elderly patients may be taking diuretics (see Chapter 7) and can easily become hypokalemic, so a potassium level must be determined on all surgical patients taking diuretics. Normal potassium levels are 3.5 to 5 mEq/L. A potassium or calcium imbalance is of special concern in surgical patients because of increased risk of cardiac arrhythmias or arrest when a general anesthetic is administered. Elective surgery may be postponed until potassium and calcium levels have been restored to a safe range.

> **NOTE:** Potassium is an electrolyte that can be added at higher concentrations in premixed IV solutions or added to the IV solution before infusion preoperatively as potassium chloride.

? MAKE IT SIMPLE

Remember to use your medical terminology skills to understand the prefixes "hyper-" and "hypo-" (as described in Chapter 8), with "hyper-" meaning excessive or above normal and "hypo-" meaning below or less than normal.

! CAUTION

IV potassium can cause severe and potentially fatal cardiac rhythm disturbances. Thus patients should be carefully monitored, and, when possible, oral potassium in liquid, tablet, or capsule form is preferable.

Sodium controls distribution of water in the body and maintains fluid and electrolyte balance. Sodium is the principal cation of ECF and vital to neuromuscular function. Normal sodium levels are 135 to 145 mEq/L. If there is too much sodium in the body, the condition is called *hypernatremia*. This condition frequently results from a relative water loss, and the cells become dehydrated. If there is too little, it is called *hyponatremia*. This results from excessive water ingestion or retention, or inadequate sodium intake.

Intravenous Fluids

Appropriate fluid and electrolyte management is an integral component of surgical patient care, both for maintaining homeostasis and for positive surgical outcomes. Nearly every surgical patient will receive IV fluids. An IV drip is "started" on the patient for two purposes: to establish direct access to the circulatory system for medication administration, and to administer parenteral

Electrolyte	Chemical Symbol	Function
Sodium	Na^+	Osmotic pressure, nerve impulse transmission
Chloride	Cl^-	Osmotic pressure, aids digestion, acid-base balance
Potassium	K^+	Osmotic pressure, acid-base balance, nerve impulse transmission, regulates heartbeat, muscle function
Calcium	Ca^{2+}	Bone growth and development, blood coagulation, enzyme activity, neuromuscular function
Magnesium	Mg^{2+}	Enzyme action in synthesis of ATP, muscle contraction, protein synthesis, nerve function
Phosphate	HPO_4^{2-}, $H_2PO_4^-$	Acid-base balance
Bicarbonate	HCO_3^-	Acid-base balance
Sulfate	SO_4^{2-}	Acid-base balance
Carbonic acid	$H_2CO_3^-$	Acid-base balance

TABLE 11.1   Major Electrolytes and Functions

ATP, Adenosine triphosphate.

fluids. IV fluids may be used at a slow rate (e.g., 30 mL/h on an adult) to keep the vein open. Parenteral fluid therapy has three objectives: to maintain daily fluid requirements, to restore previous losses, and to replace current losses. To accomplish these objectives, several fluids are available and used for specific purposes. The IV fluids most commonly used in the surgical setting are called *crystalloids*. These are solutions composed mainly of water with dissolved electrolytes, dextrose solutions, and multiple electrolyte solutions. The names of IV solutions are abbreviated on their bags and containers. The abbreviation letters indicate the components of the solution, and the numbers indicate the strength or concentration of the components in the solution. Numbers are often written as subscripts to the letters. For example, an IV solution of D5W indicates dextrose (D) is 5% of the concentration in water (W) (Table 11.2).

QUICK QUESTION

Using the information in the previous paragraph, what is the IV solution described as D10W?

Common Intravenous Fluids Administered in Surgery

Sodium chloride (NaCl) in a 0.9% solution (isotonic) is the agent of choice for fluid replacement or simple hydration and one of the most common IV fluids used in surgery. It is considered isotonic, which means its concentration of dissolved particles is similar to that of plasma and causes no shift in cell fluids. Sodium chloride is packaged in 50-, 100-, 250-, 500- and 1000-mL bags for IV administration. It comes in a variety of concentrations (the amount of sodium chloride in solution), which includes 0.225%, 0.33%, 0.45%, 0.9%, 3%, and 5% (Fig. 11.1). Sodium chloride is used when chloride loss is greater than or equal to sodium loss, for treatment of metabolic acidosis (excess acid in body fluids) in the presence of fluid loss, and to replenish lost sodium. Sodium chloride is the IV fluid used when transfusing blood products because it does not hemolyze (fill with fluid and rupture) blood cells.

TECH TIP

Normal saline (NS) and physiological saline are common terms for 0.9% sodium chloride. The concentration of sodium chloride in NS is 0.9 g per 100 mL of solution. Another common IV saline concentration is 0.45% sodium chloride. Note that 0.45% is one half the strength of 0.9% NaCl and it is sometimes written as ½ NS (for one-half NS). Other saline concentrations are 0.33% NaCl or ⅓ NS, and 0.225% NaCl or ¼ NS.

MAKE IT SIMPLE

NS is 0.9% sodium chloride. Other concentrations of sodium chloride are either hypertonic or hypotonic, and so are not considered NS.

Dextrose (D) is used in patients who require an easily metabolized source of calories: it is a natural sugar found in the body and provides energy for cellular activity. Dextrose is available in

TABLE 11.2 Common Intravenous Fluid Components

Component	Abbreviation
Dextrose	D
Lactated Ringer's (or Ringer's lactate)	LR (or RL)
Normal saline (0.9%)	NS
Saline	S
Sodium chloride	NaCl
Water	W

various concentrations in water and in NS. Dextrose in water is used to hydrate the surgical patient, spare body protein, and enhance liver function. Because the trauma and stress of surgery cause some water and sodium retention, intraoperative IV therapy often involves administration of limited amounts of dextrose 5% in water (D5W). Dextrose in water is also prepared in 2.5%, 10%, 20%, 25%, 30%, 40%, 50%, 60%, and 70% solutions.

The percentage of solution determines the clinical use of dextrose. Lower concentrations (<10%) are used for peripheral hydrations, providing calories, and assessing kidney function (if patients do not need electrolyte replacement). In higher concentrations, dextrose is used for reversing hypoglycemia, providing calories when less fluid is indicated, and with amino acids for total parenteral nutrition.

Dextrose is frequently used in saline solutions (e.g., 5% in NS [D5NS]). It is packaged in bags of 250, 500, and 1000 mL. This fluid is used for temporary treatment of circulatory insufficiency and shock caused by hypovolemia (low circulating blood volume), in the absence of a plasma extender, and for early treatment with plasma for loss of fluid caused by burns. Dextrose 10% in NS (D10NS) is supplied in 500- and 1000-mL bags and is used to replenish nutrients and electrolytes.

It should be noted that dextrose solutions given intravenously increase insulin and oral hypoglycemic requirements for the diabetic patient. Dextrose is not used in conjunction with transfusion of blood products because it causes hemolysis (breaking down) of red blood cells (RBCs).

Ionosol B (MB and T) and 5% dextrose injection are maintenance and replacement electrolyte solutions. They provide a source of water, electrolytes, and carbohydrates to cover hydration, insensible water loss, and urinary excretion. Ionosol comes packaged in 500- and 1000-mL plastic bags; Ionosol MB comes in 250- and 500-mL sizes, and Ionosol T comes in 500- and 1000-mL sizes.

Lactated Ringer's (LR), or Ringer's lactate, is a physiological salt solution used to replenish the patient's electrolytes and for rehydration to stimulate renal activity. It is the other most common IV fluid used in surgery (Fig. 11.2). LR solution, which is used to replace fluid lost from burns or severe diarrhea, closely resembles the composition of ECF. It should not be used in patients with the inability to metabolize lactate (found in the solution). Patients at high risk are those with liver disease, Addison's disease (see Insight 8.4), severe pH imbalances, shock, or cardiac failure. Hartmann's solution is very similar

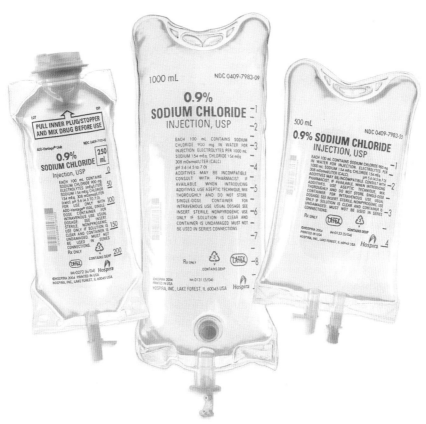

Fig. 11.1 Normal saline (0.9% sodium chloride) intravenous solutions.

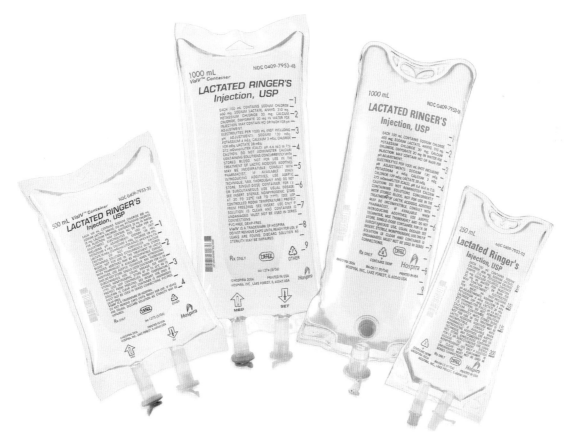

Fig. 11.2 Lactated Ringer's intravenous solutions.

to LR (except for its ionic concentration) and is often referred to as such.

Plasma-Lyte and Isolyte E are electrolyte-balanced solutions compatible with the pH of blood. They are used to treat the massive loss of water and electrolytes seen in uncontrolled vomiting or diarrhea. The composition of these solutions is similar to the plasma portion of blood.

Normosol-R is an isotonic solution with electrolytes in water used for parenteral replacement of acute losses of ECF volume. These losses could result from surgery, burns, trauma, or shock. It does not disturb normal electrolyte relationships and may be used as an adjunct to increase circulatory volume in patients with moderate blood loss. Normosol-R does not cause hemolysis of blood, so it can be used as a priming solution for the blood infusion set. It comes in 500- and 1000-mL containers. See Table 11.3 for a summary of IV fluids.

Intravenous Equipment and Supplies

An IV line is established in nearly all surgical patients before surgery. A flexible catheter, or angiocatheter (Fig. 11.3), is inserted via a needle into a vein, usually in the patient's hand

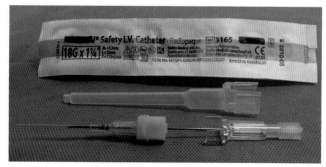

Fig. 11.3 Intravenous catheter.

or forearm. The needle is removed, leaving the catheter in the vein where it is taped securely in place. The primary IV tubing connects to the hub of the IV catheter, and the other end is connected to a container of IV solution. This tubing contains a drip chamber, injection port, and roller clamp (Fig. 11.4). Fluids and most of the medications needed during surgery are administered through the IV line. A secondary IV tubing may be used with the primary tubing when giving medications via

TABLE 11.3	**Intravenous Fluids Comparison**		
Solution	**Type**	**Uses**	**Special Considerations**
0.9% sodium chloride	Isotonic Crystalloid	Fluid loss, dehydration, hyponatremia, metabolic acidosis	Can lead to fluid overload, use with caution in patients with heart failure or edema. Often used in surgery and for blood administration
0.45% sodium chloride	Hypotonic Crystalloid	Water replacement, sodium and chloride depletion, gastric fluid loss	May cause CV collapse or increased intracranial pressure, do not use with liver disease, trauma, burns
3%, 5% normal saline	Hypertonic	Hyponatremia in critical situations, volume expander	Raises sodium levels, can cause intravascular fluid overload and PE
Lactated Ringer's or Ringer's lactate (LR or RL)	Isotonic	Dehydration, burns, lower GI fluid loss, acute blood loss, hypovolemia caused by third space shifting	Contains K+, do not use with renal failure patients, do not use with liver disease. Often used in surgery
Dextrose 5% in water (D5W)	Isotonic in bag, physiologically hypotonic*	Increase total fluid volume, hypernatremia, replace Na, Cl, and calories, enhance liver function	Not to be used in resuscitation, can cause hyperglycemia, can cause fluid overload in patients with cardiac or renal disease, cannot use with blood administration
Dextrose 5% in normal saline (D5NS)	Hypertonic	Shock if plasma expanders not available, Addisonian crisis, with plasma for burn treatment	Not to be used in patients with cardiac or renal disease, watch for fluid volume overload
Dextrose 5% in ½ normal saline	Hypertonic	Later in DKA treatment	Do not use when blood glucose falls below 250 mg/dL, use for daily maintenance of body fluids and nutrition
Dextrose 10% in water (D10W)	Hypertonic	Water replacement, conditions where some glucose is required with nutrition	Monitor blood sugar levels
Plasma-Lyte	Isotonic	Dehydration, sodium depletion	Caution with use in patients with cardiac or liver disease, risk of volume overload
Ionosol MB and 5% dextrose	Hypotonic	Dehydration, acidosis, replace electrolytes	Caution with use in patients with hyperkalemia, renal disease, congestive heart failure
Normosol-R	Isotonic	Replacement of extracellular fluid (acute) losses, replace electrolytes	Caution with use in patients with renal disease, congestive heart failure

*For explanations on isotonic, hypertonic, and hypotonic solutions, see the section on advanced practices of this chapter.
Physiologically hypotonic = the dextrose is quickly metabolized and only water remains, making it a hypotonic fluid.
Cl, Chloride; *CV*, cardiovascular; *DKA*, diabetic ketoacidosis treatment; *GI*, gastrointestinal; *K+*, potassium; *Na*, sodium; *NaCl*, sodium chloride; *PE*, pulmonary edema.

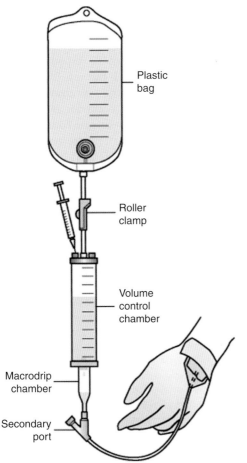

Fig. 11.4 Intravenous tubing. (From Edmunds MW: *Introduction to clinical pharmacology*, ed 7, St Louis, 2012, Elsevier.)

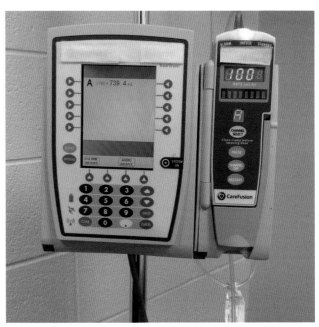

Fig. 11.5 Electronic intravenous infusion pump and controller.

"piggyback." The secondary tubing is shorter and also contains a drip chamber and roller clamp. In this setup, the secondary tubing is hung higher on the IV pole than the primary IV, so that the secondary medication infuses first. Secondary lines are used with antibiotics. At times the IV tubing may be placed in an electronic infusion pump system (Fig. 11.5).

⚡ TECH TIP

Make sure the IV tubing does not become kinked or compromised during patient positioning or during the procedure. IV fluids must be able to run at the required rate. Even from the position of scrubbed surgical technologist, you can observe the drip chamber to see that the IV fluid is moving.

BLOOD REPLACEMENT

Physiology Review

Blood is a fluid connective tissue that performs several critical functions in maintaining homeostasis. It is used to transport oxygen, nutrients, wastes, hormones, and enzymes throughout the body. Blood also maintains the body's acid-base balance (pH), its temperature, and its water content. The immune response is carried through the circulatory system as well.

Blood is so crucial to maintaining life processes that it has a self-protection mechanism—clotting—to prevent harmful loss.

Blood volume varies with the patient's body size, amount of adipose tissue, and changes in fluid and electrolyte concentrations. In an average adult, though, the circulating blood volume is approximately 70 mL/kg of body mass. For the body to be kept functioning normally, this blood volume should be maintained. Some surgical patients are at high risk of substantial blood loss during surgery; these include patients needing cardiac and peripheral vascular procedures or those with trauma. The goal of blood replacement in scheduled surgical procedures is to maintain the circulating volume of blood, and its oxygen-carrying capacity.

Blood consists of two main components: formed elements (approximately 45%) and fluid called *plasma* (approximately 55%). The formed elements include erythrocytes (RBCs), leukocytes (white blood cells [WBCs]), and platelets. Erythrocytes make up more than 99% of the body's formed elements and contain hemoglobin (Hgb), a protein responsible for transport of oxygen and carbon dioxide between the lungs and the cells. Leukocytes provide protection against foreign microbes by phagocytosis and antibody production. Platelets mediate the clotting process.

Most surgical patients undergo laboratory tests to determine the amount of Hgb present in their blood. A normal Hgb level is 12 to 16 g/100 mL of blood in adult females and 14 to 18 g/100 mL in adult males. A low Hgb level indicates reduced oxygen-carrying capacity. Because oxygen levels must be optimum during administration of general anesthesia, elective surgery may be canceled if the Hgb dips below normal levels. Another important measure of the oxygen-carrying capacity of the blood is hematocrit. Hematocrit is the volume of erythrocytes in a given volume of blood and is expressed as a percentage. Normal hematocrit levels range from 35% to 52%, varying by age and sex (Table 11.4).

In cases of known or anticipated blood loss, the patient's blood must be typed and crossmatched to administer compatible donor blood. The blood type is determined by proteins called *antigens* present on the surface of RBCs. Blood type is inherited, and there are many types and groupings based on the antigens present on the RBCs. The major groupings of concern in surgery are ABO and Rh. Patients may be type A, B, AB, or O. Type A blood contains the A antigen, type B has the B antigen, type AB contains both, and type O blood has neither. Blood is also designated as Rh positive (Rh antigen present) or Rh negative (no Rh antigen present). People also have the corresponding antibody present in their plasma; that is, type A has anti-B, type B has anti-A, type O has both anti-A and anti-B, and type AB has neither (Fig. 11.6). If type A blood is administered to a type B patient, the recipient's antibodies will attack the donor RBCs, causing a potentially fatal transfusion reaction (Insight 11.1). A blood crossmatch is performed to determine compatibility between the donor and the recipient. A sample of donor RBCs is mixed with the recipient's serum, and the results are examined to determine compatibility. See Tables 11.5 and 11.6 for more information on blood types.

Rho(D) immune globulin (RhoGAM) is a medication used to treat possible blood compatibility reactions. It is an injectable blood product manufactured from human plasma that contains anti-D to suppress the immune response of a Rh-negative mother to a Rh-positive fetus. If the anti-Rh antibody is given right after delivery, it blocks the sensitization of the mother and prevents Rh disease from occurring in the woman's next Rh-positive pregnancy. This Rh disease could result in miscarriage in subsequent pregnancies if not treated. Rho(D) immune globulin is for intramuscular injection only and is routinely given to Rh-negative mothers who deliver Rh-positive babies. (See Insight 8.2 for more information of medications used in labor and delivery.)

TABLE 11.4   Blood Values

Parameter	Females	Males
Circulating blood volume	4–5 L (4.2–5.3 qt)	5–6 L (5.3–6.4 qt)
Hemoglobin	12–16 g/100 mL	14–18 g/100 mL
Hematocrit	35%–46%	40%–52%
RBCs	4.2–5.4 million cells per mcL	4.7–6.1 million cells per mcL
Platelets	150,000–4 million/mm³	150,000–4 million/mm³

These values vary slightly depending on the source.
RBC, Red blood cell.

> **INSIGHT 11.1   Hemolytic Transfusion Reaction**
>
> If blood is not properly typed and matched before being transfused, a serious and sometimes fatal reaction, called *hemolytic transfusion reaction* or *hemolytic anemia,* can occur. This can result from incompatible blood types or Rh factors and must be treated immediately. If the patient is under general anesthesia, the symptoms are a generalized diffuse blood loss, red-colored urine, and lowered blood oxygen saturation levels (because the red blood cells are being destroyed by the patient's immune system). If any suspicious reactions occur during blood transfusion, the following steps should be taken:
> 1. Stop the transfusion and maintain venous access.
> 2. Report immediately to the surgeon and the blood bank.
> 3. Send a sample of the patient's blood to the blood bank (to rule out a mismatch).
> 4. Return any unused portion of the blood unit and blood tubing to the blood bank.
> 5. Begin appropriate medication therapy, which usually includes steroids and prophylactic measures to reduce risk of kidney failure, as soon as possible.
> 6. Send urine samples to the laboratory to check for kidney function.
>
> In some cases, the patient may have to undergo renal dialysis to rid the system of mismatched blood.

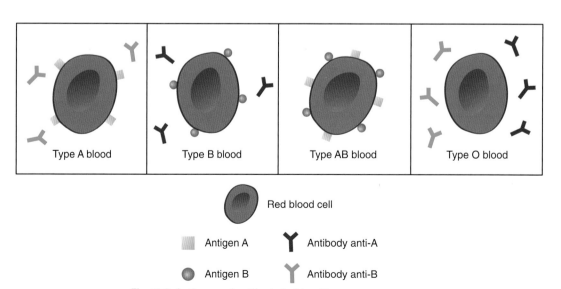

Red blood cell

Antigen A   Antibody anti-A

Antigen B   Antibody anti-B

Fig. 11.6 Antigen and antibody in blood types.

TABLE 11.5 Blood Types—Percentage in Populations

Blood Type	Caucasian (%)	African American (%)	Hispanic (%)	Asian (%)
O+	37	47	53	39
O-	8	4	4	1
A+	33	24	29	27
A-	7	2	2	0.5
B+	9	18	9	25
B-	2	1	1	0.4
AB+	3	4	2	7
AB-	1	0.3	0.2	0.1

The Rh+ factor indicates the presence of Rh surface antigen that is also referred to as the *D antigen*.
Data from the American Red Cross.

TABLE 11.6 Blood Types—Donor

Your Blood Type	Patients Who Can Receive Your Red Blood Cells	Patients Who Can Receive Your Plasma
O+	O+, A+, B+, AB+	O+, O-
O-	All blood types	O+, O-
A+	A+, AB+	A+, A-, O+, O-
A-	A+, A-, AB+, AB-	A+, A-, O+, O-
B+	B+, AB+	B+, B-, O+, O-
B-	B+, B-, AB+, AB-	B+, B-, O+, O-
AB+	AB+	All blood types
AB-	AB+, AB-	All blood types

Data from the American Red Cross.

? QUICK QUESTION

What blood type is considered the "universal donor"? Are you a universal donor?

Indications for Blood Replacement

The first fully recorded blood transfusion occurred in France in 1667, when a 15-year-old male was given lamb's blood. Amazingly, the boy did not die, perhaps because of the small amount of blood he received. This method was popular for a time until transfusion reactions were recognized and reported. France banned transfusions in 1670, and soon other countries followed. Blood transfusions did not progress for 150 years. Dr. James Blundell performed many transfusions in the early 19th century (approximately half were successful), developed instruments for the process, and published his results. Since the discovery that all human blood is not alike in 1901 by Karl Landsteiner, many advances have been made in blood transfusion therapy. Currently, blood transfusions are implemented with the knowledge that blood must be compatible in type and Rh factor. If unmatched blood is given, blood clumping, or agglutination, will occur.

The most common indication for blood replacement in surgery is hypovolemia (low circulating blood volume), seen most frequently in trauma and vascular procedures. When patients lose a certain amount of blood, they experience this syndrome, which is also called *hemorrhagic* or *circulatory shock*. The result is decreased oxygen supplied to vital organs, increased heart rate, and decreased cardiac output. This can be further complicated by the anesthetic, which may enhance the effects of hemorrhage. Other indications for blood replacement include restoration of the oxygen-carrying capacity, as seen in anemic patients or those with blood diseases, and to maintain clotting properties, as needed in patients with hemophilia.

Trauma patients may be in critical need of blood to sustain vital functions. If immediate replacement is required, and the patient's blood type is known, type-specific RBCs (packed cells) only may be administered along with fluid volume support. If the patient's blood type is unknown, O-negative blood may be administered. In either case, the surgeon must document the need for blood release without compatibility testing.

Options for Blood Replacement

There are several options available to replace blood loss in surgery; these include use of donor blood (homologous donation), which includes donor blood from friends or family for a specific patient (*directed* or *designated* donation), patients donating their own blood before surgery (autologous donation), a patient's own blood collected and used during or after surgery (autotransfusion), or use of volume expanders. Each blood replacement option has indications, advantages, and disadvantages. Some of these options may not be feasible in certain cases, depending on the situation.

Homologous Donation

A common method of blood replacement is the use of donor, or homologous, blood (this is also referred to as *allogenic blood*) (Fig. 11.7). A blood bank is responsible for collecting, processing, and releasing donor blood for use. All blood donors go through careful screening of their medical history, and those who are at risk of transmitting an infectious disease are not allowed to donate. All donor blood is tested for any signs of syphilis, hepatitis, or exposure to human immunodeficiency virus (HIV) before it is given to a patient. However, it is still possible for donor blood to present some risk of transmission of bloodborne pathogens.

Blood is separated during processing into components and then administered to treat specific needs. Component replacement therapy is an effective and efficient use of limited resources because a unit of donor whole blood separated into components can be used to treat several patients.

Whole Blood

The term *whole blood* indicates that the blood composition has not been broken down or altered. It consists of RBCs, plasma (which contains plasma proteins), stable clotting factors, and

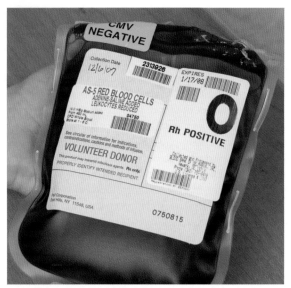

Fig. 11.7 Unit of blood with label. (From Perry AG, Potter PA, Ostendorf W: *Clinical nursing skills and techniques*, ed 8, St Louis, 2014, Elsevier.)

anticoagulants. Whole, fresh blood is rarely used for transfusion today. It is indicated only in cases of acute, massive blood loss that requires the oxygen-carrying properties of RBCs and the volume expansion provided by plasma. It is also a source of proteins and of some coagulation factors. A unit of whole blood has a volume of 500 mL/unit and raises an anemic adult's Hgb from 0.5 to 1 g/dL.

> **NOTE:** In some situations involving massive trauma and severe blood loss, the replacement of blood and fluids may be as a "1:1:1 ratio." This signifies giving equal amounts (units) of RBCs/plasma/platelets.

Packed red blood cells. Most transfusions of donor blood in surgery involve the use of packed RBCs (PRBCs), also called *packed cells*. The use of PRBCs with a synthetic volume expander has proven to be as effective as whole blood, while reducing the risks of whole blood transfusion reactions. They contain Hgb, which transports oxygen to tissues. Packed cells are obtained by removing approximately 200 mL of plasma and most of the platelets from 1 unit (500 mL) of whole blood. The infusion of PRBCs helps to restore the oxygen-carrying capacity of the patient's own circulatory system. Blood typing and cross-matching (ABO and Rh) is required. The approximate volume of one unit of PRBCs is 350 mL/unit; it can raise the patient's Hgb by 1 g/dL and the hematocrit by approximately 3%. IV fluids are administered concurrently to restore circulating volume, if needed.

Plasma. Plasma may be administered when clotting factors are needed in addition to circulating volume. This need is frequently seen when several units of blood have been replaced because the clotting factors have been removed from donor blood. Plasma is not used for volume expansion alone because albumin and synthetic expanders are as effective and eliminate the risk of transmission of bloodborne diseases. Plasma is stored as fresh frozen plasma to preserve clotting factors and thawed in

a water bath before use. It must be used within 6 hours of thawing, and blood typing is required for administration.

Platelets. Platelets are administered in surgery when large amounts of donor blood have been used to replace the patient's circulating volume. Because the platelets have been removed from donor blood, the result of massive transfusions may be an inability of the patient's circulatory system to clot properly. Platelets are infused to restore a more normal clotting process and to help to repair damaged blood vessels. They may also be administered prophylactically in patients who have low platelet counts, such as those receiving chemotherapy or radiation therapy or with leukemia. At room temperature, platelets must be continually gently agitated to prevent clumping. A unit of platelets is defined as the amount separated from a unit of whole blood. They do not have a blood type, so can be received from any qualified donor (or donors). Platelet-rich plasma, growth factors obtained from platelet concentrate, can be obtained from blood plasma for wound healing (Insight 11.2).

Cryoprecipitate. Cryoprecipitate is a plasma component used in the treatment of bleeding caused by hemophilia A, von Willebrand disease, disseminated intravascular coagulation, and lack of factor XIII. Cryoprecipitate may be administered in surgery when massive amounts of blood have been replaced, severely impacting the normal coagulation process. It is usually given in 4 to 6 unit pools at a time rather than a single unit, and blood typing is not required.

Autologous Donation

Patients scheduled for elective surgical procedures in which blood loss is anticipated, such as a total hip replacement, may be allowed to donate their own blood. This can be done up to 4 days before surgery, although a much longer period of time, such as 1 month, is preferred. This process is called *autologous transfusion* and usually involves two units of blood. Most patients can safely donate two units of whole blood over a

---

INSIGHT 11.2   Platelet-Rich Plasma for Wound Healing

From a small volume of the patient's own blood, surgeons can extract a platelet concentrate suspended in plasma that contains various growth factors (cytokines). When this platelet concentrate is reintroduced into the wound, it releases growth factors that recruit and increase the reparative cells. Thus it has the potential to greatly speed up the body's natural healing response in both soft and hard tissues. This extraction of platelet-rich plasma (PRP) is the first practical application of tissue engineering. It is used for wound healing in surgery, treatment of tendonitis, cartilage repair, cardiac care, spinal disc regeneration, and dental care. It is currently being considered for skin rejuvenation. One company, Zimmer Biomet, has developed a GPS III Platelet Concentrate System with an automated platelet collection process. The patient's blood is placed in the collection device, which is then placed within a centrifuge and spun for 15 minutes. The blood is separated into platelet-poor plasma, PRP, and red blood cells. Then the PRP is collected and placed into the wound. Another company, ConMed, has the Cascade Autologous Platelet System. This is also a kit to collect the patient's blood for producing a platelet-rich fibrin matrix that can be delivered arthroscopically and sutured into the wound. The growth factors are continually released over a 7-day period.

period of weeks just before their scheduled procedure, possibly eliminating the need for donor blood. The patient's blood is collected, processed, stored, and released for surgery by the blood bank. Patients often choose this option, if available, to protect themselves from potential bloodborne disease transmission. However, some medical conditions may make autologous donation unsafe, so not all patients are eligible.

Autotransfusion

Another form of autologous donation used intraoperatively and postoperatively is called *autotransfusion*. Autotransfusion involves the collection, processing, and reinfusing of the patient's own blood during the surgical procedure using "cell-saver" technology with little damage to the RBCs (Fig. 11.8). There are several cell-saver machines available. Some are designed specifically for emergency procedures when rapid infusion is required. Blood can be collected in a suction-type device or via bloody sponges drained into a sterile basin of saline, then aspirated into the machine. However, blood that has been exposed to collagen hemostatic agents and some medications (such as certain antibiotics) cannot be used because clotting in the machine may occur. Another method of autotransfusion, also referred to as *intraoperative autologous transfusion*, is to use a sterile blood collection and suction canister to collect the patient's blood from the operative field. When the canister is filled, the blood is washed in a red cell washer (usually found in the blood bank) and reinfused. In this method, the blood is sent out of the surgical department to be washed, and so there is time lost before reinfusion.

Autotransfusion is performed during open heart surgery, vascular procedures, major orthopedic procedures, and some trauma procedures, such as splenectomy. Autotransfusion has several advantages over the use of donor blood, including immediate replacement of blood loss without the potential for transfusion reaction or delay for blood typing and crossmatching, and no risk of transmission of bloodborne pathogens. In addition, patients with religious objections to donated blood often do not object to autotransfusion. Autotransfusion is not suitable for all patients because some trauma patients may have lost so much blood already that there is little volume left to salvage. A disadvantage of autotransfusion is that it cannot be used in the presence of cancer cells, infection, or gross contamination (e.g., open gastrointestinal tract). Autotransfusion is generally contraindicated during cesarean section because of the presence of amniotic fluid. Autotransfusion is commonplace in most operating rooms currently and is an effective option for replacement of blood lost during certain surgical procedures.

Volume Expanders

Volume expanders are used to increase the total volume of body fluid when hypovolemia occurs. By doing so, remaining RBCs can continue to oxygenate body tissues. One category is crystalloids, solutions that contain salts (electrolytes) and/or sugars. These include IV solutions, such as LR solution, NS, and hypertonic saline. Another category of volume expanders is *colloids*, solutions that contain proteins or other substances with large molecules that increase osmolarity and do not dissolve in solution. In other words, they are osmotically active and draw fluid from ECF compartments into blood plasma, increasing blood volume. Volume expanders can be used when donated blood or autotransfusion is not immediately available for emergency procedures. There are several colloid volume expanders available.

Albumin and plasma protein fraction (PPF) are plasma derivatives (and so are considered blood products) used to provide volume expansion when crystalloid solutions, such as saline and dextrose, are not adequate (as in massive hemorrhage). They are also used in the treatment of hypovolemic shock, as seen in burn patients who have lost fluid volume but not RBCs. Albumin is available in concentrations of 5%, which is equal to plasma, or as a concentrated 25% in sodium chloride solution. PPF is available as a 5% solution.

Dextran expands plasma volume by drawing fluid from the interstitial space to the intravascular fluid space. It is formed by the action of a bacterium and has osmotic properties but not oxygen-carrying capacity. Packaged as dextran 40, it is used prophylactically for thrombosis and embolism. It improves microcirculation independent of basic volume expansion and minimizes the changes that occur in blood viscosity that accompany shock. Dextran 70 or 75 is used to expand plasma volume in impending hypovolemic shock, as caused by hemorrhage, burns, or trauma.

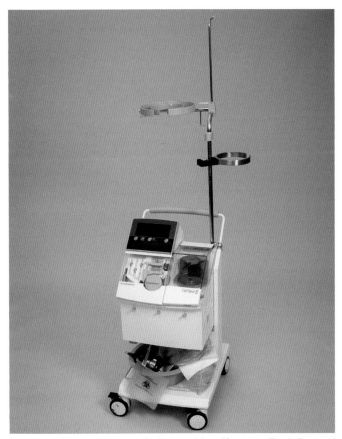

Fig. 11.8 Cell-saver/autotransfusion machine. (Courtesy Frank Pronesti T/A heirloomstudio.com.)

Hetastarch

Hetastarch (Hextend, Voluven) is also a synthetic used for its osmotic properties. It has no oxygen-carrying capacity but is needed to circulate RBCs, which carry oxygen to tissues. Hetastarch is made from hydroxyethyl starch (cornstarch). It contains electrolytes (sodium, calcium potassium, and magnesium) and acts as albumin in the management of shock. When given intravenously, it expands blood volume by 1 to 2 times the amount infused. Hetastarch comes in a 6% solution in 0.9% sodium chloride.

Growth Factors

Hematopoietic growth factors are hormone-like substances produced by the body that cause bone marrow to produce more blood cells. These growth factors can be made in the laboratory and are used with patients who have low blood cell counts. Growth factors are used in the medical setting because they can boost RBC, WBC, and platelet counts. Although they assist patients in need of transfusions, they are not used in surgery at this time, because they take days or weeks to raise blood counts and are more expensive than transfusions. Growth factors are not used in patients with severe bone marrow disease, and they could cause certain types of cancer cells to grow more quickly.

Oxygen Therapeutics

The quest continues for blood alternatives that can transport oxygen to tissues, can be given to any blood type, are safe to administer to the patient, and can be stored for long periods of time. A substitute is also needed for those with religious objections to blood transfusion. "Artificial blood" has been replaced with the more accurate term *oxygen therapeutics*. They are agents that enhance the oxygen-carrying capacity of the blood. They would not carry the risks associated with homologous blood transfusion and have been divided into two categories: perfluorocarbon emulsions (which so far have shown no positive clinical trials in this area) and modified Hgb solutions called *Hgb-based oxygen-carrying* (*HBOC*) solutions. Hgb is derived from humans or animals or artificially produced by recombinant technology. No product has yet been approved by the US Food and Drug Administration, but several are in some phases of development or clinical trials. These include the following:

Hemopure is a product made from highly purified bovine Hgb situated in a salt solution. It is an HBOC solution and provides a form of Hgb to aid in oxygen transport to tissues. Hemopure is smaller in size and less viscous than a typical RBC, which means it can carry more oxygen at a lower blood pressure. Because of its size, it can also carry oxygen through partially obstructed or restricted blood vessels. It has a shorter circulation time than blood (only 1–2 days) but does not require refrigeration. Its manufacturing process claims to rid the product of any risk of infection from viruses, including HIV, hepatitis C, and bovine spongiform encephalopathy (mad cow disease). Hemopure has a shelf-life of 36 months at room temperature. Hemopure was approved for use in 2001 in South Africa for the treatment of adult surgical patients who are acutely anemic. In 2010, it was approved in the Russian Federation for the treatment of acute, all-cause anemia. Currently in the United States, Hemopure is considered an investigational new drug that is not approved by the FDA and only available through a clinical trial or through expanded access (also called compassionate use).

PolyHeme began as a military project following the Vietnam War. It is an HBOC that uses human Hgb as the oxygen-carrying molecule in solution. The first step in its production is to extract and filter this Hgb from RBCs. Next is a multistep process to create a polymerized Hgb form that avoids undesirable effects, such as vasoconstriction and kidney or liver dysfunction. Polyheme's manufacturing process eliminates bloodborne diseases, and its shelf-life is approximately 12 months under refrigeration. It has a circulation half-life of 24 hours, so cannot be used to replace blood function over an extended length of time without repeated transfusions. PolyHeme reached phase III studies but has never been approved by the FDA.

Hemospan is produced in powder form, then mixed into liquid form and immediately transfused. It does not require blood typing and can be stored for years. Hemospan is said to demonstrate the capability of high-oxygen transport with a low Hgb content. Its technology uses unmodified Hgb from outdated human RBCs combined with polyethylene glycol to eliminate toxicity usually associated with free Hgb.

Procedure for Donor Blood Replacement in Surgery

It is essential for patient safety that the surgical technologist knows the procedure for obtaining and administering blood and blood components to the surgical patient, even if not directly involved. Each facility will have its own protocols for this process, which conform to standard practice. The following is a basic protocol and is not a substitute for facility policy. The process for administration of donated blood products must be carefully monitored at each step to prevent transfusion of incompatible elements. Transfusion of incompatible blood or blood products can cause a fatal transfusion reaction (see Insight 11.1). Basic steps are as follows:

- When it is determined the surgical patient needs a transfusion, the request is sent to the blood bank in the facility's laboratory. This is done via computer or with a requisition form (or both). The type of blood product for transfusion is noted, and the patient bar-coded label (or written/typed patient information) is attached/sent. Patient information includes patient name, identification number, date of birth, location, amount of blood product ordered, and who is requesting the blood. The blood type, including the Rh factor (if known), and the amount needed are also included.

- Next the patient's blood is typed and crossmatched, and the patient is identified with a special wristband. A sample tube of the patient's blood is sent to the blood bank with any additional paperwork required. The requisition must contain the patient's information and who is requesting the blood. The sample tube is also labeled with the patient's information, the signature of the person who drew the blood sample, and the date/time the sample was drawn.

- A confirmation of the requisition is sent back to surgery with each unit of released blood, which is placed in a sealed bag for transport. Each unit is also labeled with the patient's information and the ABO blood group, Rh group of the patient and of the blood, and blood's expiration date. This label must stay attached to the unit throughout the entire transfusion. The blood product (unit) must be checked to verify all information. Meticulous records are kept in the blood bank on each unit, and the transporter will be required to verify correct information with blood bank personnel and sign out each unit released.

- Once the donor unit(s) reaches the surgical suite, it is placed in an appropriate blood refrigerator, which must have continuous temperature monitoring of 1°C to 6°C. Plasma is stored frozen and thawed in the laboratory immediately before use. Platelets are stored at room temperature. Any units needed for immediate transfusion will be taken directly to the operating room. Both circulator and anesthesia care provider will verify the patient and donor unit information before administration. In addition, the product itself is checked for any clots, discoloration, and leaks or damage to the bag, which might result in contamination. Platelets are checked for any clumping or unusually cloudy appearance. If this occurs, the unit should not be used and must be returned to the blood bank. The blood should be returned to the laboratory unless transfusion is completed within 4 hours. The patient's vital signs (temperature, pulse, respirations, and blood pressure) are checked during transfusion at 15 and 30 minutes, then at 1, 2, 3, and 4 hours or immediately on completion. Then the vital signs are checked again 1 hour post-completion. These are documented along with any signs of transfusion reaction by the nurse or anesthesia care provider on a form that is kept with the patient's chart.

When multiple units of blood are to be administered during a short period of time or when cold blood is rapidly administered through a central venous line, the blood must be warmed to prevent transfusion complications. Blood warmers are used that have a temperature alarm and visible temperature monitor for patient safety. If blood must be transfused rapidly, a blood pump will be used. Different types of blood pumps are available, from simple pneumatic pumps to complex electric or battery-operated units that calibrate the infusion rate precisely. Pressure cuffs are also used for rapid infusion; however, care must be taken not to exceed designated pressure. All blood components must be filtered during administration, so blood administration sets containing an in-line filter are recommended for use. There are large numbers of filter sets available; their instructions are given and must be followed. Isotonic saline (0.9%) is recommended for use with blood components.

> **NOTE:** A special informed consent is required for blood transfusion. It is possible the patient may refuse, in which case there is a "Refusal of Blood Transfusion" form used to document the patient's decision.

IRRIGATION SOLUTIONS

Irrigation is an essential aspect of most open and endoscopic surgical procedures. These solutions assist in clearing the surgical field of active bleeding and improving visualization during the procedures. Irrigation is gentler on tissues than sponging

for preventing desiccation and dryness, which can lead to adhesion formation (Insight 11.3). Endoscopic procedures use irrigation solutions to distend hollow organs, such as the bladder and uterus, and joint spaces, such as the knee and shoulder. These solutions also wash out blood, bits of resected tissue, and stone fragments, while allowing for specimen collection, such as in transurethral resection of the prostate (TURP) gland. It has been demonstrated, though, that irrigation solutions may enter systemic circulation in large volumes, so they must be regarded as systemic medications.

> **! CAUTION**
>
> Test the temperature of all irrigation solutions, especially those recently taken from the warmer, because too hot of a solution can cause tissue damage. If it feels hot to your gloved hand, it is too hot for the patient and should be mixed with cooler solution. Some solutions are used chilled, such as for cardiac and transplant surgery. These solutions are maintained as "slush" for use during the procedure.

Basic Irrigation Solutions

Sodium chloride 0.9% (NS) is traditionally the irrigation solution of choice for open and some endoscopic surgical procedures. It is an isotonic, sterile, topical, conductive,

> **INSIGHT 11.3 Adhesion Barriers**
>
> Abdominal and pelvic surgery sometimes results in the formation of adhesions from scar tissue. Scar tissue forms around the incision and can cling to the surface of organs. Adhesions mature into fibrous bands, often with small calcifications and containing blood vessels. They can obstruct or distort organs, causing pain; necessitating doctor's visits, pain medication, and subsequent surgery; and lead to lost work time. An approach to preventing adhesion formation, in addition to excellent surgical technique, has been to use mechanical barriers and fluids. A barrier agent for prevention of adhesions should be nonreactive in tissue, maintain itself as the peritoneum and other structures regenerate (heal), and then be absorbed by the body.
>
> Hyskon, a 32% solution of dextran 70 suspended in glucose, is used as a distention medium and has also been used as a fluid barrier to adhesions. The concept is of a viscous solution that is absorbed in 5 to 7 days and draws fluid equal to 2.5 to 3 times the original volume into the abdomen or pelvis. This action produces a hydroflotation effect on internal structures to prevent adhesion formation. SprayGel is a synthetic absorbable adhesion barrier that consists of two polyethylene glycol–based liquids that are mixed during spraying. They form an adherent absorbable hydrogel, which remains intact for 5 to 7 days during the critical healing period. The agent then degrades into an absorbable, easily excreted by-product. SprayGel is available in a laparoscopic spray system, and as an open surgery applicator.
>
> Mechanical barriers include Interceed and Seprafilm. Interceed is a knitted fabric that comes in sheets and is placed over the wound. It dissolves in approximately 30 days. Its action is to keep the tissues apart (that would otherwise stick together) and prevent adhesions from forming. Complete hemostasis is required before applying Interceed. Seprafilm is a bioabsorbable membrane derived from sodium hyaluronate and carboxymethylcellulose. Once applied, it breaks down into a hydrated gel that is absorbed within 7 days. Adept is a solution that contains a carbohydrate polymer. It is instilled into the abdominal cavity after surgery and causes the tissues to "float." This prevents adhesions by providing a physical separation of tissue surfaces during the early phases of healing.

electrolyte-containing solution that is not administered by parenteral injection (there is a separately packaged sodium chloride solution for injection). It provides a transparent fluid medium with good optical properties that make it suitable for endoscopic surgery, such as arthroscopy. Sodium chloride is used to rinse indwelling urethral catheters and surgical drainage tubes. It can be used to wash or rinse tissues or soak surgical dressings and can serve as a diluent or vehicle for administering other pharmaceutic preparations (as antibiotics in sodium chloride irrigation). Sodium chloride, if systemically absorbed, can result in alteration of cardiopulmonary and renal function. Excessive volume of the solution or pressure during irrigation, especially in small areas or closed cavities, can result in distention or tissue disruption. If this occurs, the irrigation solution should be discontinued immediately. Sodium chloride comes in 50-, 100-, 250-, 500-, 1000-, 2000-, and 3000-mL fluid bags and in 250-, 500- and 1000-mL pour bottles. It also comes in 0.45% concentration in a variety of sizes depending on the manufacturer.

> ### 📌 TECH TIP
> At the end of the surgical procedure, the surgeon will require a "wet one" and a "dry one," meaning a sponge saturated with clean, sterile sodium chloride irrigation solution and then a dry sponge. These are used to wipe off any blood from the patient's incision site and any that has splattered or run on the patient's skin. The wet sponge also wipes any residual Betadine prep solution from the area. Then the second, clean, sterile sponge is used to dry the area and prepare it for the surgical dressings. Also note to check the surgeon's face for any splattered blood, which must be removed before talking with the patient's family.

> ### ❗ CAUTION
> Saline is a conductive solution and so is used with caution in the presence of the electrosurgical unit (ESU). The danger comes from the transfer of heat and current to adjacent tissues. When used in open surgical procedures, most fluid is suctioned from the field, so saline can be used with little risk. In endoscopic procedures, though, the ESU is applied within the fluid in a confined space, so other irrigation solutions that do not have conductive properties are used.

Sterile water is used more often to rinse instruments to cool them after autoclaving, remove residual disinfectant before coming into contact with patient skin, soak blood from hinges and serrations before terminal cleaning and autoclaving, and cool saw blades or burrs when drilling. It is also used in splash basins to remove powder from surgical gloves immediately preoperatively, and to remove blood from surgical gloves intraoperatively. It is used to dilute prep solutions (Betadine scrub solution) and to fill the balloon on Foley catheters. Like saline, sterile water can be used to cleanse indwelling urethral catheters and surgical drainage tubes and soak surgical dressings. Sterile water is nonconductive and can be used for transurethral resection of bladder tumor because it is not absorbed through the bladder. If it is used for TURP, fluid pressure is carefully monitored because it can result in intravascular hemolysis of erythrocytes. This can also result in absorption in large amounts through vascular openings. Sterile water comes packaged in

250-, 500-, 1000-, 2000-, and 3000-mL containers. Note: there is also a sterile water packaged separately for injection.

> ### ❗ CAUTION
> Sterile water is not used for irrigation in procedures using the cell saver because it would also be suctioned up into the machine. If this occurs, hemolysis of the blood cells may result, thus they cannot be reinfused. This principle also applies in cardiovascular procedures because of the possibility of water being absorbed into the vascular system. Sterile water may not be used to irrigate in the presence of cancer cells because the solution is hypotonic and would cause the cells to swell and possibly rupture, spilling their cancerous contents onto other tissues, but some surgeons require sterile water irrigation for that same purpose—to destroy any free-floating cancer cells in the area before they spread. Therefore, always ask surgeons for their preference.

> ### 📌 TECH TIP
> If not using powder-free gloves, it is good practice to remove any powder from your sterile surgical gloves before procedures (such as middle ear surgery) because it can lead to granulation tissue growth. Studies have shown that the surgical wound retains amounts of residual powder granules after surgical procedures. Use the sterile basin with water or a moistened sponge to rinse or wipe gloves, and then remove the sponge from the sterile field.

PhysioSol is a balanced electrolyte solution used as sterile irrigation for wounds and also for washing and rinsing purposes. It can be used as irrigation for body joints because its pH and electrolyte composition closely resemble that of synovial fluids. In addition, it provides a transparent fluid medium with optical properties for good visualization during arthroscopy. It is not for injection and should not be used during electrosurgical procedures. PhysioSol is packaged 1000-mL pour bottles.

Irrigation Solutions Used in Specialty Procedures

Urologic irrigation solution of 3% sorbitol is sterile, nonelectrolytic, nonhemolytic, and electrically nonconductive. It is used as an irrigating fluid for the urinary bladder because it provides a high degree of visibility without conducting heat and current from the ESU to tissues. During transurethral procedures, it removes blood and tissue fragments. During this procedure, venous sinuses may be opened, and varying amounts of irrigation solutions are absorbed into the bloodstream. Thus the patient should be monitored for altered cardiopulmonary and renal dynamics and hyperglycemia (Insight 11.4).

> ### ❗ CAUTION
> During all procedures with a distention medium, the rate of flow and total fluid volume of the irrigation solutions must be carefully monitored. Also important is the height at which the IV pole is set because this determines the rate of flow (via gravity) and pressure of the solution.

Sorbitol is sometimes used in combination with mannitol as Purisole (sorbitol 2.5% or 3%, mannitol 0.54%) for transurethral procedures and in hysteroscopy. Mannitol 5% is also used in hysteroscopy, when the ESU is used, and is indicated to prevent hydrolysis and Hgb build-up during TURP.

Glycine 1.5% is a sterile, nonconducting, nonhemolytic fluid used to irrigate body cavities. Its active ingredient is glycine, a naturally occurring amino acid, and like the other irrigants, it is nonconductive and nonelectrolytic and can be used with ESU. Thus it can be used in TURP and is also used in hysteroscopy, but overabsorption during this procedure can result in water intoxication with hyponatremia and acid-base imbalance (metabolic acidosis). Glycine comes packaged in 1500-mL pour bottles and 2000-, 3000-, and 4000-mL flexible plastic bags.

Hyskon is a 32% solution of dextran 70 suspended in glucose. A water-soluble glucose polymer, it was originally used as a plasma expander. Hyskon is used to distend the uterus during hysteroscopy and to irrigate blood and tissue debris from the surgical site. It is electrolyte-free and nonconductive, so it can be used with ESU. When large amounts of Hyskon are used, the possibility of systemic effects, such as plasma volume expansion, can occur.

Synovial Fluid Replacement

There are other body fluids that are being replaced, thanks in part to the advancement of arthroscopic surgery. Viscoseal is a 0.5% concentration isotonic solution of hyaluronan of fermentative origin. Hyaluronan is a vital component of hyaline cartilage and synovial fluid. Viscoseal is used to irrigate joints during arthroscopic surgery and as a synovial fluid substitute. During arthroscopic procedures, synovial fluid is "washed away" by irrigating fluids. Viscoseal, when introduced into the joint, displaces any irrigating solutions left in the space and leads to the reestablishment of the normal protective hyaluronan coating on the surface of the articular cartilage and synovial membrane.

Irrigation Equipment and Supplies

Irrigating syringes are bulb-shaped or bulb/barrel syringes (Asepto). They can also be larger standard syringes with special needle attachments for use in vascular surgery. The Asepto syringe is the most commonly used irrigator in open procedures. It is packaged sterile and holds approximately 120 mL. The regular bulb syringe, also called an *ear syringe*, does not have a barrel, and is designed to irrigate smaller areas, such as the ear canal. It is also used to aspirate (remove) fluid from the nose and mouth of an infant, such as during cesarean sections.

Evacuators are syringes used to insert and remove irrigation solutions in closed areas, such as the bladder. Examples are an Ellik or a Toomey syringe used for TURP. The Ellik is a double-bowl–shaped glass or plastic container that is filled with irrigation solution and used to "flush" the prostate area. It aspirates blood clots and resected tissue as the solution is returned back into the evacuator. The Toomey is a large syringe-type container, usually used with a metal adapter inserted onto a catheter for irrigating the bladder and prostate areas. It can also be used with an endoscope (Fig. 11.9).

Continuous irrigation, such as for cystoscopy or hysteroscopy procedures, requires a closed, disposable irrigation system. Tubing is either straight, as used for IV lines, or more commonly Y-shaped, to allow attachment of two bags or bottles of irrigation solution. The Y-tubing may be hooked up to suction along with the bags, and irrigation works via gravity. They are referred to as *suction-irrigators* (Fig. 11.10). Continuous irrigation is also used with Coblation devices. These consist of a wand, cord for power source, tubing for suction, and tubing to be hooked up to a conductive irrigation solution, such as NS (Insight 11.5 and Fig. 11.11).

Irrigation for endoscopic procedures is accomplished through irrigating channels built into endoscopes or by irrigating systems inserted into an opening or port. Irrigation solutions can also be manually inserted into endoscopes with a syringe,

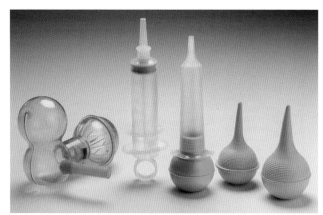

Fig. 11.9 Irrigating syringes used in surgery: Ellik evacuator, Toomey syringe, Asepto syringe, and baby and regular bulb syringes. Courtesy Frank Pronesti T/A heirloomstudio.com.

for small amounts; or a syringe and stopcock can be attached to irrigation tubing hooked up to bags of solution when larger amounts are required. There are also pumps available that supply more fluid under pressurization (a pulse lavage system that uses a battery pack). With these systems, the irrigation solutions can be introduced with more force over a longer period of time, and the pressure is adjustable (Fig. 11.12).

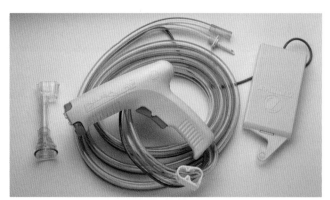

Fig. 11.12 Pulse lavage system. (From Nemitz R: *Surgical instrumentation: an interactive approach*, ed 2, St Louis, 2014, Saunders/Elsevier. Photos by Frank Pronesti.)

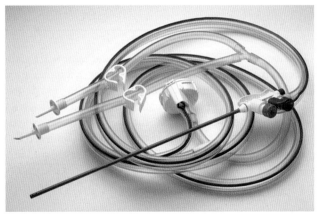

Fig. 11.10 Gravity suction irrigation system. (From Nemitz R: *Surgical instrumentation: an interactive approach*, ed 2, St Louis, 2014, Saunders/Elsevier. Photos by Frank Pronesti.)

INSIGHT 11.5   Coblation Technology

Coblation is a trademarked term for technology that uses radiofrequency energy to excite electrolytes in a conductive irrigation medium, such as normal saline. It is a controlled, nonheat-driven source of focused plasma that breaks down molecular bonds within tissue. This causes tissue to dissolve at low temperatures (usually 40°C–70°C) and results in minimal damage to the surrounding tissues. The various devices are also designed to coagulate or seal bleeding vessels. Coblation technology is used in arthroscopy, spine surgery, neurosurgery, otolaryngology, head and neck surgery, urology, gynecology, plastic surgery, and laparoscopy/general surgery.

KEY CONCEPTS

- The human body's makeup includes fluid electrolytes and nonelectrolytes distributed into ICF and ECF compartments.
- Blood and fluid replacement to normal levels are essential for survival.
- Major electrolytes are sodium, chloride, potassium, calcium, phosphate, and magnesium.
- Too much of the electrolyte in the blood is "hyper-" and too little is called "hypo-"; for example, too much potassium is hyperkalemia and too little is hypokalemia.
- Most surgical patients receive an IV to administer and maintain fluids and to establish a direct access to the circulatory system for medication administration.
- Common IV fluids used in surgery are sodium chloride, dextrose in water and sodium chloride, and LR solution.
- NS, which is 0.9% sodium chloride, is the most common IV fluid used in surgery.
- Blood serves many functions in the body, such as transporting oxygen, nutrients, waste, hormones, and enzymes, and maintaining the acid-base balance, temperature, and water content.
- In the average adult, circulating blood volume is approximately 70 mL/kg of body mass.
- Blood consists of formed elements (RBCs, WBCs, platelets) and plasma.
- Hgb is a protein responsible for carrying oxygen and carbon dioxide between the lungs and the cells.
- Hematocrit is the volume of erythrocytes in a given volume of blood expressed as a percentage.
- The most common indication for blood replacement in surgery is hypovolemia.
- Options for blood replacement include homologous donation, autologous donation, autotransfusion, volume expanders, and—in the future—oxygen therapeutics.
- There is a specific hospital protocol to follow when obtaining blood from the blood bank for the surgical patient.
- Irrigation is used to clear the surgical field of blood and tissue debris, distend hollow organs, allow for specimen collection, and act as a diluent or vehicle for the administration of other pharmaceutic preparations.
- The irrigation solution of choice for most surgical procedures is 0.9% sodium chloride (NS).
- NS is conductive and not to be used in the presence of the ESU.
- Sterile water is used for a variety of functions, including instrument care and handling, glove cleaning, cooling of instruments during surgical cases, and cleansing of urethral catheters.
- There are special irrigation solutions used for specific surgeries.
- Irrigation equipment includes bulb syringes, Asepto syringes, large standard-sized syringes, irrigating systems, and pump-irrigators.

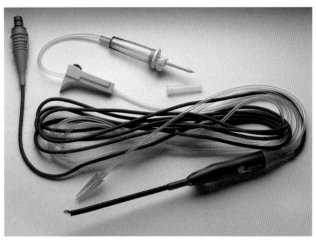

Fig. 11.11 Coblator wand and tubing. (From Nemitz R: *Surgical instrumentation: an interactive approach*, ed 2, St Louis, 2014, Saunders/Elsevier. Photos by Frank Pronesti.)

LEARNING THE LANGUAGE (KEY TERMS)

Using your textbook or a standard medical dictionary, look up and write the definitions of each term.

agglutination
antibody
antigen
arrhythmia
autologous
autotransfusion
electrolyte
hematocrit
hemoglobin
hemolysis
homologous

hypercalcemia
hyperkalemia
hypernatremia
hypocalcemia
hypokalemia
hyponatremia
hypovolemia
intravenous
isotonic
metabolic acidosis

REVIEW QUESTIONS

1. What are the basic functions of blood?
2. What is the average circulating blood volume in an adult?
3. Which surgical patients may require blood replacement?
4. What are the formed elements of blood? What is the main purpose of each?
5. What is hemoglobin? Hematocrit? What are the normal ranges in adults?
6. What are two electrolytes that have particular importance to the surgical patient? Why?
7. What common IV fluids are used in surgery? What is the purpose of each?
8. List two reasons to "start" an IV on the surgical patient preoperatively.
9. What is the primary reason for the surgical patient to receive blood replacement?
10. What is the difference between homologous and autologous donation?

CRITICAL THINKING

1. Sodium chloride 0.9% is said to be isotonic. Why is it the irrigation solution of choice for most surgical procedures?
2. What should be considered when giving a dextrose IV solution to a diabetic patient?
3. What are some of the risks involved when giving the patient a transfusion of whole blood?
4. What should the surgical technologist consider and be prepared for when the surgical patient is given large amounts of donor blood?

Scenario

You are assigned to the genitourinary room for the day. The first procedure is a TURP on a 55-year-old man with an enlarged prostate gland.

1. What type of irrigation solution will be used?
2. Why is this solution used on this procedure?
3. Why must the rate of flow and the total volume of the solution used be carefully monitored?

BIBLIOGRAPHY

Adler-Storthz K, Newland JR, Tessin BA, et al: Human papillomavirus type 2 DNA in oral verrucous carcinoma, *J Oral Pathol Med* 15(9):472–475, 1986.

Apte SS: Blood substitutes—the polyheme-trials, *McGill J Med* 11(1): 59–65, 2008.

Eppley BL, Woodell JE, Higgins J: Platelet quantification and growth factor analysis from platelet-rich plasma: implications for wound healing, *Plast Reconstr Surg* 114(6):1502–1508, 2004.

Fulcher E, Fulcher R, Soto C: *Pharmacology: principles and applications*, ed 3, St Louis, 2012, Saunders/Elsevier.

Hawary A, Mukhtar K, Sinclair A, et al: Transurethral resection of the prostate syndrome: almost gone but not forgotten, *J Endourol* 23(12):2013–2020, 2009.

Kee JL, Hayes ER, McCuistion LE: *Pharmacology: a patient-centered nursing process approach*, ed 8, St Louis, 2015, Saunders/Elsevier.

Martini R, Ober B, Nath J: *Visual anatomy & physiology*, San Francisco, 2011, Benjamin Cummings/Pearson.

Moharari RS, Khajavi MR, Khademhosseini P, et al: Sterile water as an irrigating fluid for transurethral resection of the prostate: anesthetical view of the records of 1600 cases, *South Med J* 101(4):373–375, 2008.

INTERNET RESOURCES

Abbott Laboratories: www.abbott.com.

American Cancer Society, Alternatives to Blood Transfusions, www.cancer.org/treatment/treatmentsandsideeffects/treatmenttypes/bloodproductdonationandtransfusion/blood-product-donation-and-transfusion-blood-transfusion-alternatives.

American Cancer Society, Types of Transfusions, www.cancer.org/treatment/treatmentsandsideeffects/treatmenttypes/bloodproductdonationandtransfusion/blood-transfusion-and-donation-types-of-transfusions.

ClinicalTrials.gov, Expanded Access Study of HBOC-201 (Hemopure) for the Treatment of Life-Threatening Anemia: http://clinicaltrials.gov/ct2/show/NCT01881503.

Smith+Nephew, Coblation Technology: www.smith-nephew.com/key-products/key-ent/ent-technology/coblation/.

Daily Med, 0.9% Sodium Chloride Irrigation, USP: https://dailymed.nlm.nih.gov/dailymed/archives/fdaDrugInfo.cfm?archiveid=143486.

Daily Med, 1.5 % Glycine Irrigation, USP: http://dailymed.nlm.nih.gov/dailymed/fda/fdaDrugXsl.cfm?setid=ac04939e-7641-48e6-31b3-1e6c897b5f60&type=display.

Daily Med, Hospira, Inc: 1.5% Glycine Irrigation, USP: https://dailymed.nlm.nih.gov/dailymed/drugInfo.cfm?setid=5751bfda-7cad-43e7-955d-4a850541575b.

Daily Med, Mannitol Irrigation, Sorbitol: https://dailymed.nlm.nih.gov/dailymed/drugInfo.cfm?setid=be1b2398-892c-4c5d-a045-ce12f03bea8e.

Daily Med, Normosol-R: https://dailymed.nlm.nih.gov/dailymed/drugInfo.cfm?setid=36e56b56-33c0-49e5-ddab-b55da19cae58.

Drugs.com, Conditions, Blood Disorders, *Hespan*: www.drugs.com/mtm/hespan.html.

Drugs.com, Conditions, Constipation, *Sorbitol*: www.drugs.com/mtm/sorbitol.html.

Drugs.com, Professionals, FDA PI, *Ionosol*: https://www.drugs.com/pro/ionosol-mb.html.

Drugs.com, Professionals, FDA PI, *Ionosol MB*: www.drugs.com/pro/ionosol-mb.html.

Drugs.com, Professionals, FDA PI, *Isolyte S pH* 7.4: www.drugs.com/pro/isolyte-s-ph-7-4.html.

Drugs.com, Professionals, FDA PI, Physiosol irrigation: www.drugs.com/pro/physiosol-irrigation.html.

Drugs.com, Professionals, FDA PI, *Sodium chloride irrigation Hospira*: www.drugs.com/pro/sodium-chloride-irrigation-hospira.html.

Drugs.com, Professionals, FDA PI, *Sorbitol*: www.drugs.com/pro/sorbitol.html.

Drugs.com, Professionals, Medfacts, *Albumin human*: www.drugs.com/ppa/albumin-human-normal-serum-albumin.html.

Hemoglobin Oxygen Therapeutics, Hemopure: https://www.hbo2therapeutics.com/our-product.

Hospital for Special Surgery, HSS Education, Platelet-Rich Plasma (PRP) Injections: www.hss.edu/condition-list_prp-injections.asp.

Lippincott Nursing Center, IV fluids, What nurses need to know: www.nursingcenter.com/cearticle?tid=1157503.

MedicineNet.com, Hemoglobin: www.medicinenet.com/hemoglobin/article.htm.

RhoGAM: Ortho-Clinical Diagnostics, Inc.: www.rhogam.com.

Royal Society of Chemistry, Artificial Blood: www.rsc.org/chemistryworld/Issues/2010/October/ArtificialBlood.asp.

RxList, Plasma-Lyte A. (Multiple Electrolyte Injection) Drug Information: www.rxlist.com/plasma-lyte-a-drug.htm.

Sandler S.G., Johnson V.V.: Transfusion reactions treatment & management, Medscape: http://emedicine.medscape.com/article/206885-treatment.

Semenovskaya Z., Sinert R.H., Stephanides S.L.: Hypernatremia in emergency medicine, Medscape: http://emedicine.medscape.com/article/766683-overview.

ShoulderDoc: Viscoseal: www.shoulderdoc.co.uk/article/37.

The University of Michigan Hospitals & Health Centers: 5 blood transfusion guidelines and utilization review: https://www.pathology.med.umich.edu/blood-bank/blood-transfusion-guidelines-and-utilization.

University of Michigan Health: Blood Transfusions: Your Options: www.med.umich.edu/1libr/Pathology/BloodTransfusionOptions.pdf.

Very Well Health, What is TURP Syndrome? http://surgery.about.com/od/aftersurgery/g/TURPSyndrome.htm.

KEY TERMS

central line

hypertonic

hypotonic

osmolarity

osmosis

peripheral line

PICC line

solute

solution

solvent

When a patient's treatment necessitates intravenous (IV) medication and infusion therapy, it is the responsibility of the surgical first assistant to know why such interventions are essential and how they will affect the patient. As the surgical first assistant, you should have an understanding of the pathophysiology of fluids and how they work in the body and be able to relate this to the need for IV therapy.

As mentioned earlier in the chapter, body fluids are primarily made up of water, in which a variety of substances are dissolved. The total volume of water in the body is distributed between two large compartments, the intracellular and the extracellular. These two compartments are separated by a semipermeable cell membrane. The intracellular compartment includes all water and electrolytes within the cell, called *intracellular fluid*. The extracellular compartment is subdivided into three compartments: the blood vessels (plasma) and lymphatic vessels (lymph), interstitial (within tissue spaces), and transcellular. The transcellular compartment includes cerebrospinal fluid, aqueous and vitreous humors, synovial fluid, serous fluid within body cavities, and exocrine gland secretions. This is extracellular fluid. The compositions of the fluid contained within the two compartments are distinctive in chemical formulation. Even though the two compartments have structural differences and carry out completely different tasks, they are in constant interaction with each other to maintain homeostasis. Osmosis governs the movement of body fluids between these two compartments. Osmosis is the passage of water through a semipermeable membrane from an area with a lower concentration of solutes to an area with a higher concentration.

> **NOTE:** For the cell membrane to be semipermeable, it has to be more permeable to water than to solutes (thus it controls the passage of solutes). In the body, water acts as a solvent, able to hold substances, as well as acting to dissolve them. Solutes are substances dissolved in water (the solvent), and the combination of the solute and the solvent forms the solution.

EVALUATION FOR BLOOD REPLACEMENT

Evaluation of the surgical patient's blood/fluid balance begins preoperatively and is monitored intraoperatively and postoperatively. Identifying fluid and/or clotting deficiencies will help to avoid potential hemostatic risks during the surgical procedure. Assessment includes reviewing the patient's medical records and a patient interview. Preoperative laboratory tests, such as hemoglobin (Hgb), hematocrit, and coagulation profile, may assist in predicting the need for blood transfusion. The patient may be instructed to discontinue or modify any anticoagulant therapy; prophylactic administration of drugs that promote coagulation and minimize blood loss may be used on some procedures. Keeping blood loss to a minimum and avoiding the need for blood transfusion are the goals of the surgical team. The surgical first assistant contributes to minimizing intraoperative blood loss by taking immediate and accurate actions, such as immediate direct pressure to the site until bleeding is controlled, clamping or coagulating bleeding vessels, providing an unobstructed view of the surgical site for the surgeon, and using delicate tissue handling. Other methods, such as the harmonic scalpel, laser, electrosurgical unit, or Coblator, may mechanically decrease blood loss. Cell savers, if appropriate, can also be used, but it may be necessary for the surgical patient to receive fluid/blood replacement. According to the American Society of Anesthesiologists, transfusion is rarely indicated when the Hgb is greater than 10 g/dL and is often indicated when the Hgb is less than 6 g/dL. Determination of giving blood/blood products should be based on the potential or actual ongoing blood loss, blood volume status, signs of organ ischemia, and adequacy of the patient's cardiopulmonary reserve.

OSMOLARITY OF FLUIDS

In the chapter, the composition and concentration of IV fluids were discussed. The concentration of the solute in the solution will determine its osmolarity (tonicity, measured in osmoles [Osm] per liter of solution [Osm/L]). Normal saline (NS, 0.9% sodium chloride) is an isotonic solution. This is defined as occurring when fluid that surrounds the cell membrane has the same tonicity and osmotic pull as inside the cell. Therefore, the cell remains unchanged. A hypotonic solution is when the fluid on the outside of the cell membrane has a lesser tonicity and osmotic pull than the fluid on the inside of the cell membrane. Therefore, more fluid will flow into the cell, causing it to swell and possibly burst. The opposite of this is a hypertonic solution, in which fluid on the outside of the cell membrane has a greater tonicity and osmotic pull than on the inside of the cell membrane. Thus more fluid will be pushed out of the cell causing it to shrink and shrivel (Fig. 11.A and Table 11.A.)

INTRAVENOUS SITES AND COMPLICATIONS

The surgical first assistant is not responsible for starting IV (without additional, verified training) but should be aware of IV sites, protocols, and terminology to assist in patient comfort and safety. IV fluids may be administered via a peripheral line (PIV), the most commonly used site for patients, such as

TABLE 11.A Osmolarity of Sodium Chloride Solution		
Solutions	**Concentration**	**Treatment**
Hypertonic	3% and 5%	Cerebral edema and hyponatremia
Isotonic	0.9%	Intravenous fluids
Hypotonic	0.225%, 0.33%, 0.45%	Dehydration and hypernatremia

into a vein in the arm, leg, or scalp (of an infant). A PIV should not be used in an arm with an arteriovenous fistula, in an area of flexion, or where circulation is compromised. The blood circulation through these veins can dilute the components in the IV fluids, and the rate of infusion should not exceed 200 mL in 1 hour. Most transparent IV fluids can flow safely and smoothly through peripheral veins. If blood transfusion or replacement is administered, a larger vein is preferred to facilitate blood flow. Whole blood and especially packed cells can be viscous and are often infused within a short time frame. IV fluids can also be administered over a longer period time via a central line, whereby a special catheter is placed into a large vein, such as the subclavian vein. Central lines are accessed directly (through the chest wall) or indirectly via a neck vein or peripheral vein in the arm. If a peripheral vein is used, this is referred to as a *peripherally inserted central catheter* (PICC line). Larger veins can accommodate higher concentrations of nutrients and components with faster IV flow rates (>200 mL in 1 hour). Central lines are often used when the patient needs IV therapy over an extended period of time.

Major complications of IV therapy are phlebitis, infiltration, and infection at the site. Phlebitis results when the vein becomes red, irritated, or painful. If the vein is fragile, it may rupture, with blood and IV fluids leaking into the tissue. This is known as *"blowing a vein."* Infiltration also occurs when the IV catheter dislodges from the vein and fluid escapes into the surrounding tissue. It results in coolness and pallor to the skin, edema, and swelling. Any break in the skin's integrity can result in infection. Infection at the site is characterized by redness, swelling, fever, and pain. Complications of central lines include infection, bleeding, gangrene, and thromboembolism. Central lines are more difficult to insert and maintain, and complications can result in septicemia.

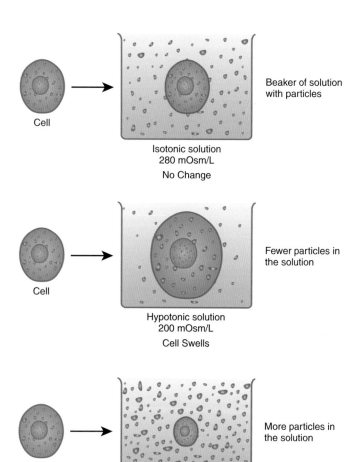

Fig. 11.A Osmotic solutions.

Beaker of solution with particles

Cell

Isotonic solution
280 mOsm/L
No Change

Fewer particles in the solution

Cell

Hypotonic solution
200 mOsm/L
Cell Swells

More particles in the solution

Cell

Hypertonic solution
360 mOsm/L

CONTINUOUS AND INTERMITTENT IRRIGATION

As described in the chapter, irrigation and IV fluids are used for a multitude of tasks in the surgical setting. Both IV fluids and irrigation solutions can be administered by two methods: continuous or intermittent. Continuous IV therapy is performed to replace and maintain fluids in the body. Continuous irrigation is fluid instilled into an area of the body through a steady flow. An example of this is distending the bladder for transurethral resection of the prostate (TURP) or to ensure visualization during an arthroscopy. Intermittent infusions are used for medication administration and secondary fluid replacement. Examples of intermittent administration are IV piggybacks, IV push (bolus), and heparin or saline locks. Intermittent irrigation is also introduced onto an area or into a cavity of the body that is then suctioned or sponged. This is performed for the removal of blood and debris from the site as during a debridement (with the Pulsavac) or after a laparotomy, by pouring irrigation from the sterile pitcher into the abdomen.

ASSISTANT ADVICE

The surgical first assistant should constantly monitor the patient's tissue status. Irrigation fluids (i.e., NS) are applied to prevent drying during the procedure and to prevent overheating of saw blades and burrs, which can cause thermal damage to surrounding tissues. In addition, any time the incision and/or tissues are exposed to room air, drying occurs. The surgical first assistant should dampen (irrigate) the tissues on a regular basis and/or place a wet sponge over the areas, if possible, to prevent desiccation.

ADVANCED PRACTICES: REVIEW QUESTIONS

1. Why is NS considered an isotonic solution?
2. Which type of solution will make the cell shrink? Why?
3. What is the difference between continuous and intermittent IV administrations? Give examples of each.

ADVANCED PRACTICES: BIBLIOGRAPHY

Kee JL, Hayes ER, McCuistion LE: *Pharmacology: a patient-centered nursing process approach*, ed 8, St Louis, 2015, Saunders/Elsevier.

Martini R, Ober B, Nath J: ,. In *Visual anatomy & physiology*, San Francisco, 2011, Benjamin Cummings/Pearson.

Skidmore-Roth L: *Mosby's medical dictionary*, ed 9, St Louis, 2012, Mosby/Elsevier.

Rothrock JC, Seifert PC: *Assisting in surgery: patient-centered care*, Denver, 2010, CCI.

ADVANCED PRACTICES: INTERNET RESOURCES

Abbott Laboratories: www.abbott.com.

American Society of Anesthesiologists Standards and Guidelines: https://anesthesiology.pubs.asahq.org/article.aspx?articleid=2088825&_ga=2.161421949.111044045.1572811892-625665852.1572811892.

Anesthesiology: The Journal of the American Society of Anesthesiologists, Inc.: http://anesthesiology.pubs.asahq.org/article.aspx?articleid=1923206.

Clinical Guidelines (Nursing): Peripheral Intravenous (IV) Lines, The Royal Childrens Hospital Melbourne: www.rch.org.au/rchcpg/hospital_clinical_guideline_index/Peripheral_Intravenous_IV_Device_Management/.

Drugs.com, Professionals, FDA PI, *Ionosol and Dextrose*: www.drugs.com/pro/ionosol-and-dextrose.html.

Drugs.com, Professionals, FDA PI, *Isolyte P in Dextrose*: www.drugs.com/pro/isolyte-p-in-dextrose.html.

Drugs.com, Professionals, FDA PI, *Plasma*-Lyte 56: https://www.drugs.com/dosage/plasma-lyte-148.html.

UpToDate, *Peripheral venous access in adults*: www.uptodate.com/contents/peripheral-venous-access-in-adults.

Anesthesia

As a surgical technologist, you will observe the administration of anesthesia in the operating room nearly every day. Why is it necessary to learn about anesthesia? After all, administration of anesthetic agents is far outside the realm of the technologist's clinical practice. The fact is that understanding the terminology, methods, and agents of anesthesia will give you a more complete picture of surgical patient care. You will be a more effective member of the surgical team if you know the names and classification of anesthetic and supplemental agents and their purposes. As a team member, you will be asked to obtain medications with whose generic and trade names you must be familiar. To facilitate a smooth flow of patient care, you will need to understand preoperative and intraoperative anesthesia routines and medications. In both routine and emergency situations, all team members must contribute maximum effort to achieve the best possible patient outcome. For the surgical technologist, part of that effort includes learning the rudiments of pharmacology as it relates to anesthesia.

12

Preoperative Medications

OBJECTIVES

After completing this chapter, you should be able to do the following:

1. Define terms and abbreviations related to preoperative medications.
2. State the purposes of preoperative anesthesia evaluation.
3. List the components of a preoperative evaluation.
4. Define and discuss preoperative medications.
5. Explain the purpose and state examples of each group of preoperative medications.

OUTLINE

Preoperative preparation is necessary to maximize the safety and comfort of every surgical patient. The surgical technologist may on occasion work in a preoperative care unit or assist in preoperative preparation of patients requiring elective or emergency surgery. To effectively assist the anesthesia care team, surgical technologists should understand the classifications, purposes, and common pharmacological agents used to prepare the patient for surgery.

PREOPERATIVE EVALUATION

A preoperative anesthesia evaluation, or assessment, is performed on all surgical patients and is conducted by the anesthesia care provider. The anesthesia care provider may be a certified registered nurse anesthetist, an anesthesiologist, or an anesthesiologist assistant. The purpose of a preoperative anesthesia evaluation is to gather pertinent patient information and to determine the optimal anesthetic plan. Information is gathered from several sources, including the patient's medical records, a preoperative patient interview, physical examination, and preoperative testing results. The preoperative anesthesia evaluation is used to confirm the patient's surgical diagnosis and to assess concurrent medical conditions that might increase the risk of anesthesia-related complications. It also identifies medications the patient may be taking (including herbal and other over-the-counter [OTC] medications) or drugs of abuse and any allergies the patient may have.

The evaluation usually consists of a questionnaire (Fig. 12.1) to be completed by the patient and a follow-up interview with the anesthesia care provider, who completes a preanesthesia evaluation form (Fig. 12.2). The interview provides an opportunity for the anesthesia care provider to answer the patient's questions and to establish a therapeutic relationship, which also serves to reduce the patient's anxiety. When the interview concludes, written, informed anesthesia consent is obtained from the patient.

The preanesthesia physical examination is a complete assessment of the patient's physical status. Special emphasis is placed on assessment of diabetes and diseases of the cardiovascular and respiratory systems. In addition, the patient's upper airway is evaluated to assess the potential risk of difficult airway management. The airway is evaluated for all patients, even when a local or regional anesthesia plan is intended.

Additional preoperative testing may be ordered depending on the findings of the preoperative evaluation. A panel of routine preoperative tests for all patients has not been shown to accurately predict anesthesia-related complications, so tests are ordered only when the patient's condition(s) indicate a necessity. For example, a potassium level is assessed for patients taking diuretics (see Chapter 7), and a blood glucose level is determined for patients with diabetes. Examples of other preoperative tests that may be indicated for select patients include electrocardiogram (ECG), pulmonary function studies, hemoglobin and hematocrit measurements, coagulation studies, and

Preanesthesia Health History Questionnaire

Your medical and anesthesia health history is important as we partner with you and your healthcare team to optimize your health to develop your plan for anesthesia. We appreciate your time to complete this questionnaire.

Patient Name _____ Age_____ Weight _____ Height _____ Date _____

Allergies (drugs, environment) _____

_____

Current Medications (prescribed, vitamin, herbal, over the counter)_____

_____

Procedures with Anesthesia _____

_____

Do you have a history of the following?	Yes	No		Yes	No
Angina/Chest Pain			Kidney Failure/Dialysis		
Heart Attack/Stent			Kidney Stones		
Congestive Heart Failure			Urinary Tract Infection		
Hypertension			Frequent Headaches/Migraine		
Irregular Heart Beat			Numbness/Tingling/Weakness		
Pacemaker/Internal Defibrillator			Seizure		
Murmur/Mitral Valve Prolapse			Stroke/TIA		
Peripheral Vascular Disease			Arthritis/Fibromyalgia		
Blood Clot/Pulmonary Embolus			Back or Neck Pain/Injury		
Smoker packs/day___ years ___ quit ___			Glaucoma/Macular Degeneration		
Asthma/Emphysema/Home Oxygen			Retinal Detachment/Cataracts		
Chronic Cough/Frequent Bronchitis			Contact Lenses		
Recent Cold/Flu			Hearing Impaired/Hearing Aids		
Pneumonia/TB			Muscle/Nerve Disease		
Short of Breath at Rest			Chemotherapy/Radiation Therapy/Cancer		
Short of Breath One Flight of Steps			Anxiety/Panic Attacks/Depression		
Sleep Apnea/CPAP/BiPAP/Snore			Blood Transfusion		
Alcohol/Recreational Drugs			Oral Piercing (tongue, lip)		
NSAIDS			Bleeding Disorder/Anemia		
Latex Allergy			Sickle Cell Trait or Anemia		
Heartburn/Esophageal Reflux			Diabetes		
Hepatitis/Yellow Jaundice			Insulin Pump		
Hiatal Hernia			Hypo/Hyperthyroid		
Stomach Ulcer			HIV		
Taken steroids in the last year			Isolation in the Hospital for Infection		
Loose, Chipped Teeth/Dentures/Partial/Crowns			Anesthesia Issues		
			Pregnant If yes, due date _____		

Original AANA 1991, Revised November 2022

Fig. 12.1 Sample preoperative patient questionnaire. (Modified from American Association of Nurse Anesthetists: Preanesthesia Questionnaire.)

serum chemistry panels. When all the necessary information is obtained, the patient's preoperative physical status is classified according to criteria established by the American Society of Anesthesiologists (Table 12.1).

PREOPERATIVE MEDICATIONS

During the preoperative evaluation, the anesthesia care provider will determine the patient's need for preoperative

Preanesthesia Evaluation	Name		DOB		Height	Weight	BMI
			Age				
Procedure			BP	Pulse	Resp	SpO$_2$	Temp
			Allergies	☐ None			
			Medications ☐ None			☐ Medication list attached	

Procedures/Anesthesia History	Medication	Dose	Frequency	Last Dose

Patient/Family Anesthesia Issues	Patient	Family	None				
Malignant hyperthermia							
Difficult airway							
Nausea/vomiting							
Other							

Airway Assessment Dentures ↑ ↓ Partial ↑ ↓

Missing, loose, chipped teeth ☐ No ☐ Yes   Nares Patent R L

Mallampati I II III IV   Neck mobility ☐ Adequate ☐ Limited

Previous difficult airway/obstruction ☐ No ☐ Yes   TMJ ☐ No ☐ Yes

Comment

System	Comment	System	Comment
Respiratory ☐WNL	Tobacco Use: ☐ No ☐ Yes	**Neuro/Musculoskeletal** ☐WNL	
Asthma Productive cough Bronchitis Recent URI Pneumonia TB COPD OSA Dyspnea CPAP/BiPAP Orthopnea	___PPD for ___ years Quit _____ CPAP with patient ☐ No ☐ Yes	Seizures Arthritis Headaches Back/joint pain CVA/TIA Chronic pain Disoriented/dementia Neuromuscular Loss of consciousness disease Syncope/vertigo Paralysis Paresthesia	
Cardiovascular ☐WNL		**Renal/Endocrine** ☐WNL	FBS _____ @_____

Angina   Hypertension
ASHD   MI
CHF   Murmur
PVD   Pacemaker/ICD
Dysrhythmia   Rheumatic fever
		UTI Diabetes
		Urinary retention Type ☐I ☐II
		Renal failure Weight gain/loss
		   Hypothyroid
		   Hyperthyroid
			Dialysis Last _____ Next_____

GI/Hepatic ☐WNL		**Hematology/Oncology** ☐WNL	
GERD/Hiatal Hepatitis/Jaundice Hernia Liver failure Ulcer Cirrhosis Bowel obstruction		Anemia Cancer Bleeding/bruising Immunosuppressed HIV Chemotherapy Hemophilia Radiation therapy Transfusion history Steroid use	
Reproductive ☐ N/A	UPT/SPT ☐ Neg ☐ Pos Date_____	**Ethanol** ☐ No ☐ Yes Social ____/day ___/week	
LMP ____/____	Signed refusal of test ☐ N/A ☐ Yes	**Drug Use** ☐ No ☐ Yes/day ____ Last ____Drug(s) In Recovery ☐ Yes	
G ___ P ___ LC ___		**Exam:**	
Tubal Ligation Planned ☐ No ☐ Yes		**Plan:** **Physical Status** 1 2 3 4 5 6 E	

Diagnostic			Results Reviewed ☐ Yes	
WBC	Hb/Hct	Plts		
Na	Cl	Glucose	BUN	
K	CO$_2$		Cr	
INR	PT	PTT		
EKG				
CXR				
ECHO/STRESS/CATH			**Comorbidity Summary:**	
Other				

Date/Time	Signature	Date/Time	Signature

AANA Original 1991 Revised November 2015

Fig. 12.2 Sample preanesthesia evaluation. (Modified from American Association of Nurse Anesthetists: Preanesthesia Evaluation.)

medications. Preoperative medications are given, as needed, to prepare the patient for surgery, both psychologically and physically. Preoperative medications can be classified by action, each group having a specific purpose. The preoperative administration of antibiotics to reduce the risk of surgical site infections has been discussed in Chapter 5.

Sedatives

Sedatives are given to relieve anxiety, which is common in surgical patients. In most patients, these drugs produce a mild drowsiness, and they may have amnestic (pertaining to amnesia) and antiemetic effects. The most common sedatives used preoperatively are the benzodiazepines, a chemical classification

TABLE 12.1 American Society of Anesthesiologists

Classification	Definition
ASA I	A normal healthy patient
ASA II	A patient with mild systemic disease
ASA III	A patient with severe systemic disease
ASA IV	A patient with severe systemic disease that is a constant threat to life
ASA V	A moribund patient who is not expected to survive without the operation
ASA VI	A declared brain-dead patient whose organs are being removed for donor purposes
E	The addition of "E" denotes Emergency surgery: (An emergency is defined as existing when delay in treatment of the patient would lead to a significant increase in the threat to life or body part)

Excerpted from (American Society of Anesthesiologists Physical Status Classification System 2020) of the American Society of Anesthesiologists. A copy of the full text can be obtained from ASA, 1061 American Lane Schaumburg, IL 60173-4973 or online at www. asahq.org.

of drugs used to control anxiety. In low doses, benzodiazepines produce anxiolysis (relief of anxiety); at higher doses, they produce sedation and anterograde amnesia. The patient will remain conscious but may not remember events that occur once the sedative is administered. This effect may explain why some patients have the perception that they were anesthetized in the preoperative preparation area.

MAKE IT SIMPLE

Use medical terminology to help understand the terms anterograde and retrograde amnesia. The prefix "retr/o-" means backward or behind, so people with retrograde amnesia do not remember events that led up to a particular event, such as the time immediately before a motor vehicle accident. Those events occurred backward in time. The prefix "anter/o-" means in front of, so patients with anterograde amnesia do not remember events that occur from a point forward—forward in time.

The benzodiazepine family of drugs includes diazepam (Valium), lorazepam (Ativan), and midazolam. One characteristic of benzodiazepines is high-lipid solubility, which means that the chemicals are absorbed quickly and completely and are easily able to cross the blood-brain barrier to exert their effects. Benzodiazepines are highly bound to plasma proteins.

QUICK QUESTION

What does it mean that a drug is "highly bound" to plasma proteins? How does that affect a drug's ability to exert its effects? See the sections on pharmacokinetics and plasma protein binding in Chapter 1 to check your answers.

These three agents vary in their affinity for receptor-binding sites, which accounts for differences in potency. Benzodiazepines are administered intravenously in weight-dependent dosages

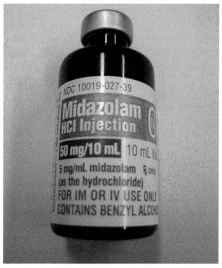
Fig. 12.3 Injectable midazolam, 5 mg/mL. (From Malamed SF: *Medical emergencies in the dental office*, ed 7, St Louis, 2015, Elsevier.)

(mg/kg) for preoperative sedation. Adverse effects of benzodiazepines are minimal in healthy patients. Midazolam is the most common benzodiazepine administered preoperatively (Fig. 12.3).

Analgesics

Some patients may require analgesia (pain relief; literally "without pain") preoperatively. Examples include trauma patients and those patients who will require insertion of invasive monitors (see Chapter 13) before surgery. When indicated for analgesia, opioids may be administered preoperatively. The term *opioid* (literally, resembling opium) refers to all drugs (natural, semisynthetic, or synthetic) having morphine-like actions. Opioids cause analgesia and mild sedation in usual doses and may reduce the amount of anesthesia needed for the surgical procedure. Nausea and vomiting may occur and are thought to be a result of opioid-induced stimulation of the nausea trigger zone in the medulla. Slowing of respiration and reduced intestinal motility are expected. Because of slowed respiration, the patient is monitored with a pulse oximeter (see Chapter 13) and supplemental oxygen may be given. Respiratory depressant effects of opioids are significantly enhanced when benzodiazepines are administered. The patient's level of consciousness should be assessed frequently when opioids are administered. Preoperative use of opioids may be contraindicated for outpatient surgery because of the prohibitively intense patient monitoring required. The sedative effect of benzodiazepines may preempt the need for opioids in some instances.

Morphine (Duramorph) is a *natural* opioid, derived from the poppy plant *Papaver somniferum* (see Chapter 1), that may be used preoperatively for analgesia. Morphine may be indicated for patients experiencing significant pain who are expected to be admitted as inpatients after surgery. Morphine is given intravenously with onset of action expected in 2 to 5 minutes, peak in 10 to 15 minutes, and effects often lasting 2 to 4 hours or more.

The most common *synthetic* opioid used in surgery is meperidine (Demerol). Meperidine is administered intravenously to provide preoperative analgesia. Onset of effect occurs in 1 to

3 minutes, peaks at 5 to 20 minutes, and provides analgesia for 2 to 4 hours.

> ### ⚠ CAUTION
>
> Opioids are covered under federal and state-controlled substances acts (see Chapter 2) and must be handled according to hospital policy. The surgical technologist must be thoroughly familiar with and adhere to institutional procedures regarding controlled substances.

Anticholinergics

Anticholinergics are agents that block the action of the neurotransmitter acetylcholine (ACh), inhibiting the transmission of parasympathetic nerve impulses (Fig. 12.4). ACh is a key neurotransmitter in the autonomic nervous system, so these agents exert systemic effects.

Anticholinergics are not routinely used preoperatively, but may be indicated in specific instances to inhibit mucous secretions of the respiratory and digestive tract (antisialagogue effect). Most anesthetic agents in use today do not cause significant salivation, so anticholinergics are less frequently indicated. Decreased oral secretions may be desired when an endotracheal tube is in place for a general anesthetic or for intraoral procedures, such as bronchoscopy or maxillofacial surgery. These medications may also be administered preoperatively to block certain receptors on the vagus nerve (vagolysis). A common side effect is an increased heart rate, which is an example of the systemic effects of anticholinergics.

When indicated, anticholinergics most frequently used preoperatively are atropine, scopolamine, and glycopyrrolate. Both atropine and scopolamine cross the blood-brain barrier, so they can also cause sedation and amnesia. Atropine is administered intravenously, and onset is almost immediate with a duration of 15 to 30 minutes. At routine clinical doses, atropine does not cause significant sedation or amnesia. Scopolamine is 3 times more potent an antisialagogue than atropine and is given when both an antisialagogue effect and sedation are desired. Scopolamine is an anticholinergic that is administered intravenously with immediate onset and effect lasting for 30 to 60 minutes. It is a drug that has multiple therapeutic effects, so it is classified in several categories. Scopolamine is also classified as an antisialagogue, a sedative, and an antiemetic. Scopolamine is also presented in the next section of gastric agents because of its therapeutic classification as an antiemetic. Glycopyrrolate is twice as potent an antisialagogue as atropine and has a longer duration. It is administered intravenously; onset occurs within 1 minute and lasts 2 to 3 hours. Glycopyrrolate does not cross the blood-brain barrier, so it does not cause sedation or amnesia.

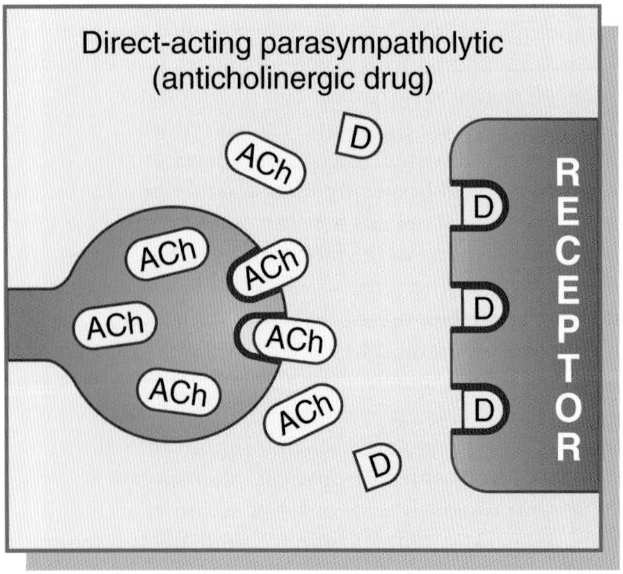

> ### ✎ TECH TIP
>
> Anticholinergics may also be used intraoperatively to block the vagal response (called *reflex bradycardia*) to certain stimuli, such as stretching the peritoneum during open abdominal procedures, bowel manipulation, cervical traction in gynecologic cases, carotid artery dissection, or stretching eye muscles during retinal procedures. Alert the anesthesia care provider when you are about to increase retraction pressure on any of those structures. Pay close attention to ECG sounds during those types of procedures to detect reflex bradycardia.

Gastric Agents

Anxiety and fear, so often seen in surgical patients, initiates a stress response mediated by the sympathetic nervous system, which may slow down or stop the digestive process (Insight 12.1). The presence of food in the stomach, as may be found in trauma patients, and the acidic nature of gastric contents may present significant risk to patients requiring general anesthesia. During induction of general anesthesia, the lower

Fig. 12.4 Anticholinergic response. The anticholinergic drug occupies the receptor sites, blocking acetylcholine. *ACh,* Acetylcholine; *D,* anticholinergic drug. (From Kee JL, Hayes ER, and McCuistion LE: *Pharmacology: a nursing process approach*, ed 7, St Louis, 2012, Elsevier.)

> ### INSIGHT 12.1   **Gastric Physiology Review**
>
> The digestive system is responsible for intake and processing of nutrients and elimination of nutrient waste. The stomach, which is part of the digestive system, processes food by two means—mechanical and chemical. The mechanical process of digestion is caused by the peristaltic motions of the muscles and folds (rugae) of the stomach, which mix food with gastric secretions. This mixture becomes a thin liquid, called *chyme*, which is propelled in small amounts through the pylorus into the duodenum. The chemical process of digestion is caused by the action of an enzyme called *pepsin*. In the presence of hydrochloric acid (HCl), pepsin becomes active and breaks down protein contained in the ingested food. HCl is produced by the parietal (oxyntic) cells of the stomach and is the chemical responsible for the acidic nature of gastric contents. It is interesting to note that the stomach contains 1 billion parietal cells, each capable of secreting 3.3 billion hydrogen ions per second. Secretion of these chemicals is controlled by both the nervous and endocrine systems. The nervous system regulates production of gastric chemicals via stimulation of the parasympathetic fibers of the vagus nerve. The sight and smell of food also initiates stimulation of gastric glands to produce digestive chemicals. Ingestion of food causes stretching of the stomach, which is transmitted through the nerves, and a response is generated that produces more stimulation of gastric glands. For further explanation of digestion, consult a physiology textbook.

esophageal sphincter may relax to an extent that a reflux of gastric contents may occur. In addition, some agents administered at this time may cause nausea, with an increased risk of vomiting. If the patient vomits or gastric reflux occurs during induction of anesthesia, gastric contents can enter the lungs, causing mild to severe damage. This complication is called *aspiration*, which may result in aspiration pneumonitis—the body's inflammatory response to the presence of foreign substances in the lungs. Severe aspiration pneumonitis is extremely rare in healthy patients undergoing elective surgery, so routine preoperative administration of gastric agents in patients without risk factors is not indicated.

Even though elective surgical patients are expected to be NPO (*nil per os*, or nothing by mouth) for a period before surgery (Insight 12.2), gastric secretions are still present. Patients at increased risk of aspiration include those with gastrointestinal (GI) obstruction, history of gastroesophageal reflux disease (GERD), diabetes, obesity, or pregnant patients in labor or scheduled for cesarean section. In addition, patients presenting with a need for emergency surgery may have a full or partially full stomach. Risk of aspiration is highest at intubation and extubation (see Chapter 14). Damage to the lungs is dependent on the volume and acidity of the contents aspirated. When indicated in patients with risk factors for gastric reflux and possible aspiration, several different gastric agents may be used for preoperative prophylaxis, alone or in combination with other agents. Clinical studies are ongoing to determine which agents, alone or in combination, are proving to be most effective.

Antacids

Antacids are used to chemically neutralize gastric acid already present in the stomach. Several antacids, such as Tums, are available OTC (see Chapter 2). Preoperative administration of an antacid is intended to minimize damage to the lungs from gastric acid, should aspiration occur. Unfortunately, recent studies have shown that preoperative administration of these agents to reduce gastric acidity has not significantly reduced lung damage caused by aspiration. If indicated, sodium citrate with citric acid is a nonparticulate liquid antacid that may be administered preoperatively to neutralize the acidity of stomach contents. Gastric acid normally has an acidity, or pH, of 2 to 3. Sodium citrate is metabolized to sodium bicarbonate—a base that chemically neutralizes gastric acid. When indicated,

sodium citrate is given orally in a dose of 15 to 30 mL. Effects are immediate, and the duration is approximately 2 hours.

Histamine Receptor Antagonists

Histamine (H2) receptor antagonists are antacids named for their physiological action on the receptors found on parietal cells in the stomach. By blocking H2 receptors, these agents temporarily interfere with the production of gastric acid by parietal cells. These antacids are also available in oral form OTC, for occasional use.

The most common H2 blocker given preoperatively is famotidine (Pepcid). Famotidine may be given orally the night before or the morning of surgery or intravenously. Onset of effects is noted in 20 to 45 minutes, and effects last for 7 to 9 hours. To be the most effective at intubation, H2 blockers should be administered 2 to 3 hours before procedure start time. These agents are not used in emergency surgery because they do not change the acid already present in the stomach.

Proton-Pump Inhibitors

Proton-pump inhibitors (PPIs) are medications that bind irreversibly with the acid pump of parietal cells and prevent the release of HCl (gastric acid). Most commonly prescribed for oral administration to treat symptoms of GERD, these agents are also used preoperatively. PPIs are examples of *prodrugs*.

> **❓ QUICK QUESTION**
>
> What are prodrugs? How is their action different from other drugs? See the sections on pharmacokinetics and biotransformation in Chapter 1 to check your answers.

PPIs are unique in that they are not converted to active drugs in the liver but in the parietal cell canaliculus (tubular canals into which hydrochloric acid is secreted). These drugs prevent the final step of gastric acid production by interfering with hydrogen (H+) and potassium (K+) ion exchange in the H+, K+-ATPase (adenosine triphosphatase) proton pump, which is located on the surface of parietal cells (Fig. 12.5).

The prototype drug in this category is omeprazole (Prilosec), but it is not commonly used preoperatively because it takes days to become fully effective. Other drugs in this category are lansoprazole (Prevacid), esomeprazole (Nexium), pantoprazole (Protonix), and rabeprazole (AcipHex). Prevacid IV, Nexium IV, and Protonix IV are available in freeze-dried powder form that must be reconstituted before intravenous (IV) administration. IV administration of pantoprazole (Protonix IV) will reduce gastric acid in 20 minutes.

Antiemetics and Gastrokinetics

Antiemetics are agents administered preoperatively to reduce nausea and minimize the possibility of postoperative nausea and vomiting (PONV) in at-risk patients. The types of patients most at risk for PONV are pediatric (especially preadolescents); those patients who have or will receive opioids, barbiturates, or etomidate; and female patients (females are 2–3 times more likely to experience PONV than males, particularly after

---

> **INSIGHT 12.2 "NPO After Midnight" or Fasting Before Elective Surgery**
>
> It has long been thought that if we reduced gastric fluid volume, we would reduce the risk of pulmonary aspiration of stomach contents on induction of anesthesia. Gastric emptying times vary though, by what is in the stomach (solid food vs. clear liquids). Recommendations have been modified so that clear liquids (such as water, carbonated beverages, clear tea, or black coffee) are allowed up to 2 hours before induction of anesthesia. Oral medications can now be taken with up to 150 mL of water in the hour preceding induction. Gum chewing is not allowed preoperatively because of resulting increases in gastric fluid volume.

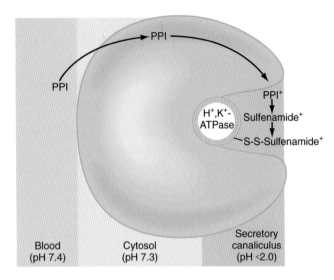

Fig. 12.5 Model illustrating the mechanism of action of proton-pump inhibitors (PPIs). PPIs reach the parietal cell from the bloodstream, diffuse through the cytoplasm, and accumulate in the acid environment of the secretory canaliculus. In the canaliculus, the PPI becomes protonated and trapped as a sulfenic acid, followed by dehydration to a sulfenamide. The sulfenamide binds covalently by disulfide bonds to one or more cysteines of the hydrogen-potassium adenosine triphosphatase (H+,K+-ATPase) to inhibit the enzyme. Whereas all PPIs bind to cysteine 813, omeprazole also binds to cysteine 892, lansoprazole to cysteine 321, and pantoprazole to cysteine 822. (From Feldman M, Friedman LS, Brandt LJ: *Sleisenger and Fordtran's gastrointestinal and liver disease*, ed 10, St Louis, 2016, Elsevier.)

intraabdominal surgery). Obesity has been thought to be associated with increased risk of PONV, but a systematic review of research failed to demonstrate significant influence of body weight on PONV. Recent evaluation also failed to demonstrate obesity as a predictor of PONV.

Certain procedural factors also contribute to the incidence of PONV, such as length of procedure (longer procedures increase the risk for PONV) and type of procedure. Types of procedures associated with a greater risk of PONV include abdominal procedures (especially female laparoscopic) and procedures usually performed on children, such as strabismus correction, tonsillectomy and adenoidectomy, orchiopexy, and middle ear procedures. Research studies continue to better determine which patients are most likely to benefit from the administration of preoperative antiemetics.

Three main categories of medications that are used to prevent PONV are the following:
- Gastrokinetics (metoclopramide)
- Neuroleptics (droperidol)
- Serotonin antagonists (ondansetron)

Metoclopramide (Reglan) is classified as a gastrokinetic agent, and it is used to reduce gastric fluid volume in at-risk patients, such as those with delayed gastric emptying (most associated with diabetes), pregnant patients, those with anticipated difficult airway, and emergency patients who have not been NPO. It stimulates motility of the upper GI tract (and thus gastric emptying) without stimulating gastric acid secretion,

but administration of metoclopramide does not ensure complete emptying of the stomach. In addition, metoclopramide reduces the risk of postoperative nausea because it also works as a peripheral and central dopamine receptor antagonist. It is administered intravenously with onset expected in 1 to 3 minutes and a duration of 1 to 2 hours (Table 12.2).

Droperidol is an antiemetic drug with sedative properties that is less frequently used in current practice. It is also classified as a neuroleptic agent (see Insight 14.3). The US Food and Drug Administration (FDA) requires a "boxed" warning (formerly known as "black box" warnings) on droperidol, the most serious warning for an FDA-approved drug. Indications for use of droperidol have been limited, and its use is restricted to second line only, because of an increased risk of fatal cardiac arrhythmias. When indicated, droperidol is administered intravenously, with effects seen in 3 to 10 minutes and a duration of 2 to 4 hours.

The most commonly used antiemetic agent used preoperatively is ondansetron (Zofran). It is classified as a serotonin antagonist, also known as a 5-HT3 receptor antagonist. This category of medications also includes granisetron and dolasetron, which are most often used to manage chemotherapy-induced nausea and vomiting. Dolasetron is a prodrug (see Chapter 1) that must be metabolized or broken down to an active metabolite, hydrodolasetron, to exert its effect. These agents are relatively free from side effects compared with metoclopramide and droperidol, but they are more costly.

Ondansetron (Zofran) is given intravenously over a period of 2 to 5 minutes immediately before induction. Its effects last from 12 to 24 hours, and it has been very effective in reducing the incidence of PONV, especially in patients undergoing ambulatory gynecologic or middle ear procedures. Ondansetron may also be given in combination with dexamethasone (see Chapter 8) for an additive effect noted in the first 3 hours after surgery.

TABLE 12.2	**Gastric Agents Used Preoperatively**
Generic Name	**Trade Name**
Antacid	
sodium citrate	N/A
H2 blockers	
famotidine	Pepcid
cimetidine	Tagamet
Proton-Pump Inhibitor	
pantoprazole	Protonix IV
Antiemetics	
ondansetron	Zofran
metoclopramide	Reglan
scopolamine	Transderm Scop
promethazine	Phenergan

Another drug that may be given to prevent PONV is scopolamine. In some reports, it has been shown to be as effective as ondansetron in preventing PONV. It is usually administered by dermal patch, which may be applied the night before or just before surgery. Side effects include visual disturbances, dizziness, and dry mouth. The patch contains 1.5 mg of scopolamine, and it is left in place for approximately 72 hours.

<table>
<tr><td>

KEY CONCEPTS

- A preoperative assessment is made by the anesthesia care provider to determine the optimal anesthesia plan.
- A preoperative evaluation consists of a patient interview, physical examination, and medical records review.
- Several general categories of medications may be used to prepare the patient both physically and psychologically for surgery. These include antibiotics, sedatives, analgesics, anticholinergics, and several types of gastric drugs.
- To assist the anesthesia care provider, the surgical technologist should be familiar with drugs administered preoperatively and their purposes.

</td></tr>
</table>

LEARNING THE LANGUAGE (KEY TERMS)

Using your textbook or a standard medical dictionary, look up and write the definitions of each term.

amnestic
analgesia
anterograde
anticholinergic
antisialagogue
anxiolysis

aspiration
benzodiazepine
NPO
opioid
vagolysis

REVIEW QUESTIONS

1. Why is a preoperative evaluation conducted?
2. What are the categories of preoperative medications?
3. What is the purpose of each category of preoperative medication?

4. Can you state an example of a medication in each category of preoperative medication?

CRITICAL THINKING

Scenario

Mr. O'Neill is a very nervous, obese, 61-year-old man with a history of diabetes and GERD. He is scheduled for an open reduction and internal fixation of a distal tibial fracture. He received a preoperative dose of 2 mg of midazolam 15 minutes before being brought into the operating room. As he is settled on the operating room bed, the novice circulator begins to explain the importance of postoperative wound care to Mr. O'Neill.

1. In addition to midazolam, which other categories of preoperative medications do you think Mr. O'Neill will have received and why?
2. Is this the appropriate time to instruct Mr. O'Neill regarding his wound care? Why or why not?

BIBLIOGRAPHY

Bardal S, Waechter J, Martin D: *Applied pharmacology*, St Louis, 2011, Saunders/Elsevier.
Duke JC, Keech BM: *Duke's anesthesia secrets*, ed 5, St Louis, 2016, Saunders/Elsevier.
Fulcher EM, Fulcher RM, Soto CD: *Pharmacology: principles and applications*, ed 3, St Louis, 2012, Saunders/Elsevier.
Key JL, Hayes ER, McCuistion LE: *Pharmacology: a patient-centered nursing process approach*, ed 8, St Louis, 2015, Elsevier.
Nagelhout JJ, Plaus KL: *Handbook of anesthesia*, ed 5, St Louis, 2014, Elsevier.

Nagelhout JJ, Plaus KL: *Nurse anesthesia*, ed 4, St Louis, 2010, Saunders/Elsevier.

INTERNET RESOURCES

American Society of Anesthesiologists, ASA Physical Status Classification System: www.asahq.org/resources/clinical-information/asa-physical-status-classification-system.
Drugs.com, Professionals, AHFS Monographs, Scopolamine: www.drugs.com/monograph/scopolamine.html.

KEY TERMS

bowel prep
cathartics
convulsions

hypertension
idiopathic

MEDICATIONS FROM THE MEDICAL SETTING TO THE SURGICAL SETTING

In addition to the preoperative medicines described in this chapter, there are others that must be considered before the patient undergoes a surgical procedure. Medications are prescribed either for surgical preparation or as part of a current therapy for an unrelated condition. One of the most common preparations for all patients undergoing elective GI procedures is the "bowel prep." Healthcare workers often discount this procedure, even though it affects the patient systemically. Other medicines that patients may be taking preoperatively are antihypertensive or anticonvulsive drugs. Patients may remain on these medicines throughout the surgical procedure, usually under the advice of the anesthesia care provider. The surgical first assistant should be aware of these medicines and preparations and their effects upon the surgical patient.

BOWEL PREPARATIONS

All patients undergoing abdominal surgical procedures in which the small bowel, colon, or rectum may be involved will be required to perform a preoperative bowel preparation (evacuation). A thorough bowel prep will eliminate any bowel content before surgery to provide a clear view of the mucosa. Poor preparation may result in missed pathology, such as polyps, lesions, or tumors. This could result in incorrect diagnosis, longer procedures, and the need for repeated procedures. Each surgeon may order a slightly different type or version of the bowel prep, depending on the surgeon's preference and the patient's age and health. The standard prep includes instructions for a clear liquid diet and drinking a bowel-cleaning solution, or cathartic, at designated times before the procedure. Previously, the bowel prep was a two-phase procedure: a mechanical phase of emptying the bowel and a chemical phase using an antibiotic. It was thought the antibiotic would help to eliminate resident bacteria (*Escherichia coli*, or *E. coli*) from the bowel. This is no longer common practice; however, prophylactic antibiotics may be given before the procedure to patients with specific conditions, such as cystic lesions along the gastrointestinal tract. The mechanical phase of the prep is performed by the patient, at home, usually the day before the procedure. It consists of medications to evacuate all feces from the colon. An example of one such medication is GoLYTELY, which is polyethylene glycol–electrolyte solution (PEG-ES), sodium chloride, sodium bicarbonate, and potassium chloride taken orally and is administered in a 2-L dose. This solution may be combined with two or four bisacodyl (Dulcolax) laxative tablets taken by mouth with 8 ounces of water, at home, and begins working within an hour. The patient must drink large amounts of these fluids within a short period of time, usually 4 L within 2 to 3 hours. Depending on the time of the procedure, the patient may be instructed to divide the solution into two different doses that can be taken over a longer period of time. PEG-ES is available in the pharmacy under trade names such as Colyte and NuLYTELY. Another solution used is polyethylene glycol 3350 (Miralax). These may be prescribed without the bisacodyl tablets and are called *MoviPreps*. These preparations increase the amount of water in the intestinal tract, which stimulates bowel movements. They contain potassium, sodium, and other minerals, which replace the electrolytes that are eliminated from the body during the bowel evacuation. They can also be used before a barium x-ray examination or other intestinal procedures. (Note: there are also medications given in tablet form, as enemas, or as bowel suppositories to achieve the same purpose.) Because these preparations cause diarrhea to evacuate fecal material, patients undergoing bowel preparation will experience a significant fluid loss. This fact combined with the patient's NPO status will require administration of more fluids intraoperatively and postoperatively. Patients with other medical problems may not tolerate this fluid shift and will require hospitalization to complete the prep. The PEG-ES preparation may cause nausea in some patients. Metoclopramide (Reglan), 10 mg orally, may be prescribed to decrease the nausea to retain the prep.

ANTICONVULSANTS

Millions of people in the United States have active epilepsy, which causes abnormal electrical discharges in the cerebral neurons that lead to loss of consciousness, convulsions, and seizures. They are treated with medications referred to as *anticonvulsants*. These medications act on the neurons in the brain by depressing their discharge and preventing seizure activity. Other conditions for seizures include injuries at birth, head trauma, tumors, and idiopathic (unknown) causes. Patients require a continuous level of anticonvulsants to prevent a seizure event. Therefore, surgical patients may need to remain on this therapy throughout the procedure and postoperatively. Anticonvulsants can be placed in several categories, which include benzodiazepines, barbiturates, hydantoins, and succinimides. There are also several miscellaneous anticonvulsants that are available. Examples of specific medicines are found in Table 12.A.

HYPERTENSION MEDICINES

Hypertension is defined as a blood pressure greater than 140/90 mm Hg and affects approximately 25% of the population. The effects of hypertension kill 2500 Americans every day. In most cases, the etiology is unknown. This is referred to as *essential* (or *primary*) *hypertension*. The vast majority of patients with hypertension require antihypertension drug therapy to control the blood pressure. Any interruption of this therapy will cause the patient's blood pressure to rise and may have an adverse effect on the outcome of the surgical procedure. Therefore, patients being treated for hypertension may

TABLE 12.A Anticonvulsants	
Category	**Examples**
Benzodiazepines	Diazepam, clonazepam, clorazepate, lorazepam
Barbiturates	Phenobarbital, primidone
Hydantoins	Fosphenytoin, phenytoin
Succinimides	Ethosuximide, methsuximide
Miscellaneous	Valproic acid, carbamazepine, gabapentin

be instructed to take their daily medications with a sip of water 2 hours before surgery. Physicians today have many medicines in their arsenal to control hypertension. These medicines are grouped according to their effects on the body. They are diuretics, β-blockers, angiotensin-converting enzyme (ACE) inhibitors, calcium-channel blockers, and α-blockers. Another group of medications being used is called *angiotensin II receptor blockers* (ARBs). They are similar to ACE inhibitors because they help dilate arteries. This action lowers blood pressure and makes it easier for the heart to pump blood throughout the body. Like ACE inhibitors, ARBs can improve congestive heart failure symptoms and prolong life.

Patients may require a combination of several medications to control the hypertension. When hypertension is treated, it is best to take the staged approach. The patient is prescribed one type of medicine, while the blood pressure is monitored. Additional medications from other groups are added until the blood pressure returns to a normal level.

ADVANCED PRACTICES: REVIEW QUESTIONS

1. Which procedures will require a preoperative bowel prep? Why?
2. How does the patient cleanse the bowel before the procedure?
3. Name two preparations for bowel cleansing.
4. How do anticonvulsants work?
5. Name the groups of medications used to treat hypertension.

ADVANCED PRACTICES: BIBLIOGRAPHY

Fulcher EM, Fulcher RM, Soto CD: *Pharmacology: principles and applications*, ed 3, St Louis, 2012, Saunders/Elsevier.

Kee JL, Hayes ER, McCuistion LE: *Pharmacology: a patient-centered nursing process approach*, ed 8, St Louis, 2015, Saunders/Elsevier.

ADVANCED PRACTICES: INTERNET RESOURCES

About.com, Bowel Prep During Bowel Surgery: https://www.verywellhealth.com/bowel-prep-what-you-need-to-know-3157016.

Colonoscopy.com, Antibiotics: www.colonoscopy.com/medical-information/antibiotics.

Drugs.com, Gabapentin: www.drugs.com/gabapentin.html.

Drugs.com, MoviPrep: www.drugs.com/moviprep.html.

BowelPrepGuide: Colorectal Cancer in 2018: The Good, the Bad and the Ugly: https://bowelprepguide.com/colorectal-cancer-2018/.

Mayo Clinic, High Blood Pressure (Hypertension), Symptoms: www.mayoclinic.org/diseases-conditions/high-blood-pressure/basics/symptoms/con-20019580.

RxList, Drugs A-Z, Celontin (Methsuximide): www.rxlist.com/celontin-drug.htm.

UpToDate.com, Antibiotic Prophylaxis for Gastrointestinal Endoscopic Procedures: http://www.uptodate.com/contents/antibiotic-prophylaxis-for-gastrointestinal-endoscopic-procedures.

WebMD, Drugs & Medications, Miralax: www.webmd.com/drugs/2/drug-17116/miralax-oral/details.

13

Patient Monitoring and Local and Regional Anesthesia

OBJECTIVES

After completing this chapter, you should be able to do the following:

1. Define terms and abbreviations related to patient monitoring and anesthesia.
2. Explain types of patient-monitoring devices, including components and purposes.
3. Discuss monitored anesthesia care (MAC) and its levels of sedation.
4. Discuss local anesthesia, including applications, common agents used, examples, and safety considerations.
5. Discuss regional anesthesia, including applications, common agents used, examples, and safety considerations.
6. Explain types of regional blocks.

OUTLINE

Surgical intervention and administration of anesthetic agents are complex and challenging processes that place enormous physiological stress on the patient. The administration of anesthesia requires continuous monitoring of the patient's vital signs. Intraoperative monitoring has become more comprehensive and precise, enabling continuous assessment of critical indicators. The surgical technologist must become familiar with the various types of patient monitoring, components of the devices, and purposes. Although the primary focus of the scrubbed surgical technologist is at the surgical site, it is crucial that each team member be aware of the patient's wellbeing at all times and be prepared to provide support to the anesthesia care provider and patient when necessary.

Both the American Association of Nurse Anesthesiology and the American Society of Anesthesiologists (ASA) have published standards of care regarding patient monitoring.

In addition, the Council on Surgical and Perioperative Safety (CSPS), an incorporated multidisciplinary coalition of professional organizations, whose members are directly involved in the care of surgical patients, has published a Safe Surgery Principle regarding patient monitoring. It states the following:

> **NOTE:** "The CSPS endorses perioperative monitoring of patient physiologic parameters appropriate to patient comorbidities, the anesthetic technique used, and the complexity of the procedure. Physiologic alarms should be audible."
> Adopted July 16, 2006, modified July 15, 2007, February 5, 2009. Available at http://www.cspsteam.org/

In the second part of this chapter, we begin a discussion of anesthesia. The term *anesthesia* literally means "without sensation." Surgical patients may be conscious or unconscious, but while receiving any type of anesthesia, they should not perceive pain. The precise chemical and physiological means by which anesthetics work are not yet fully clear, but we do know that the mechanism depends on the type of agent being administered. For example, some drugs induce amnesia, whereas others induce unconsciousness or change the perception of pain. There are four major types of anesthetic techniques: sedation/monitored anesthesia care (MAC), local, regional, and general. This chapter presents a brief description of sedation/MAC and basic information on local and regional anesthesia. Basic concepts of general anesthesia are covered in Chapter 14.

PATIENT MONITORING

Each of the patient's vital signs is continuously monitored during surgical intervention. Continuous monitoring provides a means to rapidly identify changes in the patient's physiological status. The first line of patient monitoring is direct observation of the patient by the anesthesia care provider, and its importance cannot be underestimated. The patient's oxygen saturation is monitored by direct observation and by use of the pulse oximeter. Respiration is monitored by patient observation and, when the patient is under heavy sedation or general anesthesia, by measurement of levels of expired carbon dioxide. Circulation is monitored by continuous electrocardiography (rate and rhythm) and by frequent measurement of blood pressure (BP). Temperature is assessed by various methods, as indicated by the patient's situation. During general anesthesia, the patient's neuromuscular function and level of awareness are monitored when indicated. Certain patient conditions and some particular surgical procedures may require advanced or invasive monitoring methods, such as placement of arterial or central venous pressure lines. See Box 13.1 for a summary of the most common physiological functions monitored in the surgical patient.

BOX 13.1 Summary of the Most Common Physiological Functions Monitored in Surgical Patients

Function	Value
Electrocardiogram (ECG)	Adult resting: 60–100 beats per minute Children (1–10 years): 70–130 beats per minute Infants (1–11 months): 80–120 beats per minute Newborns (0–30 days): 70–190 beats per minute
Pulse oximetry	Oxygen saturation should be >95% in healthy patients
Blood pressure	<120 mm Hg systolic and <80 mm Hg diastolic
Temperature	37°C or 98°F
Capnometry	Sustained carbon dioxide waveform of >30 mm Hg indicates correct placement of endotracheal tube
Consciousness	A scaled number between 45 and 60 indicates an appropriate depth of general anesthesia
Neuromuscular function	Zero of the four twitches indicates complete muscle relaxation
Arterial pressure	Establish patient baseline waveform and monitor changes; digital values range: 90–140/60–90 mm Hg
Central venous pressure	Establish patient baseline waveform and monitor changes; digital values are inconsistent and less reliable than waveform analysis
Pulmonary artery pressure	Establish patient baseline waveform and monitor changes; digital values range: 15–25/8–15 mm Hg but are less reliable than waveform

The complex nature of surgical patient monitoring can be simplified by applying the principles of cardiopulmonary resuscitation: *a*irway, *b*reathing, and *c*irculation. While under local or regional anesthesia, the patient maintains his or her own *airway* (oxygenation), and it is confirmed by pulse oximetry. With the patient under general anesthesia, the airway is secured with an endotracheal tube or laryngeal masked airway. In some instances of general anesthesia, the patient's airway is controlled via bag/mask ventilation by the anesthesia care provider. *Breathing* (respiration) is monitored by direct observation, confirmed with the pulse oximeter and capnography, and controlled or assisted by an anesthesia care provider, when the patient is under general anesthesia. *Circulation* is monitored by electrocardiography and BP.

Electrocardiography

The patient's heart rate and rhythm will be continually assessed with electrocardiography. Electrocardiography is the process of recording the electrical impulses of the heart. Electrodes that sense the electrical activity of the heart are placed on the patient's skin and attached to leads, which transmit those electrical impulses to the electrocardiograph (ECG) device (Fig. 13.1). The electrical activity of the heart is recorded and displayed on a screen. The ECG may be set to record a tracing of the electrical activity on a strip of paper. The ECG device is also set to emit an audible signal to indicate heart rate and rhythm.

! CAUTION

For patient safety, the audible ECG signal must be set loud enough to be heard by the anesthesia care provider over extraneous operating room noise.

The ECG may be recorded with three- or five-lead systems. The surgical technologist in the circulating role may assist the anesthesia care provider in placing the electrodes, which should be securely adhered to areas of clean, dry skin. The electrodes should be protected from preparation solutions and placed so

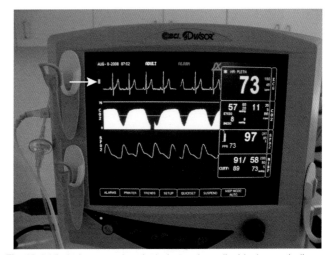

Fig 13.1 Vital signs monitor, includes carbon dioxide (*arrow* indicates electrocardiogram). (From Malamed SF: *Sedation*, ed 5, St Louis, 2010, Elsevier.)

that a change in the patient's position (e.g., supine to lateral) will not disrupt electrode contact. In a five-lead system, electrodes are placed on each shoulder, each hip, and in the fifth intercostal space near the left anterior axillary line. A baseline reading is obtained, and the ECG is used to monitor changes in the heart rate and rhythm during surgery.

The ECG is supplemented by auscultation (listening to the sounds of the chest [e.g., the heart rate, rhythm, and pulmonary sounds]) with a precordial stethoscope. A modified version of a standard stethoscope, the precordial stethoscope is taped onto the patient's chest at the left sternal border or in the suprasternal notch. Alternatively, an esophageal stethoscope may be used, particularly if the chest is prepped into the sterile field. A long piece of tubing extends from the stethoscope to a specialized earpiece, placed in the anesthesia care provider's ear, thus enabling continuous auscultation. Auscultation is also used to assess respiratory rate and lung sounds and to verify placement of airway devices used in general anesthesia.

> **⚑ TECH TIP**
>
> A review of basic physiology of the electrical conduction system of the heart is highly recommended. The surgical technologist should be able to interpret a normal ECG cycle, including the meaning of the P wave, QRS complex, and T wave. By listening to the audible ECG in the background noise of the operating room, the surgical technologist should be able to appreciate various types of dysrhythmias, including bradycardia, tachycardia, and asystole. In addition, the surgical technologist should be able to identify a premature ventricular contraction and the presence of an active pacemaker by its characteristic spike. Each of these abilities contributes to the surgical technologist's value as a surgical team member. The ability to recognize and appreciate the importance of changes in heart rate and rhythm enables the surgical technologist to provide assistance to the anesthesia care provider and patient when necessary.

Pulse Oximetry

Pulse oximetry is a noninvasive measure of the oxygen saturation of blood. A two-sided sensor probe is attached to a finger, toe, or earlobe (Fig. 13.2). The probe emits red and infrared light, which is absorbed while passing through tissue. Remaining light is detected by the opposite side of the sensor probe and used to calculate the saturation of peripheral oxygen. Ideally, the saturation should be above 95%. When indicated, pulse

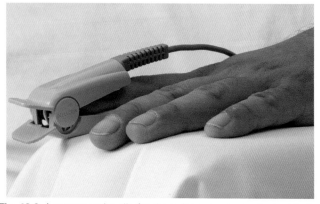

Fig. 13.2 A sensor probe clip for the pulse oximeter is attached to the patient's finger. (Courtesy Frank Pronesti T/A heirloomstudio.com.)

oximetry readings are confirmed with a measurement of arterial blood gases. Readings may be affected by administration of intravenous (IV) dyes, such as methylene blue (see Chapter 6), but most devices currently used are capable of adjusting to such conditions. Vasoconstriction caused by hypothermia can affect readings when a finger sensor is used.

An audible signal reflects pulse rate, and the signal tone indicates saturation. A deeper tone indicates lower oxygen saturation. For patient safety, this audible signal must be loud enough to be heard by all members of the operating room team.

> **⚑ TECH TIP**
>
> Even while cleaning up the back table after a procedure, the surgical technologist should be alert to the rate and tone of the pulse oximeter. A patient's slow pulse or dropping oxygen saturation during emergence from anesthesia may signal an emergency situation, such as laryngospasm (see Chapter 15). The surgical technologist must be able to identify such a situation, stop clean-up duties, and turn full attention to the patient and the needs of the anesthesia care provider, until the crisis has been resolved.

Blood Pressure

BP is a measure of the force of blood against the vessel walls. BP is typically measured at the brachial artery. An inflatable cuff is placed on the patient's upper arm. The cuff is inflated to a pressure that occludes the pulse, and the pressure is gradually released. The point at which the pulse is first detected is the systolic pressure, and the point at which the pulse can no longer be detected is the diastolic pressure. Automated BP devices have replaced the old mercury-based sphygmomanometers, but readings are still reported in millimeters of mercury (mm Hg). For an accurate reading of BP to be obtained, the cuff must be an appropriate size for the patient. The cuff should be long enough to cover the circumference of the patient's upper arm, plus approximately 40%. The width of the cuff is important too. A cuff that is too narrow may record higher pressure, and a cuff that is too wide may record lower than the accurate pressure.

Normal BP in a healthy adult is considered to be less than 120 mm Hg systolic and less than 80 mm Hg diastolic. Opinions are changing regarding what is considered a normal BP measurement. In adults older than age 50 years, a measurement that was once accepted as normal BP is now considered prehypertensive. Multiple variables affect BP, including ventricular contraction strength, capillary resistance, vessel wall elasticity, and blood volume.

The BP cuff is placed on the patient's arm that does *not* have the IV cannula in place, whenever possible. The cuff is connected to a device that automatically measures BP at specified intervals. During induction of general anesthesia, BP is monitored more frequently. The machine may be set to emit an audible alarm if the BP is not within preset parameters.

An invasive measure of BP may be obtained through placement of an arterial line, discussed later in this section.

Temperature

All surgical patients are at risk of mild-to-significant hypothermia, so continuous temperature monitoring is indicated for most surgical procedures. Some patients, particularly pediatric and geriatric patients, are more vulnerable to changes in body temperature that necessitate continuous temperature monitoring. Temperature may be assessed from any number of locations, including skin, axilla, bladder, esophagus, and ear. Simple liquid crystal temperature strips can be placed on the patient's forehead for basic monitoring of skin temperature. More precise measurements of core temperature are indicated in some patients and for some types of surgical procedures. In such cases, a lower esophageal probe may be used because it offers the most accurate reading of core temperature with the least risk of patient injury. Normal body temperature varies from patient to patient, and it also varies by the time of day. Oral temperature is usually within a limited range near 98 °F (approximately 37°C). A patient's baseline temperature measurement is obtained, and changes are monitored and assessed. Core temperatures lower than 36°C indicate hypothermia. Hypothermia alters several normal body functions, and it is associated with an increased risk of surgical site infections. Several precautions are taken to minimize heat loss, such as a forced-air warmer (Fig. 13.3), and the patient's body temperature is continually monitored to verify the effectiveness of those precautions.

Capnometry

Capnometry is a measurement of carbon dioxide (CO_2) exhaled by the patient, called *end-tidal CO_2*. This monitor is used to verify adequate ventilation whenever the patient is under heavy sedation or general anesthesia. In general anesthesia, an adapter is connected to the breathing circuit, and a small-diameter piece of tubing extends from the adapter to the analyzer. An oxygen cannula with a CO_2 sampling tube is available to monitor the sedated patient. The concentration of expired CO_2 is measured and displayed as a continuous graph and in numerical value. An audible alarm is set to indicate when preset levels are exceeded. Capnometry is an extremely valuable tool in the assessment of respiratory function and can serve a critical role in early detection of problems, such as an esophageal intubation, compromised ventilation, or malignant hyperthermia (see Chapter 15).

Monitoring Consciousness

Traditionally, the depth of various components of general anesthesia has been monitored in several ways, including basic vital signs and nerve stimulation, but traditional monitoring methods may not have been sufficient in some patients to adequately assess the level of patient awareness under anesthesia. Patient awareness while under anesthesia is a rare, but significant,

concern (see Chapter 14), estimated to occur in approximately 1 to 2 of 1000 patients undergoing general anesthesia. In an effort to assist the anesthesia care provider in assessing the depth of consciousness under anesthesia, a modified electroencephalogram (EEG) may be used to determine the level of consciousness by recording electrical activity in the brain (Fig. 13.4). It provides a direct measure of the effect of general anesthetic agents on the brain. EEG information is obtained from a sensor placed on the patient's forehead. The monitor interprets the information and displays a reading between 0 and 100, a scale used to indicate the patient's level of consciousness. A number near 100 indicates that the patient is fully awake and responsive, and a number between 45 and 60 indicates an appropriate depth of general anesthesia with a low probability of explicit recall (see Chapter 14).

Neuromuscular Function

During general anesthesia, muscle relaxants are administered to facilitate endotracheal intubation and a relaxed surgical site (see Chapter 14). A nerve stimulator (Fig. 13.5) is used to assess neuromuscular function and the extent of blockade. A stimulus

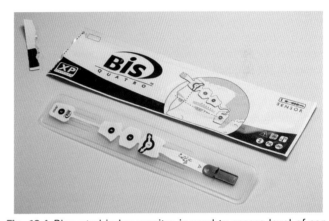

Fig. 13.4 Bispectral index monitor is used to assess level of consciousness. (Courtesy Frank Pronesti T/A heirloomstudio.com.)

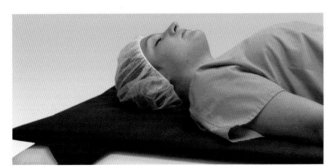

Fig. 13.3 KOALA Warming Mattress. (Courtesy NOVAMED USA.)

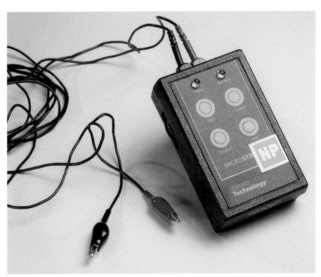

Fig. 13.5 A nerve stimulator is used to assess level of muscle relaxation. (Courtesy Frank Pronesti T/A heirloomstudio.com.)

is delivered to the nerve from a surface electrode or probe, often placed at the ulnar nerve or a branch of the facial nerve. Four stimuli (called a "*train-of-four*," or *TOF*) are administered, and the extent of the block is estimated based on the twitch response. The presence of four of the four twitches indicates no muscle relaxation, whereas zero of the four twitches indicates complete muscle relaxation. Nerve stimulation is used to determine if the patient's jaw and vocal cords are adequately relaxed for intubation and to determine when additional muscle relaxants should be administered during a surgical procedure. Nerve stimulation is also used to assess the extent to which muscle relaxants are wearing off and the patient is becoming ready to breathe on his or her own after surgery.

Advanced Monitoring

Certain patient conditions and surgical procedures may require additional monitoring. These invasive monitoring techniques include arterial catheterization and pressure monitoring, central venous catheterization and pressure monitoring, and pulmonary artery (PA) catheterization (Swan-Ganz catheter). An arterial pressure–monitoring catheter (often referred to as an *arterial line* or *art-line*) is usually placed in the radial artery and connected to a transducer that records continuous, immediate, and highly accurate measurement of BP. Placement of an arterial line is indicated for a number of reasons, including potential for rapid changes in BP, frequent sampling of arterial blood for blood gas analysis, or when routine BP measurement is inaccurate.

When indicated, a central venous pressure–monitoring catheter (CVP line) is positioned in the superior vena cava and is used to assess the volume of blood returning to the heart. A CVP line is also used to assess the need for fluid replacement and to prevent fluid overload.

A PA catheter (such as a Swan-Ganz catheter) is guided through the heart into a branch of the PA to obtain measurements of central venous pressure, PA pressure, pulmonary capillary wedge pressure, and cardiac output (Fig. 13.6). PA catheters are most frequently used in adult patients during cardiac surgery, lung transplantation, and liver transplantation.

During heart surgery, transesophageal echocardiography (TEE) may be used to assess cardiac function. A probe is placed into the esophagus, and high-frequency sound waves are emitted through the tissue. An image of the heart is obtained and interpreted. TEE can be used to observe cardiac wall motion and valve function, to assess intravascular fluid volume, and to identify the presence of air in the heart. Blood flow through the heart can be assessed with echocardiography and pulse-wave, continuous, or color Doppler technology.

When the patient has been admitted to the operating room and all the appropriate basic monitoring devices are in place, baseline measurements are recorded, and the patient is ready for administration of anesthesia. Invasive monitoring devices may be placed before or after the administration of general anesthesia.

SEDATION AND MONITORED ANESTHESIA CARE

The ASA has defined the term MAC as a specific anesthesia service for a diagnostic or therapeutic procedure that includes all aspects of anesthesia care—before, during, and after the procedure. According to the ASA Position on Monitored Anesthesia Care (as updated in 2018), MAC may include varying levels of sedation, analgesia, and anxiolysis as needed. The levels of sedation for diagnostic or therapeutic procedures range on a scale from minimal sedation (anxiolysis) to moderate sedation/analgesia (conscious sedation) to deep sedation/analgesia to general anesthesia. The anesthesia care provider continuously monitors all vital signs, including the patient's heart rate and ECG, BP, respirations, and oxygen saturation, during these procedures.

Indications for MAC include the nature of the procedure, the patient's clinical condition, or the potential need to convert to a general or regional anesthetic. There are many diagnostic or therapeutic procedures that are conducted with MAC, including colonoscopy and esophagogastroduodenoscopy. Agents that may be administered during MAC include midazolam, fentanyl, alfentanil, meperidine (Demerol), and propofol (Diprivan).

Local Anesthesia

For anesthesia to be accomplished, transmission of the sensation of pain through nerve impulses can be interrupted at several locations, including nerve endings, groups of nerves, or at the level of the brain. Local anesthesia is the parenteral administration of an anesthetic agent to nerve endings in the immediate surgical site.

> ### ❓ QUICK QUESTION
>
> What does the term *parenteral* administration mean? Check your answer in Chapter 1.

Whether anesthetics are injected (infiltrated) into tissue or applied topically to mucosal membranes, local anesthesia affects a small, circumscribed area. Local anesthetics, such as lidocaine, interfere with sensory nerve endings in the operative area; thus they block transmission of pain impulses to the brain.

When local anesthesia is used without an anesthesia care provider present, it is imperative that a registered nurse (RN) be assigned to monitor the patient's vital signs during the surgical procedure. The RN assesses the patient's physical condition and

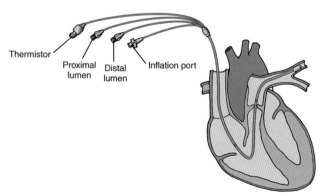

Fig. 13.6 Swan-Ganz catheter. (From Buck CJ: *Step-by-step medical coding 2016*, St Louis, 2016, Elsevier.)

Thermistor

Proximal lumen   Distal lumen   Inflation port

psychological status, so that appropriate measures can be taken to maintain patient safety and comfort. Heart rate and rhythm are measured by ECG, and BP, respirations, and oxygen saturation are also monitored continuously. The RN may administer sedatives as ordered by the surgeon. Only physically healthy and psychologically stable patients undergoing brief, uncomplicated surgical procedures are appropriate candidates for local anesthesia without monitoring by an anesthesia care provider.

Applications for Local Anesthesia

Local anesthesia is the method of choice for several types of surgical procedures. It may be used with or without sedation, depending on the patient's condition or the extent of the procedure. Some of the common surgical applications for local anesthesia with MAC include breast biopsy, transvenous pacemaker insertion, venous access port or catheter insertion, or placement of a dialysis access graft. Cataract surgery is usually performed with the patient under local anesthesia with MAC; topical drops and intracameral (meaning within a chamber, anterior chamber in this case) injections are used, as needed (see Chapter 10).

A specialized type of local infiltration requiring MAC is called *tumescent anesthesia*, and it is widely used in aesthetic surgery for liposuction. Tumescent anesthesia is a technique that involves injection of a large volume of a dilute solution into subcutaneous tissues to facilitate fat suctioning, provide local anesthesia, and reduce blood loss. The solution commonly contains 0.05% to 0.1% lidocaine, epinephrine 0.5 to 1.5 mg/L, and normal saline. Sodium bicarbonate may be added to increase absorption and shorten onset time. Glucocorticoids, such as triamcinolone, may also be added to reduce inflammation and potential scarring.

If the patient's condition and the extent of the surgical procedure do not require MAC, a number of procedures may be performed with an RN to monitor the patient. For example, in general surgery, local anesthesia may be appropriate for excision or biopsy of small soft tissue masses, such as excision of lipomas, nevi, or other skin lesions. In urology, cystoscopy may be performed with a topical anesthetic agent. In orthopedic surgery, local anesthesia may be used for limited work on digits, such as repair of finger lacerations or toenail excisions. Local anesthesia is used in plastic surgery for procedures, such as excision of small lesions or minor scar revisions.

TECH TIP

It is important for surgical technologists to be aware of the fact that although local anesthesia blocks sensory nerve pain impulses at the site of injection or application, the patient is still able to move muscles and feel pressure. Do not be alarmed if patients move their fingers during a finger laceration repair, while you are holding retractors. In addition, if patients remark that they can "feel" something during local anesthesia, it is necessary to determine whether what they are feeling is actually pain or, for example, simply the pressure of retractors or the surgeon's hand.

Agents Used for Local Anesthesia

Local anesthetic agents are chemically classified as either aminoesters or aminoamides. The pharmacokinetic action of

INSIGHT 13.1 Pharmacokinetics of Local Anesthetic Agents

It may be helpful to review the processes of pharmacokinetics applied to local anesthetics. It is interesting to note that pharmacokinetics is different for local anesthetics than it is for other medications. Recall that absorption is the process in which medications are taken into the body, and the process of distribution takes the drug to its site of action. Local anesthetics are different in that they are injected or applied topically directly to the intended site of action. The pharmacokinetic processes of absorption and distribution by the circulatory system actually cause a reduction in the intended effect of local anesthetics at the site of action. Dilute epinephrine may be added to a local anesthetic to cause vasoconstriction and thus slow the absorption of the agent into systemic circulation.

The pH of tissues at the site of action also affects the action of local anesthetics. When an infection is present, the tissue is slightly acidic, which reduces the ability of these agents to exert their effects.

Plasma protein binding is another important aspect of the distribution phase of pharmacokinetics. Local anesthetic agents vary widely in the extent of plasma protein binding, which impacts availability for metabolism and excretion. Procaine (Novocain, an aminoester) is only 6% bound, lidocaine is 64% bound, mepivacaine is 65% bound, ropivacaine is 94% bound, and bupivacaine is 97% bound to plasma proteins.

Because the chemical structures are different, the two types of local anesthetic agents are also metabolized in different ways. Aminoester local anesthetics are metabolized in the blood. These chemicals are hydrolyzed by enzymes circulating in the plasma (plasma cholinesterase) and are rapidly excreted in urine. Aminoamides are almost completely metabolized by hepatic enzymes in the liver, and very little of the unchanged drug molecules is excreted in urine.

local anesthetics is significantly different from that of other drugs, and it differs between the two chemical classes of agents (Insight 13.1). The duration of action of local anesthetics is caused by the differences in their plasma protein–binding capacity and their individual lipid-binding affinity, which also accounts for variations in duration, depending on the area of the body to be anesthetized.

QUICK QUESTION

How does plasma protein binding affect a drug's duration of action? Check your answer in Chapter 1.

The first local anesthetic agents, topical cocaine and injectable procaine (Novocain), were aminoesters. Cocaine is a naturally occurring alkaloid derived from coca leaves. It has long been known to have anesthetic effects when used topically on mucous membranes. It may be used in nasal surgery but is less frequently used today because acceptable alternatives are available.

! CAUTION

Cocaine is for topical use only; it is never injected.

Cocaine comes in 4% solutions; thus it may be administered on cotton applicators or nasal packing, or it may be sprayed directly on the mucosal surface. In addition to its anesthetic properties, cocaine is also a powerful vasoconstrictor. This means it reduces bleeding and helps shrink mucous membranes.

Thus it is particularly useful in nasal surgery because it allows better visualization in the nasal cavity. Dosages are carefully calculated to the patient's age and physical condition, and the lowest dose necessary is used to achieve the required anesthetic effect. Concentrations greater than 4% increase potential for systemic toxic reactions. Adverse effects are seen primarily in the central nervous system (CNS). These include excitement and depression and may lead to respiratory arrest. Because of these complications, cocaine is less often used in nasal surgery today. Nasal local anesthesia is currently more commonly accomplished with injection of lidocaine (Xylocaine) and the topical application of either phenylephrine (Neo-Synephrine) or the nasal spray oxymetazoline (Afrin), to shrink mucous membranes.

> **⚠ CAUTION**
>
> Cocaine is a controlled substance (see Chapter 2). It should never be left unattended in the operating room, and any cocaine solution dispensed but unused should be returned to the pharmacy or destroyed. At least two people should witness the destruction of unused cocaine to verify that it has not been used for illicit purposes.

Two other aminoester local anesthetic agents are also used in surgery. Benzocaine (14%, contained in Cetacaine spray) is a topical agent with rapid onset and a duration of 30 to 60 minutes. It may be applied before bronchoscopy or fiberoptic endotracheal intubation. Tetracaine (Pontocaine) is a potent and long-acting local anesthetic. A 0.5% solution may be used for topical anesthesia before cataract surgery (see Chapter 10). Tetracaine may also be used in spinal anesthesia, a type of regional anesthesia, because it provides rapid onset and excellent motor and sensory block lasting 90 to 120 minutes.

> **❓ MAKE IT SIMPLE**
>
> The names of all the local anesthetic agents end in "-caine." It is easy to identify the amide anesthetics when you remember the "*i.*" The letter *i* occurs in am*i*de and in the first part of the generic name of each amide agent—l*i*docaine, bup*i*vacaine, rop*i*vacaine, and mep*i*vacaine. The letter "*i*" does not occur in the first part of the generic names of ester anesthetics—cocaine, benzocaine, and tetracaine. Another option is to look at the entire generic name and see that the letter "*i*" will be in the name of the amides twice (e.g., bup*i*vaca*i*ne), whereas aminoesters have only one "*i*" in the generic names (e.g., coca*i*ne).

The most common local anesthetic agents used in surgery are aminoamides: lidocaine (Xylocaine), bupivacaine (Marcaine), and ropivacaine (Naropin). A less commonly used local anesthetic agent is mepivacaine (Carbocaine). All of these agents, except ropivacaine, may be combined with dilute epinephrine (see Chapter 8). Most local anesthetics (except ropivacaine) cause some vasodilation, which speeds absorption. Recall that epinephrine is a potent vasoconstrictor. When combined with a local anesthetic agent, epinephrine causes local vasoconstriction, slowing the absorption of the agent into the circulatory system. This action keeps the local anesthetic in the surgical site longer, thus increasing the duration of effect. Some manufacturers will

call attention to local anesthetic agents mixed with epinephrine by adding red print or a red band on the vial label for rapid identification (Fig. 13.7). Local anesthetics without epinephrine may have a blue band on the label. This practice helps staff visually identify the correct formulation, but it is not a substitute for thorough reading of the entire label before delivery to the sterile field.

> **⚠ CAUTION**
>
> Local anesthetic agents with epinephrine should *not* be used for peripheral infiltration anesthesia on fingers, toes, tip of the nose, or penis because of vasoconstriction caused by epinephrine.

> **⚠ CAUTION**
>
> Epinephrine premixed in a local anesthetic agent is present in very tiny amounts (most commonly 1 part of epinephrine to 100,000 or 200,000 parts of solvent). The surgical technologist must be aware that epinephrine is also available separately in the very high concentration of 1 mg/mL (1:1000), 100 or 200 times stronger than the dose intended for injection (see Chapter 4 and Insight 13.2). It is vital to administer epinephrine in the correct concentration for the correct purpose and by the correct route. If the high 1 mg/mL (1:1000) concentration of epinephrine is inadvertently injected, severe tachycardia (rapid heart rate) and hypertension will result, increasing the potential for cardiac arrest. All medications present on the sterile field must be correctly labeled (name and dose) and identified when passing to the surgeon to avoid medication administration errors (see Chapter 4).

The most common local anesthetic agent in use today is lidocaine. Lidocaine is fast acting and rapidly metabolized. The duration of anesthesia with infiltrated lidocaine is approximately 30 to 60 minutes. If epinephrine is added to a lidocaine solution, the duration of effect is approximately 2 to 3 hours. The prolonged effect occurs because epinephrine slows systemic absorption, keeping more of the drug at the site of action. Lidocaine is available for injection in solutions of 0.5%, 1%, 1.5%, and 2%, with and without epinephrine 1:100,000 and 1:200,000. It is also available in a 4% topical solution for nasal

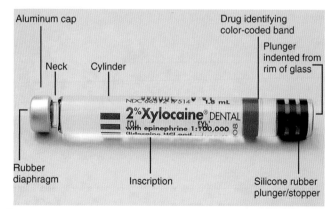

Fig. 13.7 Components of the glass cartridge, including a red band indicating that the local anesthetic agent has been mixed with epinephrine. (From Malamed SF: *Handbook of local anesthesia*, ed 6, St Louis, 2013, Mosby.)

INSIGHT 13.2 Practical Mathematics and Lidocaine with Epinephrine Dosages

Basic mathematics is used in the calculation of strength, dosage, and ratios of medications. Local anesthetics, with and without epinephrine, are examples of the daily use of mathematics in the operating room.

For example, lidocaine is available in a 1% solution. This means that 1 g of solute (the medication) is contained in 100 mL of solvent (the diluent). Multiply this dose by 10, and the result is 10 g/1000 mL or 10 g/L—or this figure can be divided by 1000 to obtain the equivalent, which is 10 mg/mL. If the patient receives an injection of 20 mL of 1% lidocaine, the dosage of lidocaine is 200 mg (20 mL times 10 mg).

When combined with a local anesthetic, epinephrine dosages are expressed as a ratio. For example, dilute epinephrine (1:100,000 or 1:200,000) may be added to lidocaine. The ratio indicates a solution of 1 part epinephrine (the solute) to 100,000 or 200,000 parts of solvent (the diluent). A 1:1 solution means there is 1 g of solute per gram (mL) of solvent. Thus a 1:100,000 solution of epinephrine contains 0.01 mg/mL or 10 mcg/mL. In contrast, epinephrine is also available separately in a 1:1000 solution. Divided by 1000, it can be expressed as 1 mg/mL. The dosage is dramatically different if a 1:1000 (1 mg/mL) solution is used instead of the 1:100,000 (0.01 mg/mL) solution. Inject 30 mL of epinephrine 1:100,000, and the dose is 0.3 mg, but inject 3 mL of 1:1000 epinephrine and the dose is 30 mg—a 100-fold increase.

Understanding principles of basic mathematics can make a significant difference in protecting the surgical patient from medication errors.

---

and oral mucosal applications. Lidocaine 2% jelly (URO-jet) is packaged in a sterile, prefilled syringe used for topical urethral application for cystoscopy.

NOTE: Some people may mistakenly refer to lidocaine as "Novocain," which is a completely different agent. Novocain is the trade name for procaine, which was used by dentists for many years, but is seldom used currently. Procaine is classified chemically as an aminoester-type anesthetic. Aminoester-type anesthetics cause more allergic reactions than aminoamide-type anesthetics. Patients who are allergic to Novocain do not usually have allergies to lidocaine because these agents have different chemical structures and metabolic pathways.

Bupivacaine (Marcaine) is an aminoamide anesthetic that is approximately 4 times more potent than lidocaine and has a longer duration, from 3 to 7 hours. Bupivacaine is available in solutions of 0.25%, 0.5%, and 0.75%, with and without epinephrine 1:200,000. Bupivacaine is more highly bound to plasma proteins than lidocaine, and it is more lipid soluble, which help account for its longer duration. Unlike other local anesthetics, bupivacaine's duration of action is not prolonged by the addition of epinephrine but adding epinephrine to bupivacaine does limit vascular uptake. Bupivacaine 0.25% is also frequently used near the end of some surgical procedures to provide postoperative analgesia. It may be used to block nerves after inguinal herniorrhaphy or laparoscopic port sites after cholecystectomy.

Bupivacaine also binds to cardiac muscle, so its chief adverse effect is cardiotoxicity. It is contraindicated for IV regional anesthesia (IVRA) because toxicity is most closely associated with intravascular administration.

⚠ CAUTION

The product package insert contains a warning that the use of 0.75% bupivacaine is *not* recommended for obstetric epidural anesthesia. Cardiac arrest with difficult resuscitation or death has been reported in patients receiving bupivacaine (generally the 0.75% concentration) for obstetric epidural anesthesia.

Ropivacaine (Naropin) is an aminoamide local anesthetic agent released for use in 1996. It is similar in duration to bupivacaine but is generally less cardiotoxic. It is available in concentrations of 0.2%, 0.5%, 0.75%, and 1%. Naropin is packaged in vials and plastic ampules of 10 mL, 20 mL, and 30 mL. Plastic ampules (Fig. 13.8) of 10 mL and 20 mL are available in "Sterile-Pak" for delivery to the sterile field. This type of packaging enables the surgical technologist to fill a syringe with the agent at the sterile back table rather than requiring the circulator to hold the container for delivery to the field (see Chapter 4).

Mepivacaine (Carbocaine) is another aminoamide anesthetic that has a similar potency to lidocaine, with a similar duration. Mepivacaine is available in solutions of 1%, 1.5%, 2%, and 3% solution and may be combined with epinephrine. It is not available for topical use. Mepivacaine is used less often, because it does not have a significant advantage over lidocaine, which is used more frequently and thus is more readily available. See Table 13.1 for a comparison of common local anesthetic agents.

Adverse reactions to amide local anesthetics are primarily dose-related and affect both the CNS and the cardiovascular system.

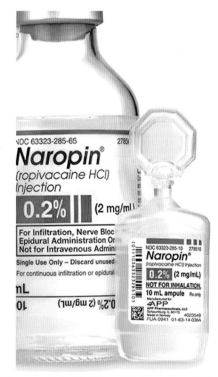

Fig. 13.8 Naropin is available in sterile polypropylene ampules. (Courtesy APP Pharmaceuticals, LLC., a company of the Fresenius Kabi Group, Schaumburg, IL.)

TABLE 13.1   Comparison of Common Local Anesthetic Agents

Generic Name	Trade Name	Solutions Available (%)	Duration (h)
lidocaine with epinephrine	Xylocaine	0.5, 1, 1.5, 2	2–3
mepivacaine with epinephrine	Carbocaine	1, 1.5, 2, 3	2–3
ropivacaine	Naropin	0.2, 0.5, 1	2–6
bupivacaine	Marcaine	0.25, 0.5, 0.75	3–7

🔧 TECH TIP

For the prevention of dose-related toxicity, it is vital that the surgical technologist keep track of the amount of any local anesthetic agent used from the sterile back table. Use a sterile marking pen (see Chapter 6) to keep a running total of the volume used, so that the concentration and final total amount can be accurately reported to the anesthesia care provider. The anesthesia care provider will use this information to calculate and record the actual dose of local anesthetic administered.

Adverse CNS effects are variable, from drowsiness at low doses to excitement or agitation at higher doses. Excitement may or may not occur, and the patient may go from a drowsy state to unconsciousness and into respiratory arrest. Nausea and vomiting may also occur. Other CNS adverse effects include visual disturbances, tingling, slurred speech, and excitability, which can lead to seizures. Cardiovascular adverse effects are also dose-related and include hypotension, bradycardia, and ventricular arrhythmias, leading to possible cardiac arrest. Systemic toxicity from local anesthetics is most commonly caused by inadvertent intravascular injection during peripheral nerve infiltration. See the section on advanced practices of this chapter (Table 13.A) for a comparison of maximum dosages of local anesthetics.

❓ QUICK QUESTION

Why are concentration and volume of a local anesthetic agent important when reporting the final total? See Chapter 4 to check your answer.

Regional Anesthesia

Regional anesthesia is a technique used to accomplish both sensory and motor block to an entire area of the body. Regional anesthesia blocks nerves (not just nerve endings) or groups of nerves (called a *plexus*) at specific locations; thus it provides a larger anesthetized area. Regional blocks can affect sympathetic, sensory, and motor nerve supply, so an anesthetized limb may be immobile, as well as numb. Any type of regional anesthesia requires continuous monitoring of the patient's vital functions, including heart rate and ECG, BP, respirations, and oxygen saturation, by a qualified anesthesia care provider.

Regional blocks are effective for many types of surgical procedures but frequently take more time to administer than a general anesthetic. Various types of regional anesthetic techniques are usually named for the nerves or areas of the body to be blocked. Although nearly any group of nerves can be blocked, we discuss only the most frequently used regional anesthetic techniques in this text. The most commonly used regional blocks are spinal and epidural, collectively referred to as *central neuraxial blockade*.

Spinal Anesthesia

For spinal anesthesia, agents are injected through the dura mater into the subarachnoid space and cerebrospinal fluid (CSF) in the lumbar area of the spine (Fig. 13.9); this is called the *intrathecal route*. Injection is at the end of the spinal cord, usually not higher than L3 to L4. This technique anesthetizes the entire lower body. Preoperative preparation may include administration of anxiolytics and analgesics (see Chapter 12) to minimize discomfort. The circulator usually assists the anesthesia care provider during injection of a spinal anesthetic by helping the patient to get into optimum position. The patient may be positioned laterally to facilitate correct needle placement (i.e., patients may lie on the side, with knees bent and chin on chest). Thus the patient is usually instructed to curl up as much as possible, pushing his or her lower back out toward the anesthesia care provider. This position spreads the vertebral bodies apart so the spinal needle may be more easily inserted, but it is difficult for some patients, especially the elderly, to curl their backs. These patients may be assisted gently into position, with caution to avoid injury. Alternatively, patients may be in a sitting position for administration of a spinal anesthetic. The patient may sit on the operating bed with his or her back to the anesthesia care provider.

Skin around the injection site area is prepped with an antiseptic agent, and a small, fenestrated sterile drape is placed over the area. Local anesthesia is injected through skin and subcutaneous tissue before insertion of a spinal needle through the ligaments and dura. The spinal needle is correctly placed when a drop of CSF appears. A syringe containing anesthetic agent is attached to the spinal needle, and a small amount of CSF is aspirated to reconfirm placement. The agent is injected, the needle and syringe are withdrawn, and the patient is placed in supine position. The level of anesthesia is verified, often with the use of an alcohol wipe. Alcohol will feel cold on an unblocked area of skin and warm or neutral on a blocked area. Another technique that may be used to assess the level of spinal anesthesia is pinprick. The patient feels a sharp pinprick on an unblocked area of skin, and a dull sensation on a blocked area.

Spinal anesthesia is usually quicker to administer than an epidural and provides more intense sensory and motor blockade. In addition, proper needle placement is clearly verified by the appearance of CSF. If continuous spinal anesthesia is indicated, a small catheter is placed for repeated dosing.

The most common local anesthetic agents used for spinal anesthesia include tetracaine, bupivacaine, and ropivacaine. Local anesthetic agents used for spinal and epidural anesthesia

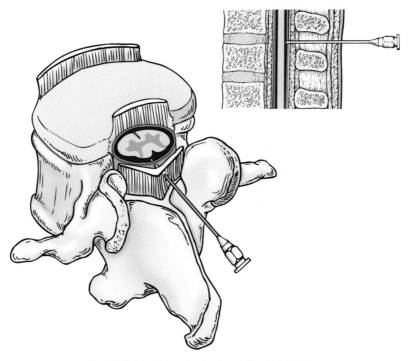

Fig. 13.9 Location of spinal anesthesia injection.

must be formulated as preservative-free, and this will be clearly indicated on the drug label. Dilute epinephrine may be added to prolong blockade, but it may also delay postoperative urination during recovery, so epinephrine is less frequently used for outpatient surgery. Instead, an opioid, such as fentanyl or sufentanil, may be added to prolong duration of spinal anesthesia without prolonging recovery time.

? QUICK QUESTION

What does the term *opioid* mean? Opioids are classified as which type of agents? See Chapter 12 to check your answer.

Spinal anesthesia is used for procedures of the lower abdomen, perineum, and lower extremities. It is often used for transurethral resection of the prostate gland or bladder tumors, for lower leg vascular procedures (such as embolectomy), for select orthopedic procedures (such as total knee arthroplasty), and for cesarean sections.

A drop in BP may occur with administration of a spinal or epidural anesthetic because of vasodilation. Younger, more athletic patients with lower resting heart rates have a higher risk for significant bradycardia under spinal anesthesia. Another complication of spinal anesthesia is postdural puncture headache (PDPH), which can be severe and is thought to be associated with the creation of a persistent tear or slit in the dura. Severe PDPH may be treated by administration of a "blood patch" (i.e., an epidural injection of 20 mL of the patient's blood at the original spinal injection site). The development and use of "pencil-point" needles for intrathecal injection has decreased the incidence of this complication (Fig. 13.10).

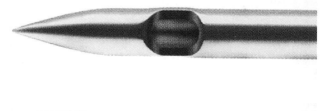

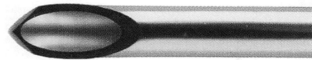

Fig. 13.10 Pencil point (*above*) and cutting bevel tip (*below*) spinal needles. (Courtesy Smiths Medical ASD Inc., St. Paul, MN. In Liu DT: *Labour ward manual*, ed 4, St Louis, 2007, Elsevier.)

NOTE: An extreme complication of neurotoxicity attributed to the use of 5% lidocaine in spinal anesthesia is cauda equina syndrome, a paralysis of nerves resulting in lower extremity muscle weakness and impaired bowel and bladder function. Lidocaine in high concentrations (5%) is not used in spinal anesthesia because of the potential for neurotoxicity.

Intrathecal catheters and pumps are used to deliver analgesics to patients with various types of chronic pain. These devices are not used for surgical anesthesia but may be placed in the surgical setting as part of the patient's treatment for chronic pain issues.

Epidural Anesthesia

In epidural anesthesia, an anesthetic agent is injected into the space surrounding the dura mater (Fig. 13.11). A single injection may be administered, or a catheter may be placed

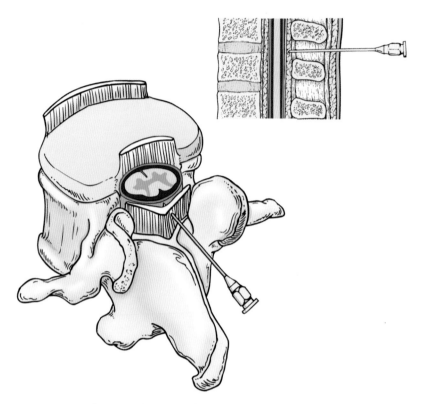

Fig. 13.11 Location of epidural anesthesia injection.

for continuous infusion or repeated injections. Sedation may be given to help relieve discomfort of injection and catheter placement (except in pregnant patients because sedation would also affect the baby). When indicated for use in pediatric patients, an epidural is placed after general anesthesia is induced. Positioning, prepping, and draping for administration of an epidural anesthetic are identical to those described for a spinal anesthetic. Local anesthesia is administered at the injection site and an epidural needle is placed. A catheter is advanced through the needle, and the needle is carefully withdrawn. A catheter-to-syringe adapter is attached to the catheter, and the catheter is taped in place on the patient's back, and an empty 3-mL syringe may be attached. Correct placement is verified when CSF does *not* enter the syringe. A test dose of agent is administered, followed by small doses at intervals over a 1- to 3-minute period. Agents can be administered intermittently or by continuous infusion. Common agents used for epidural anesthesia include lidocaine, bupivacaine, and ropivacaine. Dilute epinephrine (1:200,000) may be added to prolong duration, and small doses of opioids may be used to manage postoperative pain.

Epidural anesthesia is used to relieve the pain of labor and vaginal delivery, and to provide anesthesia for cesarean section. Bupivacaine (0.25% and 0.5%) is an excellent choice for obstetric epidural anesthesia. A motor block will almost always be obtained with a bupivacaine concentration of 0.5%. In obstetric anesthesia, concentrations of 0.125%, plus very low doses of fentanyl, are used to provide "walking epidurals" (i.e., analgesia without motor block).

Epidural blocks may also be used as an adjunct to general anesthesia in select patients to minimize the amount of general anesthesia needed; they may also be used for postoperative pain control after such procedures as thoracotomy.

Epidural anesthesia has some advantages over spinal anesthesia, including reduced risk of hypotension and less incidence of PDPH (because the dura is not intentionally punctured). In addition, epidural anesthesia may be administered at levels above L3 to L4—for example, at T4-T5 for thoracic analgesia. Epidural anesthesia requires greater volume of agent (typically 20 mL) than spinal (typically 1 to 2 mL) and has a slower but longer onset of action. Slower onset of action is caused by the time it takes the agent to cross the dura to reach the CSF, but epidural is preferred over spinal anesthesia when the surgical procedure duration is variable or extended, or when prolonged postoperative analgesia is necessary.

Caudal block. Caudal anesthesia is a type of epidural block injected into the epidural space via the sacral canal (Fig. 13.12) at the sacral hiatus (level S5). Caudal blocks are primarily used in conjunction with general anesthesia for urologic and lower extremity surgical procedures in children for postoperative pain management. Although less common now, caudal blocks may be used for vaginal childbirth, but they are administered in the obstetric unit rather than in the surgical suite.

Rectal (perianal) block. A perianal block may be used for pain management in certain types of anal procedures such as treatment for rectal prolapse, external hemorrhoids, and anorectal abscess. Although medication is not entering the epidural space, this is an option for regional anesthesia for appropriate procedures.

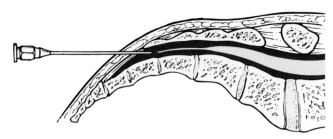

Fig. 13.12 Location of caudal block.

Peripheral Nerve Block

There are several techniques for peripheral nerve block (PNB), also called *extremity block*. These types of blocks may be used for procedures on distal arms and legs, the hand and fingers, and foot and toes. The upper extremities (arm, hand, fingers) are more frequently blocked than the lower extremities. For most surgical procedures on the lower extremities, a spinal or epidural is preferred rather than the use of several nerve blocks to achieve equal blockade. The arm may be blocked at several locations—including the brachial plexus, median, radial, and ulnar nerves—whereas the leg may be blocked at the femoral, obturator, or sciatic nerves. Depending on the surgical site, portions of the hand, foot, and digits may also be blocked.

Preoperative preparation for extremity block includes premedication with anxiolytics and analgesics to lessen discomfort during administration of the block.

When a PNB is performed, precise location of the nerve(s) to be blocked is necessary to avoid penetration of the nerve sheath, damage to nearby blood vessels, and unintended intravascular administration of the agent. Ultrasound-guided regional anesthesia is the preferred method used to identify the location for injection. Alternatively, a nerve stimulator may be used for this purpose. When correct needle placement has been verified, a syringe is used for gentle aspiration to verify that the needle is not in a blood vessel. A test dose is administered, followed by several small doses of the agent, until the intended dose is completed. Anesthetic agents typically used for extremity blocks include lidocaine, ropivacaine, and bupivacaine. The block duration may be extended by the addition of dilute epinephrine.

A brachial plexus block may be used for procedures on the hand, forearm, or elbow. A brachial plexus block may be administered in several different locations, including interscalene, supraclavicular, and infraclavicular, but the most common approach is axillary (Fig. 13.13). Approximately 30 to 40 mL of local anesthetic is injected around the nerves that are adjacent to the axillary artery, which makes the entire arm both numb and immobile. This technique may be used for surgical procedures performed from the elbow to fingers.

Most regional extremity blocks have one primary disadvantage: it takes time for them to take effect. This means they may delay surgery. Extremity blocks may therefore be administered in the preoperative holding area. Some institutions have

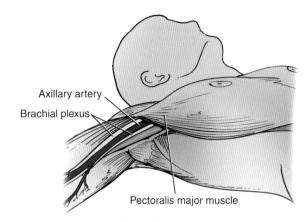

Fig. 13.13 Location of axillary block injection.

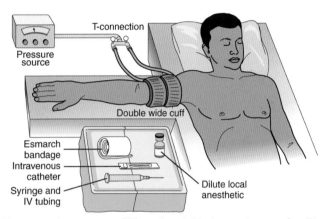

Fig. 13.14 Intravenous (IV) regional block—equipment for Bier block with double tourniquet. (From Phillips N: *Berry & Kohn's operating room technique*, ed 12, St Louis, 2013, Elsevier.)

a separate "block room", where the anesthetic agent is administered and the block is allowed time to fully take effect before transport to the operating room. It is sometimes difficult, though, to time the block so that the patient is ready when the operating room becomes available.

Intravenous Regional Anesthesia

One of the most common extremity blocks is IVRA, also called *Bier block* (Fig. 13.14). IVRA is faster and easier to administer than brachial plexus block, and its onset is immediate. This technique can be used for procedures on upper and lower distal extremities, although it is most frequently used for procedures on wrists and hands. It is particularly useful for soft tissue procedures lasting 1 hour or less, such as release of carpal tunnel, trigger finger, ganglion excision, or moderate Dupuytren contracture.

Lidocaine is the most common agent used for IVRA. Epinephrine is not used with lidocaine to prolong effect because IVRA duration is dependent upon tourniquet time rather than an agent's particular duration.

> **! CAUTION**
>
> Bupivacaine is contraindicated for IVRA because toxicity is most closely associated with intravascular administration.

For example, for a procedure on the hand, a pneumatic or electric double-cuffed tourniquet is placed around the patient's proximal (upper) arm. An IV catheter is inserted in a dorsal vein of the hand, and blood is forced from the distal limb (exsanguination), by elevating the arm, and wrapping it tightly with an Esmarch rubber bandage. The distal and then the proximal tourniquet cuff are inflated to 250 mm Hg pressure, and the bandage is removed. The distal tourniquet cuff is deflated, approximately 40 to 50 mL of 0.5% preservative-free lidocaine is injected into the catheter, and the catheter is removed. The agent diffuses out of the IV space into the nearby nerve fibers, causing analgesia. The arm may present with a blotchy appearance, because of incomplete exsanguination. The tourniquet remains inflated throughout the procedure to keep the anesthetic agent in the area. If the cuff pressure becomes too uncomfortable for the patient, the distal cuff is inflated and the proximal cuff is slowly deflated, which may provide a measure of relief. IVRA is both rapid and effective, but there may be some discomfort caused by exsanguination and tourniquet use. Often the patient requires mild sedation.

Once the surgical procedure is completed, the tourniquet cuff is released slowly and intermittently reinflated to avoid rapid infusion of the anesthetic into the systemic circulation. The most significant risk of IVRA is tourniquet failure, which could cause a toxic volume of anesthetic agent to rapidly enter systemic circulation. Discomfort caused by tourniquet pressure generally precludes use of IVRA for procedures lasting more than an hour. IVRA is not usually the technique of choice for fracture reduction because of discomfort caused by exsanguination and because IVRA does not provide postoperative analgesia. Another contraindication to IVRA is traumatic laceration, which may allow uncontrolled release of the agent from the limb.

Retrobulbar Block

Retrobulbar blocks are injected behind the eye into the muscle cone (see Fig. 10.6) to block branches of the oculomotor nerve. These blocks may be used for procedures requiring a motionless, anesthetized eye. Retrobulbar blocks may be administered by an ophthalmologist or an anesthesia care provider. A typical injection may be made up of equal parts of 0.5% to 0.75% bupivacaine and 2% lidocaine with 150 units of hyaluronidase (see Chapter 10). To minimize patient discomfort, a sedative may be given intravenously before retrobulbar injection. Once the most common anesthesia technique for cataract extraction, retrobulbar blocks are rarely used currently. A similar technique called *peribulbar block* involves injection of the anesthetic agent outside the muscle cone to avoid the optic nerve, but it requires more anesthetic agent and has a slower onset of action.

> **KEY CONCEPTS**
>
> - The vital signs of all patients undergoing surgical intervention must be closely monitored.
> - Vital signs monitored on all patients include heart rate and rhythm, oxygen saturation, BP, and respirations.
> - Additional parameters measured under general anesthesia include temperature, expired CO_2, consciousness level, and neuromuscular function.
> - Certain patient conditions and surgical procedures may require additional invasive monitoring, such as arterial pressure, central venous pressure, or PA pressure.
> - When basic monitoring parameters are established, the appropriate anesthesia method is administered. More invasive monitors may be placed after the patient is under anesthesia.
> - Four major classifications of anesthesia techniques are sedation/MAC, local, regional, and general anesthesia.
> - Several agents are used to produce local anesthesia, and the surgical technologist handles these agents on a daily basis.
> - Several techniques are used to accomplish regional anesthesia, and there are many applications for these techniques.

▌ LEARNING THE LANGUAGE (KEY TERMS)

Using your textbook or a standard medical dictionary, look up and write the definitions of each term.

auscultation
blood pressure (BP)
capnometry
electrocardiography
epidural
exsanguination

intrathecal
local anesthesia
monitored anesthesia care (MAC)
pulse oximetry
regional anesthesia

▌ REVIEW QUESTIONS

1. How is each physiological vital sign monitored in surgery?
2. Which types of monitoring are considered invasive?
3. What are the four major types of anesthesia?
4. What kinds of surgical procedures may be performed under local or regional anesthesia?

5. Which agents are used to accomplish local and/or regional anesthesia?
6. What should you know about the use of epinephrine with local anesthetic agents?
7. Can you list some types of regional anesthesia? What types of procedures may be performed under each?

CRITICAL THINKING

Scenario 1

Ms. Ortiz is a 78-year-old woman with emphysema. She has recently undergone a hysterectomy for uterine cancer. The pelvic lymph nodes were positive for cancer. She has been admitted to surgery for placement of a venous access port for chemotherapy.

1. Would you select local anesthesia with or without MAC? Justify your answer.
2. How would her medical condition affect the pulse oximetry measurements? Why?

Scenario 2

Mr. Delano is a 69-year-old man admitted to surgery for placement of a transvenous pacemaker. The surgeon's preference card indicates that you should have 50 mL of 1% lidocaine with epinephrine 1:100,000 on the back table for injection.

1. Would you select local anesthesia with or without MAC? Justify your answer.
2. Is the agent indicated on the preference card acceptable for this procedure? Why or why not?

BIBLIOGRAPHY

Bardal S, Waechter J, Martin D: *Applied pharmacology*, St Louis, 2011, Saunders/Elsevier.

Duke JC, Keech BM, editors: *Duke's anesthesia secrets*, ed 5, St Louis, 2016, Saunders/Elsevier.

Nagelhout J, Plaus K, editors: *Nurse anesthesia*, ed 5, St Louis, 2014, Saunders/Elsevier.

INTERNET RESOURCES

American Association of Nurse Anesthesiology, Standards for Nurse Anesthesia Practice: https://www.aana.com/?s=docs+default-source+practice-aana-com-web-documents-%28all%29%2Fstandards-for-nurse-anesthesia-practice.pdf%3Fsfvrsn%3De00049b1_2.

American Society of Anesthesiologists, Standards and Guidelines: www.asahq.org/standards-and-guidelines.

Council on Surgical and Perioperative Safety, CSPS Safe Surgery Resources, Patient Monitoring: www.cspsteam.org/2-patient-monitoring/?rq=patient%20monitoring.

Drugs.com, Bupivacaine Hydrochloride: https://www.drugs.com/search.php?searchterm=Bupivacaine+hydrochloride&sources%5B%5D=.

Medscape, Ropivacaine (Naropin): http://reference.medscape.com/drug/naropin-ropivacaine-343367#0.

Shelton R.M., Rokhsar C.K.: Tumescent Liposuction, Medscape: http://emedicine.medscape.com/article/1835414-overview#a01.

KEY TERMS

circumoral
erythema
paraaminobenzoic acid (PABA)
pain threshold

pain tolerance
tinnitus
urticaria

CLASSIFICATIONS OF LOCAL ANESTHETICS

Local anesthetics work by interfering with nerve conduction and pain perception from the point of pain to the central nervous system (CNS). Their duration depends on the blood supply to the affected area. In areas with good vascularity, their anesthetic effect is more rapidly carried away. Local anesthetics are classified into two groups: aminoesters (esters) and aminoamides (amides). The structural difference of these two agents is the pathway in which they are metabolized and their allergic potential. Esters are relatively unstable in solution and are rapidly hydrolyzed in the body by acetylcholinesterase at the neuromuscular junction. One of the metabolic products of hydrolysis is paraaminobenzoic acid (PABA), which is associated with hypersensitivity and allergic reactions. Ester agents include cocaine, procaine, tetracaine, and chloroprocaine.

Amides are relatively stable in solution and are slowly metabolized by the enzymes in the liver. Allergic reactions are extremely rare, so amides are more commonly used in current clinical practice. Amides include lidocaine, prilocaine, bupivacaine, ropivacaine, and mepivacaine.

? MAKE IT SIMPLE

A simple way to remember which local anesthetics are amides is to look at their generic spelling: the letter "*i*" appears twice.

! CAUTION

Because amides are metabolized in the liver, care should be used in patients with severe liver disease or patients taking medication that interferes with the metabolism. Monitoring for signs of toxicity is critical.

ADVERSE EFFECTS OF LOCAL ANESTHETICS

In the surgical first assistant role, it is imperative to understand that the principal adverse effects of local anesthetics are allergic reactions and systemic toxicity. Keep in mind that aminoamides are less allergenic than aminoesters (because of the metabolic product PABA) and, although rare, allergic reactions can be life-threatening.

Allergic reactions are classified into two categories: local and systemic. A local allergic reaction (hypersensitivity) is similar to allergic contact dermatitis. Clinical signs may include erythema, urticaria, and edema. Systemic allergic reactions (anaphylactic signs) may include generalized erythema, urticaria, facial edema, wheezing, bronchoconstriction, cyanosis, nausea, vomiting, hypotension, and cardiovascular collapse. Treatment is symptomatic and supportive (see Chapter 15).

Systemic toxicity from local anesthetics is caused by excess concentration of the medication in the blood. This effect is most often encountered after an accidental intravascular injection, administration of an excessive dose or rate of injection of the anesthetic, delayed drug clearance, or administration into vascular tissues. See Table 13.A for maximum dosages of common local agents.

Systemic toxicity from local anesthetics involves the CNS and the cardiovascular system. Signs and symptoms of CNS toxicity may include tinnitus, circumoral numbness, metallic taste in the mouth, lightheadedness, visual disturbances, nausea and/or vomiting, slurred speech, muscular twitching, drowsiness, seizures, and coma. Cardiovascular toxicity can produce reduced cardiac contractility, vasodilation, and dysrhythmias. Peripheral effects include vasoconstriction at low doses and vasodilation at higher doses, which results in hypotension. Signs and symptoms of cardiovascular toxicity include chest pain, shortness of breath, palpitations, lightheadedness, diaphoresis, and syncope. Severe systemic toxicity is treated by maintaining the patient's

TABLE 13.A   Maximum Dosages of Commonly Used Local Anesthetic Agents

Agent (Esters)	Concentration	Maximum Dosage Guidelines (Total Cumulative Adult Dose per Procedure)	Onset (min)	Duration (h)
procaine (Novocain)	0.25%–0.5% (via dilution)	7 mg/kg, not to exceed 350–600 mg (infiltrative)	2–5	0.25–1
chloroprocaine (Nesacaine)	1%–2%	11 mg/kg, not to exceed 800 mg	6–12	0.5
tetracaine (Pontocaine)	0.5%–2%	Not to exceed 20 mg (topical application)	3–8	0.5–1
Agent (Amides)				
lidocaine (Xylocaine)	1%–2%	4.5–5 mg/kg, not to exceed 300 mg	<2	0.5–1
lidocaine with epinephrine	1%–2% with epi 1:100,000 or 1:200,000	7 mg/kg, not to exceed 500 mg	<2	2–6
bupivacaine (Marcaine)	0.25%–0.5%	2.5 mg/kg, not to exceed 175 mg	5	2–4
bupivacaine with epinephrine	0.25% with epi 1:200,000	Not to exceed 225 mg	5	3–7
mepivacaine (Carbocaine)	1%	7 mg/kg, not to exceed 400 mg (infiltrative)	3–5	0.75–1.5

It should be noted that sources vary slightly in onset and duration times. *epi*, Epinephrine.

airway and administering oxygen and fluids. Seizures are controlled with diazepam or succinylcholine. Cardiac instability may be managed with vasodilators, antiarrhythmics, and inotropes. Systemic absorption of the anesthetic can be reduced by one third with the addition of a vasoconstrictor, such as epinephrine.

CONCENTRATION OR DOSAGE

Local anesthetics are presented in percent of concentration or percent of strength. They are calculated as the number of grams of medication in 100 mL of solution. Therefore a 2% lidocaine solution is 2 g of medication in 100 mL of solution. A further breakdown of this concept would be 2 g equals 2000 mg; therefore each 100 mL of solution contains 2000 mg of lidocaine. Breaking it down further, 1 mL contains 20 mg of lidocaine. A quick calculation is to move the decimal point one place to the right because this will determine milligrams per milliliters of local anesthetic. Examples are:

2.0% = 20 mg/mL
1.0% = 10 mg/mL
0.25% = 2.5 mg/mL

Local anesthetics are typically in lower concentrations when used for infiltration anesthesia. Infiltration anesthesia involves intradermal, subcutaneous, or submucosal administration across the nerve paths that supply the involved body areas. The dose depends on the type of procedure, the degree of anesthesia required, and the patient's condition. A reduced dosage of local anesthetic is indicated for patients who are debilitated, acutely ill, very young, very old, or have liver disease, arteriosclerosis, or occlusive arterial disease.

EPINEPHRINE ADDITIVE TO LOCAL ANESTHETICS

Epinephrine acts as a vasoconstrictor that not only decreases bleeding but also slows the rate of systemic absorption of the anesthetic. This allows the body more time to metabolize the anesthetic and prolongs the anesthetic effects. Given the slower absorption rate, a larger volume of anesthetic with epinephrine can be injected without causing toxicity. Epinephrine can be used in a variety of surgical procedures. An example of this would be septoplasty with turbinectomies. A local anesthetic with epinephrine is beneficial because of the vascularity of the nasal mucosa and the confined space within the nasal cavity.

Concentrations of epinephrine are described as a ratio (e.g., 1:100,000 or 1:200,000) and are calculated as the number of grams of the agent in a given volume of solution. The previous examples show 1 g of epinephrine in 100,000 mL of solution and 1 g of epinephrine in 200,000 mL of solution, respectively. If the number of grams is always 1, then the greater the number on the other side of the ratio, the less concentrated the solution becomes. A 1:100,000 solution of epinephrine is stronger than a 1:200,000 solution.

> **! CAUTION**
>
> Local anesthetics containing epinephrine should be used with extreme caution in an area where vascular supply is minimal (e.g., fingers, tip of nose, penis, and toes).

POSTOPERATIVE PAIN MANAGEMENT WITH LOCAL AND REGIONAL ANESTHETICS

Traditionally, oral or intramuscular anesthetics or opioids have been used for postoperative pain management. The patient's reaction to pain is subjective and depends on the individual's perception of pain, pain threshold, and pain tolerance, as well as the physiologic changes caused by an operative procedure. Despite the belief that opioids provide optimal pain relief, studies have shown that more than half of the surgical patients receiving opioids remain in moderate-to-severe pain. The surgical first assistant should also recognize that narcotics, such as the opioids, can cause respiratory depression to the point of respiratory arrest if the dose is too great. The recognition that unrelieved pain contributes to perioperative morbidity and mortality has inspired preemptive analgesic techniques to control postoperative pain. The surgical first assistant may be involved with implementing various techniques for pain control during the procedure.

Local anesthetics can be administered into the incision sites or intraarticular area. Local infiltration not only provides analgesia but also appears to reduce local inflammatory responses to surgery and trauma. An example is bupivacaine (Marcaine), which can provide up to approximately 4 hours of pain control (longer if it contains epinephrine). The maximum dose of bupivacaine for infiltration is 175 mg (70 mL of 0.25% solution). Another alternative is continuous local infusion therapy (site-specific infusion), when a catheter is placed in the incision site or intraarticular area, and a continuous infusion or boluses of local anesthetic can be administered with patient-controlled pumps. This is known as *patient-controlled analgesia*. The pump dispenses 2 mL or 4 mL of local anesthetic to the surgical site per hour. Depending on the type of pump, a 4-mL bolus chamber can be squeezed, providing additional medication to the site. These pumps are disposable and have 2- or 4-day duration.

Regional anesthetic techniques can block or reduce pain postoperatively, from several hours to several days. An example is peripheral nerve blocks, which can provide significant pain relief for approximately 12 to 18 hours. With additives, such as dexamethasone, the duration is longer. Greater pain control by local or regional anesthetics has the potential to allow the patient earlier discharge from the hospital/facility, the ability to tolerate physical therapy, and/or return to more activities faster.

ASSISTANT ADVICE

Local anesthetics containing epinephrine will have red labels and/or red printing noting the concentration of epinephrine.

ADVANCED PRACTICES: REVIEW QUESTIONS

1. Explain the difference between aminoesters and aminoamides.
2. Why should patients with hepatitis be closely monitored while receiving amides?
3. Name the two principal adverse effects on the patient from local anesthetics.
4. What is the difference between a local and systemic allergic reaction? Give clinical signs of each.
5. What causes systemic toxicity from local anesthetics? Give two symptoms.
6. Why can a larger volume of local anesthetic with epinephrine be injected into tissues without causing toxicity?

ADVANCED PRACTICES: BIBLIOGRAPHY

Fulcher EM, Fulcher RM, Soto CD: *Pharmacology: principles and applications*, ed 3, St Louis, 2012, Saunders/Elsevier.

Kee JL, Hayes ER, McCuistion LE: *Pharmacology: a patient-centered nursing process approach*, ed 8, St Louis, 2015, Saunders/Elsevier.

Savoie FH, Field LD, Jenkins RN, et al: The pain control infusion pump for postoperative pain control in shoulder surgery, *Arthroscopy* 16(4):339–342, 2000.

ADVANCED PRACTICES: INTERNET RESOURCES

CareFusion, Pain Management and Patient-Controlled Analgesia: Improving Safety and Quality of Care: www.bd.com/assets/documents/continuing-education/BD_Conference-Pain-Management-PCA-2005_CE_EN.pdf.

Graber R, Kraay M, Regional Anesthesia for Postoperative Pain Control, Medscape: http://emedicine.medscape.com/article/1268467-overview.

Kapitanyan R, Su M, Local Anesthetic Toxicity, Medscape: https://emedicine.medscape.com/article/1844551-overview.

McKinley Medical, ACCUFUSER Post-Op Pain Control Pump: https://www.clinicaltrials.gov/ct2/show/NCT01976494.

Medscape, Tetracaine: http://reference.medscape.com/drug/pontocaine-tetcaine-tetracaine-343373.

Medscape, Infiltrative Administration of Local Anesthetic Agents: http://emedicine.medscape.com/article/149178-overview.

RxList, Naropin: www.rxlist.com/naropin-drug.htm.

14

General Anesthesia

OBJECTIVES

After completing this chapter, you should be able to do the following:

1. Define terms and abbreviations related to anesthesia.
2. List and discuss indications for general anesthesia.
3. Identify and describe anesthesia equipment.
4. Explain the basic components of a general anesthetic.
5. List methods of inducing general anesthesia.
6. Define the phases of general anesthesia.
7. Explain options for airway management.
8. List steps in the process of endotracheal intubation.
9. Discuss the maintenance phase of the surgical procedure, including the concepts of awareness under anesthesia and muscle relaxation.
10. Discuss the emergence phase of the surgical procedure, including the process of extubation.
11. Identify the major categories of anesthesia medications.
12. Discuss intravenous induction agents, including their purpose and examples (including generic and trade names).
13. Discuss the purpose of analgesics, including a comparison of opioids used for analgesics during general anesthesia.
14. Discuss inhalation agents, including their purpose, their disadvantages, and examples.
15. Discuss neuromuscular blocking agents, including the three types of muscle tissue.
16. Compare and contrast depolarizing and nondepolarizing muscle relaxants.
17. List and describe reversal agents for various anesthetics.

OUTLINE

General anesthesia is a *systemic* state of anesthesia, rather than anesthesia in a large area (regional) or a specific site (local). General anesthesia interferes with the brain's ability to interpret pain impulses coming from anywhere in the body. The term *anesthesia* is literally defined as an absence of sensation, but in the context of general anesthesia, it is more correctly defined as a drug-induced temporary loss of consciousness, during which patients are not arousable, even by painful stimulation.

The decision to use a general anesthetic is based both on the requirements of the surgical procedure to be performed and on the individual patient. For example, a general anesthetic is used when there are multiple operative sites or for a procedure on an area that is difficult to block regionally, such as the thoracic or abdominal cavities. Examples of surgical procedures on multiple locations include skin grafts, breast reconstruction, and autologous bone grafts. Surgical procedures that require an absolutely motionless field, such as retinal surgery, are also performed under general anesthesia. In addition, the expected duration of the surgical procedure may influence the choice of general anesthesia because of patient discomfort when the patient is required to lie flat on the operating room bed for a long period.

Patient factors that influence the selection of general anesthesia include patient age, cognitive ability, mental or emotional state, and (when possible) patient preference. Patient age is a primary consideration in that children are almost never candidates for regional or local anesthesia, regardless of the surgical procedure being performed. General anesthesia is usually indicated when the patient's cognitive ability is impaired, causing an inability to understand, communicate, or cooperate with directions required in regional or local anesthesia. For example, mentally disabled patients or those with Alzheimer disease may not be capable of understanding what is happening to them, so general anesthesia is the method of choice. Patient preference is taken into account when possible; for example, if a patient is very frightened at the idea of a spinal needle being inserted into the back and is in otherwise good health, general anesthesia may be a more appropriate choice than regional.

Historically, early agents used to produce general anesthesia had unwanted side effects—they were extremely toxic to the patient or they were explosive (Insight 14.1). Modern advances in the pharmacology of anesthesia, though, have produced many agents that accomplish general anesthesia with a high degree of safety. Several classes of drugs are used to achieve general anesthesia, often in combination. The desired result is a patient who: (1) remains unconscious, (2) is pain free, (3) retains no memory of the event, (4) is immobile, and (5) maintains normal cardiovascular function. Although several theories have been suggested, the exact mechanism of agents used to induce and maintain general anesthesia is still not clearly understood. Different categories of agents affect different parts of the body at the cellular level; examples are the following:

- Drugs used to produce an unconscious state affect the reticular activating system in the brain stem.
- Agents used to produce analgesia (opioids) bind with receptors on cell membranes in the brain and spinal cord, altering the transmission of pain signals.
- Muscle relaxants work at the neuromuscular junction of skeletal muscles.

The ability to safely provide general anesthesia is an art, as well as a science. The anesthesia care provider manages a delicate balance of agents to achieve the necessary components of general anesthesia, while maintaining the patient in a stable physiological state. In addition, the anesthesia care provider manages the timing of these agents so that the anesthetic effect is wearing off as the surgical procedure is concluding. In most situations, the goal is to have patients awake, alert, and breathing on their own before transport to the postanesthesia care unit (PACU).

In addition to pharmacological agents, various pieces of equipment that assist in the process of administering general anesthesia are used by the anesthesia care provider. Much of this equipment is integrated into the anesthesia workstation (Fig. 14.1). Components of an anesthesia workstation include manual and automatic ventilation systems, breathing circuits, oxygen (O_2) and nitrous oxide (N_2O) central pipeline hoses and backup tanks, vaporizers (for volatile gases), pressure regulators and gas-mixing components, and gas-scavenging systems. Exhaled gases are routed through a carbon dioxide (CO_2) absorbent (soda lime) canister. A number of respiratory and physiological monitors are used, including electrocardiogram (ECG), pulse oximeter, blood

INSIGHT 14.1 Yesterday and Today: Anesthesia

In today's world, surgery and anesthesia are inseparable concepts, but this was not always true. Surgery can be divided into two eras: preanesthesia and postanesthesia. In the preanesthesia era, surgery was based on speed because the patient would often die from hemorrhage, shock, or the trauma of the operation. Ironically, shock may have helped to relieve some of the pain before death occurred. The postanesthesia era began in the 19th century when discoveries were finally published, accepted, and used.

Attempts to alleviate pain probably date back as far as humankind has experienced suffering. These first attempts treated pain as an evil spirit or demon, and the idea was to frighten it away. Thus early anesthesia involved tattoos, jewelry, talismans, amulets, and charms. Pain relievers existed and were used in ancient times, but they were impure, unsafe, and unreliable. Ancient pain remedies documented include a Babylonian clay tablet from approximately 2250 BC that gives the remedy for a toothache. Early Egyptian surgeons applied pressure to nerves or blood vessels, which caused insensibility to a specific part of the body for an operation.

Many early methods of pain control used drugs. Alcohol was often used in the form of spirits or wines. Along with opium and marijuana, ancient literature contains many references to the *Mandragora* (mandrake or mandragon) plant as a pain reliever that produced a confused mental state. Dioscorides, a 1st-century Greek physician, administered the Mandragora root, boiled in wine, to his patients before they went under his knife. Mandragora was also known as the *potion of the condemned* because it was given to criminals to decrease the agonies of crucifixion.

In addition to drugs, other pain-control methods were used in the preanesthesia era. One method was to produce unconsciousness by compressing the carotid arteries to decrease heart rate; another was to place a wooden bowl over the patient's head and strike the bowl to cause a concussion. Another method came from China in the form of acupuncture, which decreased pain sensations. A third method was cryothermia. This was documented in England in 1050, in an Anglo-Saxon manuscript that instructed the surgeon to wait a while before making the incision, as the patient sat in cold water "until it can become deadened."

The word *anesthesia* comes from the Greek word *anaisthesis*, which means "no sensation." *Anesthesia* appeared in *Bailey's English Dictionary* in 1721, but the term itself was reportedly coined by Oliver Wendell Holmes in a letter in 1846.

Unfortunately, many agents with anesthetic properties were known for generations but were not applied in surgery. The great alchemist Paracelsus (1493?–1541) mixed sulfuric acid with alcohol and distilled his concoction. He believed this mixture, called *sweet vitriol*, could quiet suffering and relieve pain. We know this mixture today as ether. Nitrous oxide was discovered by Joseph Priestley in 1772. Both nitrous oxide and ether were popularized by traveling "professors" as entertainment tools. Volunteers would inhale the gases and become intoxicated. This fad produced "laughing gas parties" and "ether frolics." Little known to the public at the time was the fact that in 1800 a man named Humphrey Davy had described the use of nitrous oxide to relieve pain produced by a wisdom tooth.

It was after one of these public demonstrations of ether that a young physician named Crawford W. Long contemplated its use as an anesthetic during surgery. He was inspired when he saw friends receive injuries without pain while under the vapor's influence. On March 30, 1842, Dr. Long administered ether to James M. Venable and successfully removed a tumor from the patient's neck. A dentist named Horace Wells observed a similar demonstration of nitrous oxide in 1844 and used it in his dental practice for many years to relieve pain from tooth extractions. Unfortunately, Wells' demonstration to Harvard Medical School was not a success, possibly because of incomplete administration of the gas, and nitrous oxide was not accepted. Wells' partner, Dr. William T.G. Morton, realized that although nitrous oxide was unreliable, an alternative could be found in ether vapor. After numerous experiments, Morton contacted Dr. John Warren, a senior surgeon of the Massachusetts General Hospital. A demonstration was arranged for October 16, 1846. This demonstration was a success, as a tumor was removed from the jaw of a 20-year-old male, who remained insensible throughout the procedure. Thus the postanesthesia era was officially begun with Dr. Warren's famous remark, "Gentlemen, this is no humbug."

The widespread use of anesthesia began in England on April 7, 1853, when Queen Victoria accepted the use of chloroform during childbirth. Her physician was Dr. Sir James Young Simpson. Chloroform had been discovered in 1831; however, its use by the queen led to its acceptance by the medical community. From these beginnings, anesthesia has developed into the vital branch of medicine we know today.

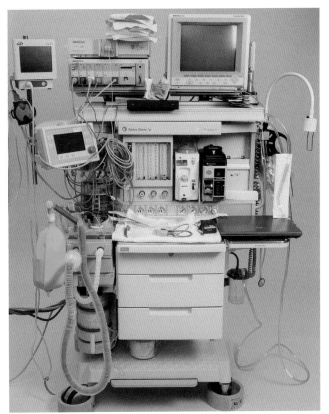

Fig. 14.1 An anesthesia workstation. (Courtesy Frank Pronesti T/A heirloomstudio.com.)

pressure (BP) monitor, level of consciousness monitor, and instruments to measure inhaled and exhaled O_2, CO_2, and anesthetic agent levels. Physiologic and respiratory monitors are equipped with audible alarm systems for additional safety. Alarms are set to emit a signal when readings occur outside preset parameters. Each component is checked for proper function before admitting the patient to the operating room. Additional equipment used to assist the delivery of anesthesia and provide physiological support to the patient includes infusion control devices (see Fig. 11.5), thermoregulatory devices, fluid warmers, and fluid pumps.

COMPONENTS OF GENERAL ANESTHESIA

General anesthesia is accomplished by administering agents to achieve four major goals. These goals, or components, of general anesthesia are unconsciousness (a state of being unaware), analgesia (painlessness), amnesia (memory impairment), and immobility (skeletal muscle relaxation) (Box 14.1). That is, the patient must remain unconscious, pain free, and immobile, while retaining no explicit memory of the event. Different

agents are used to accomplish each of these required components. The anesthesia care provider monitors the effects of the agents administered and works to maintain the patient's cardiovascular stability throughout the course of anesthesia.

Administration Methods

Two methods, or routes, are used to administer general anesthetic agents: inhalation and intravenous injection. An inhalation anesthetic is administered as a gas the patient breathes, whereas intravenous agents are administered directly into the bloodstream, through a small catheter placed in a vein. No intravenous agent in current use can provide all the required effects and only those effects, so a combination of administration methods is used. The term *balanced anesthesia* refers to the technique that uses a combination of inhalation and intravenous agents to accomplish general anesthesia. Another (but much less common) anesthesia technique uses a combination of a regional block, such as an epidural, and a light general anesthetic. This technique is useful for select patients undergoing major vascular procedures because it decreases the amount of general anesthetic agents required, helping to maintain cardiovascular stability, and provides an effective means of postoperative pain control. This technique is also valuable for use in selected orthopedic, thoracic, and other surgical specialty procedures.

PHASES OF GENERAL ANESTHESIA

There are five phases of general anesthesia: preinduction, induction, maintenance, emergence, and recovery (Box 14.2). Preinduction includes preoperative assessment and preparation of the patient, both physically and psychologically (see Chapter 12). The intraoperative phases of general anesthesia are induction, maintenance, and emergence. Recovery is the postoperative phase. Phases of general anesthesia are not to be confused with the concept of stages of anesthesia (Insight 14.2), which was based on the effects of ether.

Preinduction Phase

The preinduction phase begins as the patient is admitted to the preoperative holding area and continues up to the point of administration of anesthetic agents. In this phase, the patient is assessed and prepared for anesthesia and surgery. Part of the history and physical examination specific to anesthesia includes assessment of the patient's airway—even for patients not scheduled to undergo general anesthesia. A history is obtained regarding airway issues and a physical examination is conducted to determine neck mobility and assess other factors that might indicate potential for a difficult airway. Classification systems, such as the Mallampati score and Cormack-Lehane score, are

INSIGHT 14.2 Stages of Anesthesia

Classic texts describe four stages of anesthesia. These stages are based on the physiological effects of ether, one of the first anesthetic agents. Each stage was based on observations of body movement, respiratory rhythm, oculomotor reflexes, and muscle tone.

Stage 1. *Amnesia:* Induction to loss of consciousness.

Stage 2. *Delirium* (or excitement): Patient is unconscious but still responding reflexively and unpredictably to certain stimuli.

Stage 3. *Surgical anesthesia:* Adequate depth of anesthesia is reached so that an incision can be made and procedure performed without negative patient response (such as hypertension or tachycardia).

Stage 4. *Overdose* (or medullary depression): Level of anesthesia is so deep that cardiovascular and respiratory function is compromised to the point of collapse because of depression of those centers in the brain.

It is important to note that the stages, as traditionally described, are no longer as useful in anesthesia practice. Current anesthetic agents are able to bring the patient more quickly through stages 1 and 2 and so may exhibit different signs during induction and make the early stages more difficult to identify. These signs, based on muscular responses, are also invalidated with the current frequent practice of administration of muscle relaxants. In addition, modern anesthetic agents are much more predictable than ether, so stage 4 is less likely to occur.

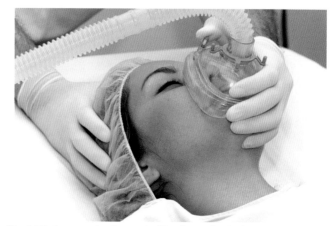

Fig. 14.3 An anesthesia mask. (iStock.com/herjua)

Heart rate and ECG, BP, respirations, O_2 saturation, expired gases (end-tidal CO_2, O_2, and anesthetic gases), and temperature are closely observed to constantly assess the physiological status of the patient. An anesthesia mask is usually placed over the patient's nose and mouth, and 100% O_2 is administered, a process known as *preoxygenation* (Fig. 14.3). This practice is performed to bring the O_2 saturation of the patient's blood to the highest possible level before induction.

Induction Phase

The induction phase begins when medications are administered to initiate general anesthesia and concludes when an adequate depth of anesthesia is reached, and the patient's airway is secured.

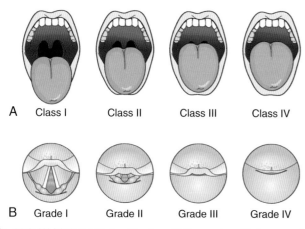

Fig. 14.2 (A) Mallampati classification. (B) Cormack and Lehane grading of laryngoscopic views. (A, From Phillips N: *Berry and Kohn's operating room technique,* ed 11, St Louis, 2007, Mosby. B, From Spiro SG, Silvestri GA, Agusti A: *Clinical respiratory medicine,* ed 4, St Louis, 2012, Elsevier.)

! CAUTION

The patient may experience a period of agitation or excitement during induction. Hearing sensitivity is also heightened (hyperacusis) during induction of anesthesia. The effect of loud noises and sudden movement may be intensified during this time, inducing a stress reaction in the patient. The stress response may be characterized by unstable cardiovascular functions, which is potentially harmful to the patient. In addition, moving the patient suddenly at this time can trigger laryngospasm. Thus the surgical technologist and all members of the surgical team must make every effort to minimize unnecessary operating room noise and movement of the patient during induction.

used to categorize the patient's risk for difficult airway management (Fig. 14.2). Appropriate medications are administered during this phase, as ordered by the anesthesia care provider (see Chapter 12). One goal of the preinduction phase is to have the patient arrive in the operating room calm, physiologically stable, and fully prepared for anesthesia.

The preinduction phase continues as the patient is transported to the operating room and transferred to the operating room bed in the supine position. The circulator secures the safety belt over the patient's thighs and obtains warm blankets for patient comfort. The anesthesia care provider begins by attaching monitoring devices to the patient and obtaining baseline vital signs. The vital functions of all patients receiving a general anesthetic are continuously monitored (see Chapter 13).

Induction agents are usually administered by intravenous injection. The option of masked induction, with an inhalation anesthetic, may be chosen for children to avoid the emotional trauma of placing an intravenous catheter. Various induction agents are used to produce an unconscious state, amnesia, and analgesia. A variation of standard induction technique called *neuroleptanesthesia* (Insight 14.3) was used in specific situations but is rarely used in current practice. When the patient becomes unconscious, the anesthesia care provider ensures that an adequate airway is maintained.

Airway Management

The exchange of O_2 and CO_2 (respiration) is a vital function that must be sustained throughout any surgical procedure.

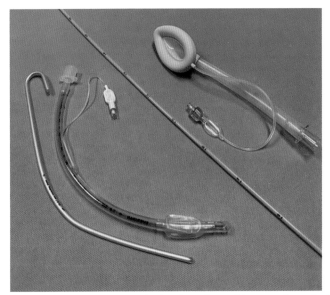

Fig. 14.4 Stylet, endotracheal tube, bougie, and laryngeal masked airway.

An unconscious patient requires additional support to ensure optimal respiratory function, and various methods of airway management are used to provide that support. The patient's airway may be managed with a mask for surgical procedures of short duration when muscle relaxation is not required, such as myringotomy with placement of pressure equalization tubes. When the patient becomes unconscious, a nasal or pharyngeal (oral) airway may be placed, as needed, to displace the tongue and facilitate air exchange through the mask. The mask is held in position with straps, and the anesthesia care provider supports the airway by maintaining the patient's head in a chin-lift position.

In select patients, the airway may be managed with a laryngeal masked airway (LMA) (Fig. 14.4), also known as a *supraglottic airway*. An LMA consists of a flexible shaft attached to a silicone mask that is inflated to seal the airway. Sizes range from 1 to 5, and the proper size is selected based on the patient's

weight. After induction of anesthesia, an LMA is inserted and positioned in the laryngopharynx to cover the epiglottis and larynx. The LMA cuff is inflated to provide a seal, and the tube is connected to the breathing circuit. Surgical patients may continue to breathe on their own (if no muscle relaxant is needed for the surgical procedure), or respirations may be controlled with the use of a ventilator or by manual ventilation (if muscle relaxants are administered). The LMA, which does not require laryngoscopy or muscle relaxation, is particularly useful for ambulatory surgical procedures. Contraindications to LMA include procedures on the oral cavity, obesity, hiatal hernia, gastroesophageal reflux disease (GERD), and low pulmonary compliance. Several variations of the LMA are available, including an intubating LMA (Fastrach), LMA CTrach, LMA Supreme, and LMA ProSeal, allowing for expanded applications in select patients.

Many patients are not appropriate candidates for management with a mask or an LMA and require more precise control of the airway. In addition, many surgical procedures are of longer duration, require deep muscle relaxation, or are performed in a lateral or prone position, all of which require a more highly controlled airway. Deep muscle relaxation is achieved by the administration of neuromuscular blockers, which cause temporary relaxation of skeletal muscles including the muscles of respiration. During a surgical procedure requiring deep muscle relaxation, patients will not be breathing on their own, so respirations are controlled by mechanical ventilation through a tube placed into the patient's trachea called an *endotracheal (ET) tube* (Fig. 14.4). ET tubes are made of clear, flexible polyvinyl chloride sized by internal diameter in 0.5-mm increments and available with or without inflatable cuffs used to provide a sealed airway. External markings on the tube are in centimeters and are used to determine the length of tube insertion. A flexible stylet may also be inserted through the lumen of the ET tube to facilitate its passage into the trachea (Fig. 14.4).

An ET tube is placed through the patient's mouth, into the trachea, to establish the most direct and precisely controlled airway. The placement of an ET tube, called *intubation*, begins after induction agents and muscle relaxants are administered to render the patient unconscious and immobile.

 TECH TIP

The circulator assists the anesthesia care provider during intubation and should be present at the patient's head as soon as induction begins.

When the patient's airway is adequately managed with masked ventilation, a short-acting muscle relaxant (neuromuscular blocker) is administered to relax the vocal cords and facilitate placement of the ET tube. When the patient is adequately relaxed to suppress the laryngeal reflex, an ET tube is inserted past the epiglottis, through the vocal cords, and into the trachea under direct visualization, with an intubating laryngoscope (Fig. 14.5). An intubating laryngoscope (somewhat similar to an operating laryngoscope) is used to retract the tongue and lift the jaw to visualize the larynx and vocal cords. Detachable laryngoscope blades, such as a Macintosh (curved) or a Miller

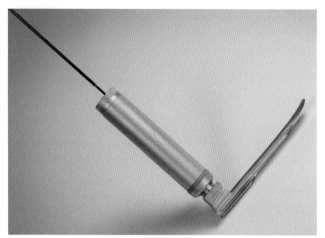

Fig. 14.5 A laryngoscope. (Courtesy Frank Pronesti T/A heirloom studio.com.)

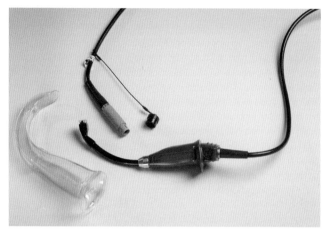

Fig. 14.6 A GlideScope video laryngoscope. (Courtesy Frank Pronesti T/A heirloomstudio.com.)

(straight), of various sizes are used to retract the patient's tongue. A flexible stylet may be placed inside the ET tube to guide the tube along the correct path, and the circulator may be asked to remove the stylet when the tube is in position. The end of the tube is placed midway between the vocal cords and the carina of the trachea (the carina is the place where the trachea bifurcates into right and left main stem bronchi), and the cuff is inflated. Correct placement of the ET tube is verified by clinical assessment, measurement of exhaled CO_2, and auscultation of bilateral breath sounds.

ET intubation may also be accomplished with the use of video laryngoscopy. This development is a significant advance in technique, and it is very useful for difficult intubations. The video laryngoscope contains a microvideo camera in the laryngoscope blade that transmits images to a viewing screen. This provides a clear, indirect view for intubation and enables tube placement with the patient's head in neutral position. Examples of video laryngoscopes include the GlideScope (Fig. 14.6), C-MAC, and McGrath. The use of a tracheal tube introducer, known as a bougie, may be used to aid tracheal intubation in poor laryngoscopic views or after failed intubation attempts. A bougie is a thin, plastic rod that is passed into the trachea, over which the ET tube is inserted (Fig. 14.4).

A variation on standard induction technique called *rapid sequence induction* (RSI) may be used for patients who are at an increased risk of gastric reflux and pulmonary aspiration. RSI is used for patients who have not been NPO (nothing by mouth [*nil per os*]) (especially trauma patients) and those with a history of hiatal hernia, GERD, previous gastrointestinal surgery, diabetes, or obesity. RSI is used to secure and control the airway quickly. The patient is preoxygenated, and an induction agent is administered. Fentanyl may be given 1 to 3 minutes before the induction agent to minimize reaction to laryngoscopy and intubation. A nonparalyzing dose of a nondepolarizing neuromuscular blocker (such as pancuronium), and a dose of succinylcholine (a depolarizing neuromuscular blocker) are administered. Cricoid pressure (also known as the *Sellick maneuver*) is applied with the thumb and index finger to the cricoid cartilage, gently compressing the esophagus downward against the cervical vertebrae

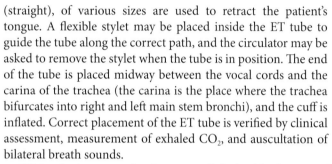

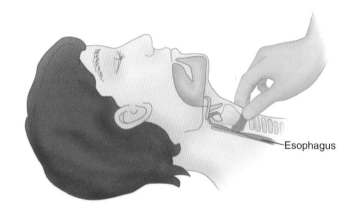

Esophagus

Cricoid pressure

Cricoid ring occluding esophagus

Esophagus

Fig. 14.7 Applying cricoid pressure. (From Rothrock, JC: *Alexander's care of the patient in surgery*, ed 15, St Louis, 2015, Elsevier.)

to prevent gastric contents from entering the trachea and lungs (Fig. 14.7). Cricoid pressure is maintained until the ET tube is in the correct position. ET tube placement is verified as described previously, and a nasogastric tube may be placed through the mouth to empty stomach contents.

In certain circumstances, other intubation techniques may be indicated. Nasal intubation may be used for particular surgical procedures performed in the oral cavity, such as repair of mandibular fractures, when the presence of the ET tube in the mouth may not be desirable. The ET tube is inserted through the nose to the oropharynx, a laryngoscope is used to visualize the vocal cords, and a Magill forceps may be used to guide the ET tube into place.

If the preoperative evaluation indicates a potential significant problem for ventilation and intubation (difficult airway), the patient may be intubated before induction using fiberoptic ET intubation. This technique is reserved for patients with specific conditions, such as morbid obesity, a history of difficult intubation, facial deformities, laryngeal cancer, unstable cervical spine fractures, or other conditions that may compromise the airway. Preparation for intubation before induction begins with administration of an antisialagogue (an agent to dry salivary secretions), such as glycopyrrolate (Robinul), approximately 30 minutes before intubation.

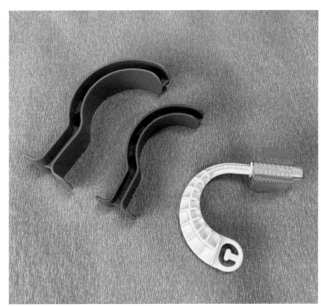

Fig. 14.8 Large oral airway, small oral airway, and bite block.

QUICK QUESTION

Robinul is also classified as which category of medication? Can you list some of its other actions? Check your answers in Chapter 12.

The patient's laryngeal reflex may be suppressed with the use of a topical anesthetic agent, such as Cetacaine (a combination of benzocaine, tetracaine, and butamben) spray. Sedation is administered so that patients can tolerate the intubation and yet continue to breathe and protect their own airway. Intubation may be accomplished by nasal or oral route, depending on the situation. If a nasal intubation is selected, topical vasoconstrictors (such as cocaine, oxymetazoline [Afrin], or phenylephrine) may be used intranasally to prevent bleeding (epistaxis). The ET tube is loaded over a flexible fiberoptic bronchoscope, and the scope is gently guided into the trachea. The ET tube is placed in position, the bronchoscope is removed, and anesthesia induction commences.

Regardless of the method, the anesthesia provider is responsible for ensuring no structures of the oral cavity are injured during the intubation process. A bite block may be placed to prevent the patient from biting the ET tube and occluding airflow or to prevent bite injuries to the structures of the oral cavity (Fig. 14.8). Once intubation is accomplished, the ET tube is connected to a breathing circuit leading to the ventilator. The ET tube position is verified by auscultation during the delivery of manual ventilations. When proper ET tube position is confirmed, respirations are controlled with mechanical ventilation set to the appropriate volume and rate. The ET tube is secured in position, and an adequate depth of anesthesia is achieved to begin the surgical procedure, concluding the induction phase of anesthesia.

Maintenance Phase

The maintenance phase begins as the patient's airway is established and secured and continues until the surgical procedure has been completed. Additional anesthetic agents are administered during the maintenance phase, as needed, to maintain a depth of anesthesia appropriate to the surgical procedure. For example, abdominal and thoracic procedures require a much deeper level of anesthesia than superficial procedures. The patient is maintained in an unconscious state with a combination of intravenous and inhalation agents, some of which also produce amnesia and analgesia. Muscle relaxants are administered, as needed, to keep the patient immobile and facilitate retraction and visualization of the surgical site. Opioids and adjunctive agents are administered, as needed, for analgesia. The anesthesia care provider maintains the delicate balance of administering the appropriate agents, in the appropriate amounts, at the appropriate times, to achieve a level of anesthesia neither too deep nor too light for the surgical procedure, while maintaining a stable cardiovascular state in the patient.

The anesthesia care provider uses direct measurements of vital signs and clinical observation to continually assess the patient's status and need for additional anesthetic agents. For example, if the analgesic agents are wearing off, most surgical patients demonstrate a measurable physiological response to pain, such as an increase in BP or heart rate. Indirect measures (clinical observations), such as sweating and lacrimation (the production of tears), are also considered reliable indicators of a pain response, but these signs may also indicate an insufficient depth of anesthesia. In addition, specific conditions may cause some of these responses as well. For example, an increased heart rate may be caused by hypovolemia rather than a painful stimulus. Some medications (e.g., β-blockers and calcium channel blockers [agents administered for specific heart conditions]) can prevent the normal heart rate increase in response to pain. Each patient and each surgical situation present unique challenges in assessing and responding to patient needs under anesthesia.

Awareness Under Anesthesia

A disturbing phenomenon known as *awareness under anesthesia* has emerged as one of the most challenging problems in current anesthesia practice. It is important to note that dreams or fleeting perceptions on induction or emergence are *not* considered true awareness under anesthesia. For reasons that remain unclear, some patients do not demonstrate characteristic (measurable or observable) physiological responses to pain or have inadequate depth of anesthesia during surgery. The result is that the patient may have direct recall or explicit memory (Insight 14.4) of intraoperative events. When muscle relaxants are used, the patient is unable to move or speak, and therefore is unable to communicate this awareness to the anesthesia care provider. An average of 0.1% to 0.2% of all patients undergoing general anesthesia experience some form of awareness (1–2 per 1000 anesthetics). Because approximately 21 million patients in the United States receive general anesthesia each year, an estimated 20,000 to 40,000 cases of awareness under anesthesia may be occurring yearly. The risk of awareness appears to be greater when it is necessary to use the lowest possible dose of anesthesia medications to avoid undesirable side effects. Patients who are hemodynamically unstable (such as trauma patients) are also at greater risk of awareness under

anesthesia, as are those undergoing cardiac and emergency obstetric procedures. Patients with a history of substance abuse and patients with chronic pain are also at greater risk. Although the extent of awareness is highly variable, approximately half of these patients report auditory recall, half report a sensation of being unable to breathe, and one third recall pain. A number of these patients reportedly go on to have posttraumatic stress disorder as a result.

🏃 TECH TIP

Previously, the surgical team was periodically reminded that the patient's hearing is the last sense to go and the first to return. Inherent in that statement is a belief that what was said during a patient's surgical procedure did not affect the patient. What we now understand about explicit and implicit memory and the number of patients who experience auditory recall (explicit memory) should motivate us to try to effect significant change in surgical team behaviors. We can no longer assume that the patient is unaffected by our conversations and comments during surgery. As surgical technologists we can support the anesthesia care providers in their efforts to bring this understanding to the attention of all surgical team members.

INSIGHT 14.4 Explicit and Implicit Memory Under Anesthesia

The term *explicit memory* refers to the ability to recall events (i.e., conscious recollection). When a patient has explicit memory of events during surgery, it may be traumatic. Although explicit memory may be somewhat vague, some patients have been able to recall specific comments and conversations that took place during their surgical procedure. Much effort is being directed at preventing such occurrences.

But what is *implicit* memory? *Implicit memory* is the term used to describe subconscious processing of information by the brain, demonstrated by changes in the performance of tasks. For example, you know how to tie your shoelaces, but you may not remember exactly how or when you learned to do so. Another example of implicit memory is posthypnotic suggestion. Popular nightclub acts offer hypnosis to audience volunteers. The volunteer is hypnotized and asked to perform some particular behavior when a cue is given. The volunteer is awakened from the hypnotic state and the cue is given, causing the volunteer to display the suggested behavior. The experience occurred, and the behavior was displayed, but the volunteer has no conscious recollection (explicit memory).

A few experiments have shown that some learning (similar to hypnotic suggestion) is possible while under anesthesia, indicating that implicit memory during anesthesia exists in some form. Surgical patients who agreed to participate in these studies were routinely anesthetized for surgery. During the surgical procedure, verbal instructions were given, asking the patient to perform a simple task (such as scratching the nose) on cue, during the postoperative interview. On the prearranged cue, a surprising number of patients displayed the suggested behavior, yet without remembering why they were doing so. These studies seem to indicate that a significant number of surgical patients hear and remember what is said (implicit memory), but without conscious recall (explicit memory). The potential impact of implicit memory and the surgical patient is enormous, and much remains unknown. Could pessimistic comments made by the surgeon and other surgical team members during surgery have a negative effect on the patient's recovery? Could positive suggestions given under anesthesia speed recovery? Until the impact of implicit memory is clearly identified, all surgical team members should consider making only positive, affirming comments, and keeping conversations on an encouraging and professional level during surgery. After all, it appears that our patients may be hearing and implicitly remembering everything we say throughout their operations.

Prevention measures include administration of midazolam for amnesia (provides anterograde amnesia only) and avoidance of the use of neuromuscular blocking agents whenever possible.

❓ QUICK QUESTION

What does the term *anterograde amnesia* mean? Check your answer in Chapter 12.

Additional methods of patient monitoring have been developed to predict and prevent awareness under anesthesia. Rather than measure physiological responses, these devices monitor brain activity and are modified types of electroencephalography. These devices may be known as *level-of-consciousness* or *anesthesia-depth monitors* (see Chapter 13). Brain function monitoring is not indicated for all patients but may be used for select patients on the basis of procedural and physiological risk factors. It is important to note, though, that although these monitors may provide additional information on patient consciousness, there is not yet a perfect system for preventing awareness under anesthesia.

Muscle Relaxation

Whereas a short-acting muscle relaxant is administered to allow intubation, a long-acting muscle relaxant is often given during the maintenance phase to facilitate exposure of the surgical site. The amount of muscle relaxation required depends on the surgical procedure, with abdominal procedures requiring the deepest relaxation. In addition to depth, timing of relaxation is a crucial factor. The duration of a long-acting muscle relaxant and the anticipated length of the surgical procedure are taken into consideration when selecting and administering the appropriate agent.

The depth of neuromuscular blockade is monitored with the use of a peripheral nerve stimulator. The peripheral nerve stimulator administers an electrical stimulus to a nerve-muscle group, and the motor response is assessed, indicating the extent of muscle blockade. Electrodes are placed at the desired location, usually the wrist, and connected to the unit. Alternatively, the unit may be placed directly over a branch of the facial nerve. Different stimuli patterns may be used as indicated, but one of the most common is the train-of-four pattern, a series of four electrical stimuli delivered approximately 0.5 seconds apart. Recall from Chapter 13 that the presence of four of the four twitches indicates no muscle relaxation, and zero of the four twitches indicates complete muscle relaxation. The patient's motor response is assessed and used to determine when and how much additional muscle relaxant is necessary to maintain optimal surgical exposure. Ideally, muscle relaxation is present through closure of the deep wound layers and wears off as the superficial layers are closed.

Emergence Phase

As the procedure is completed, the emergence phase begins, during which anesthetic agents are discontinued and allowed to wear off. If indicated, the duration of certain anesthetic agents may be shortened by the administration of reversal agents to permit the patient to gradually awaken. The emergence phase ends when the patient is transported to the PACU.

! CAUTION

The emergence phase of anesthesia is another time when the patient is hypersensitive to loud noises and movement. Because the surgical procedure has concluded and pressure exists to minimize the operating room turnover time, surgical technologists in the scrub role are busy with various tasks to break down the sterile back table. These tasks involve manipulation of instruments and metal pans and basins, which can produce loud noises. In addition, the surgical technologist in the circulating role may be performing various duties around the patient, such as dressing application, replacement of blankets, and preparation for patient transfer. Each of these activities may cause a sudden movement of the patient, which in turn may cause laryngospasm. The surgical technologist must always maintain an awareness of the surgical patient's status and make every effort to minimize movement of the patient and noise during the emergence phase of anesthesia.

As patients awaken and become able to maintain their own airway, the items used to provide airway support are removed. In masked airway the pharyngeal airway is removed (if present), but the mask may be left in place to administer O_2. If an LMA was used, it is removed and replaced with a regular mask for O_2 administration, as needed. If the patient has been intubated, particular care is used to assess the appropriate timing for removal of the ET tube, a process called *extubation*. Patients must be breathing on their own, with airway reflexes present, and must demonstrate sufficient muscle strength to be able to maintain the airway independently. A mask may be used to administer O_2 if necessary. An oral airway may be placed to maintain or open the patient's airway by preventing the tongue from covering the epiglottis (Fig. 14.8). When vital signs are stable, the patient is carefully moved to a transport stretcher and taken to the PACU for the recovery phase. The anesthesia care

provider gives a detailed report to the PACU staff nurses, who closely monitor the patient during the recovery phase. When it is deemed safe, the patient is discharged from the PACU to the appropriate care location.

AGENTS USED FOR GENERAL ANESTHESIA

Several different classes of drugs have been used to achieve general anesthesia. Multiple agents are used to provide an unconscious state, analgesia, amnesia, and muscle relaxation. These medications are presented by category, and the phases of general anesthesia in which they are administered are indicated. The broad categories covered are intravenous induction agents, analgesics, inhalation agents, neuromuscular blocking agents, and reversal agents (Box 14.3).

Intravenous Induction Agents

Intravenous induction agents are administered to produce a rapid loss of consciousness. Agents used to induce unconsciousness are classified as either sedatives or hypnotics. Benzodiazepines are sedatives (see Chapter 12) that may be used for induction. Hypnotic agents used for induction include barbiturates (methohexital), ketamine (Ketalar), etomidate (Amidate), and propofol (Diprivan). These agents may also be used during maintenance of general anesthesia.

Benzodiazepines, which have both sedative and amnestic effects, are used preoperatively and occasionally as induction agents in combination with other agents. Benzodiazepines are not commonly used for induction because of the high doses required to induce an unconscious state. Recall that the benzodiazepines include midazolam, diazepam (Valium), and lorazepam (Ativan). Lorazepam is used to treat anxiety but not for induction and/or maintenance of anesthesia. Midazolam may be administered for induction, but it causes a greater drop in BP than diazepam. Fentanyl may be given 3 minutes before midazolam to speed the onset of unconsciousness. Benzodiazepines do not provide analgesia.

Barbiturates are ultrashort-acting hypnotic agents derived from barbituric acid. Before the development of propofol (Diprivan), the most frequently used induction agents were barbiturates including Pentothal and methohexital (Brevital). For example, Pentothal takes only seconds to travel from the injection site to the brain; thus it is rapidly taken up by the brain, but it is also rapidly eliminated. For example, thiopental takes only seconds to travel from the injection site to the brain; thus it is rapidly taken up by the brain, but it is also rapidly eliminated. Methohexital is ultrashort-acting and is more often used for

---

BOX 14.3 Major Categories of Anesthesia Medications

Intravenous induction agents
Analgesics
Inhalation agents
Neuromuscular blocking agents
Reversal agents

procedures that take place outside the operating room, such as cardioversion. Both agents are alkaline (pH >10) and will cause precipitation when administered with acidic agents, such as some neuromuscular blocking drugs. Barbiturates induce anesthesia but have no analgesic effect; patients may therefore be agitated and disoriented during the emergence phase because of the pain they experience.

Ketamine (Ketalar) is a dissociative hypnotic agent used for induction of general anesthesia. Chemically related to the drug phencyclidine, or "angel dust," ketamine is a powerful amnestic and analgesic—the only hypnotic agent with this property. Onset of action is 30 to 60 seconds after intravenous injection. When ketamine is used, patients appear to be awake and their eyes may be open; however, they are dissociated from their environment, and they do not consciously recall surgical events. Ketamine can cause hallucinations and distorted visual, auditory, and tactile sensations. It also exaggerates the effect of sudden loud noises. Involuntary movements may be present, and the dissociative state may make patients difficult to handle. It may be combined with a benzodiazepine to increase amnesia and reduce emergence reactions. Ketamine is not commonly used for maintenance of anesthesia but may be used as part of a balanced analgesia plan (Insight 14.5), or it may be used for superficial procedures of short duration, such as painful dressing changes, debridement, or skin grafts. Ketamine does not produce skeletal muscle relaxation.

Etomidate (Amidate) is a hypnotic agent that produces an unconscious state in less than a minute but provides no analgesia and no muscle relaxation. This agent is often used for patients with compromised myocardial contractility, who cannot tolerate the myocardial depression often seen with other induction agents. Rapid onset and a minimal effect on BP make etomidate an excellent alternative to propofol and the barbiturates. Etomidate is also ideal for brief procedures, such as cardioversion. It is particularly useful for induction in trauma patients, who may be hypovolemic and hence unable to tolerate any additional hypotension.

INSIGHT 14.5 Managing Postoperative Pain

A number of methods have emerged to better manage postoperative pain, reduce the amount of opioid analgesics needed in the immediate postoperative period, and shorten the patient's recovery time. Administration of a combination of agents for this purpose is referred to as *multimodal pain management* or *balanced analgesia*. An example of multimodal treatment is intravenous infusion of acetaminophen as an adjunct to opioids. Ketorolac (Toradol), a nonsteroidal antiinflammatory drug, may be administered intravenously in certain situations for short-term postoperative analgesia. Ketamine, an intravenous induction agent with strong analgesic action, may be administered as a single dose and/or an infusion as part of a multimodal surgical pain management plan. In addition, a regional block, such as a transverse abdominis plane block, may be administered as part of a multimodal pain management plan for general abdominal or gynecological surgical procedures. Multimodal pain management is a dynamic concept with new options emerging—watch for innovations in your facility and dialogue with your anesthesia care providers to learn more.

Propofol is a hypnotic agent chemically unrelated to any other anesthetic agent. The active drug is 2,6-diisopropylphenol suspended in an emulsion of 10% soybean oil, 2.25% glycerol, and 1.2% lecithin (a protein found in egg yolk).

? QUICK QUESTION

What is an emulsion? How is it different from a solution or a suspension? Check your answers in Chapter 1.

The most commonly used agent for induction, propofol is injected intravenously and produces an unconscious state within a minute. It does not provide analgesia or muscle relaxation. Propofol has a characteristic milky white appearance. Strict aseptic technique must be maintained when handling propofol because it contains no antimicrobial preservatives and can support rapid growth of microorganisms. Unused portions of propofol, and intravenous lines or solutions containing propofol injection, must be discarded at the end of the procedure or within 12 hours (6 hours if propofol was transferred from the original container).

! CAUTION

Patients with allergies to soy or eggs should not receive propofol because these substances are part of the emulsion.

Potential adverse effects include hypotension, bradycardia, and apnea. Many patients (40%–90%) report a stinging sensation at the injection site. A continuous propofol infusion may be used for maintenance of general anesthesia. Because of its brief duration (4–6 minutes), patients recover alert and free of the usual side effects of an anesthetic agent.

See Box 14.4 for a summary of intravenous induction agents used in general anesthesia.

Analgesics

Analgesic agents are given during maintenance of general anesthesia to prevent pain during surgery. If adequate pain control is achieved, the amount of other anesthetic agents required may be reduced. Analgesics are administered before the anticipated pain stimulus for optimum effect.

BOX 14.4 Intravenous Induction Agents Used in General Anesthesia

Sedatives (Benzodiazepines)
midazolam (N/A)
diazepam (Valium)

Hypnotics (Barbiturates)
methohexital (Brevital)

Hypnotics (Various Chemical Categories)
propofol (Diprivan)
ketamine (Ketalar)
etomidate (Amidate)

Apply what you already know to assist you in learning pharmacology. The term *analgesia* literally means "without pain." Thus an analgesic is an agent given to prevent or treat pain. You are already familiar with many examples of analgesics available over the counter, such as aspirin (Bayer, Excedrin, etc.) and acetaminophen (Tylenol). Remember, just as you take aspirin or acetaminophen (analgesics) to relieve the pain of a headache (e.g., that caused by studying so hard to learn all this pharmacology information), analgesics are administered to our patients to relieve the pain of surgery.

An intravenous formulation of acetaminophen is indicated for preemptive surgical analgesia, in combination with opioid analgesics (discussed later). Onset of action is approximately 10 minutes, and the duration of action is approximately 4 to 6 hours. It is packaged in a 100-mL vial and contains 1000 mg of acetaminophen (10 mg/mL). Studies have indicated that use of intravenous acetaminophen with opioids may decrease the amount of opioids required during and after surgery to control pain (see Insight 14.5).

The most common analgesic agents administered for anesthesia are classified as opioids. Recall from Chapter 12 that the term *opioid* refers to drugs (natural and synthetic) that produce morphine-like effects. The brain has its own natural pain suppression system, in part consisting of neurochemicals called *endorphins* (or endogenous opioids) and specific receptor sites for these chemicals. Opioids used in anesthesia are able to bind with the brain's natural receptor sites, initiating pain suppression. These agents are most effective when administered before a painful event.

> **NOTE:** Previously the term *narcotic* was used to describe analgesics used for anesthesia and was associated with the production of a state of stupor. In current use, though, the word narcotic is used to indicate any drug that can cause dependence. Thus the term *narcotic analgesic* is no longer used in reference to anesthesia.

Opioids are available from several drug sources, such as the following:

- Plants (also known as a natural source; from the opium poppy, *Papaver somniferum*)
- Semisynthetic (modified from the natural alkaloids found in the poppy)
- Synthetic (manufactured from chemicals)

Natural opioids are morphine and codeine. Morphine will have an onset of action in 15 to 30 minutes, reach a peak in 45 to 90 minutes, and has a duration of action lasting approximately 4 hours. A combination of acetaminophen and codeine may be prescribed for postoperative pain relief.

> **NOTE:** Although *not* an analgesic, another natural derivative of the opium poppy is papaverine (Insight 14.6), a smooth-muscle relaxant that may be administered from the sterile back table.

INSIGHT 14.6 **Papaverine**

Papaverine is a chemical derived from the opium poppy (*Papaver somniferum*) that is used as a smooth-muscle relaxant during surgery. Papaverine may be administered from the sterile field during procedures on small blood vessels (such as coronary artery bypass grafts). It is injected at the vessel wall to prevent vasoconstriction from vascular muscle spasms caused by surgical manipulation.

Synthetic opioids used for anesthesia are fentanyl, alfentanil, sufentanil, and remifentanil (Ultiva). These drugs are useful in anesthesia because of their relatively short action and intense analgesic effect. Synthetic opioids are more potent analgesics than morphine, but at equivalent analgesic doses, they cause the same degree of respiratory depression.

Fentanyl is 100 times more potent than morphine. This drug has a rapid onset, approximately 30 seconds, with a duration of 20 to 40 minutes. Fentanyl provides analgesia plus some sedation. Alfentanil has one fourth the potency of fentanyl, and its onset of action is rapid. Lasting only 10 to 15 minutes, alfentanil is classified as an ultrashort-acting opioid. Sufentanil is 5 to 10 times more potent than fentanyl, but it is more rapidly cleared from the body, providing a very rapid recovery. Onset is rapid, with effects lasting 20 to 45 minutes. Remifentanil (Ultiva) is the newest ultrashort-acting opioid and is 20 to 40 times more potent than alfentanil. Onset of effects occurs in 1 to 3 minutes, but duration is only 5 to 10 minutes. If used for maintenance of the analgesia component of general anesthesia, remifentanil is given as a continuous infusion.

See Table 14.1 for a comparison of opioids used for analgesia during general anesthesia.

Inhalation Agents

Inhalation agents are gases or vaporized liquids that induce anesthesia when administered in the air the patient breathes. The first inhalation anesthetics used were ether, chloroform, N_2O, and cyclopropane. Of these, only N_2O gas is in use currently. Ether and cyclopropane are explosive, and chloroform is toxic to the liver, so use of these agents was discontinued as new agents were developed. Introduced in 1956, halothane (Fluothane) was the first nonexplosive inhalation agent. Additional inhalation agents have been developed, with each generation of new agents improving on previous agents.

Inhalation anesthetics (also called *volatile anesthetics*) are distributed in liquid form packaged in bottles. The liquid agent is poured into the appropriate vaporizer on an anesthesia

TABLE 14.1 **Comparison of Opioids Used for Analgesia During General Anesthesia**

Generic Name	Trade Name	Onset	Duration (min)
fentanyl	N/A	30 sec	45–60
alfentanil	N/A	30 sec	10–15
sufentanil	N/A	30 sec	20–45
remifentanil	Ultiva	1–3 min	5–10

machine, and the administration rate is adjusted as needed. The vaporizer turns the liquid agent into a gas that is relatively easy to administer via breathing mask, LMA, or ET tube. Inhalation agents, which are measured by the percentage of vapor present in the mixture the patient inhales, diffuse into the blood from the air in the alveoli, then rapidly diffuse out of the blood and into the brain—the site of action. Inhalation anesthetics are eliminated from the body quickly, most via the pulmonary, hepatic, and renal systems. The potency of inhalation agents is compared using a measurement called *minimum alveolar concentration* (MAC). The MAC is the concentration that at one atmosphere of pressure stops the motor response to incision in 50% of patients.

 TECH TIP

Do not confuse the concept of monitored anesthesia care (MAC), discussed in Chapter 13, with minimum alveolar concentration (MAC). If the abbreviation MAC is used in reference to an anesthesia method involving administration of sedation, anxiolysis, and/or analgesia and patient assessment provided by an anesthesia professional, it stands for "monitored anesthesia care." If the abbreviation MAC is used in reference to an inhalation agent (used in general, not local, anesthesia), it stands for "minimum alveolar concentration."

The disadvantages of inhalation agents include an increased potential for cardiovascular depression and lack of postoperative analgesia. The selection of an inhalation agent is influenced by factors such as solubility of the gas and the patient's cardiac output. The most common inhalation agents in use currently include the gas N_2O and three volatile liquid anesthetics, isoflurane (Forane), desflurane (Suprane), and sevoflurane (Ultane) (Fig. 14.9).

N_2O—a colorless, odorless, tasteless gas—is one of the most widely used inhalation anesthetics in clinical practice. N_2O provides rapid onset and emergence and is eliminated by the lungs. Its mild analgesic and amnestic characteristics make it an excellent adjunct to volatile liquid inhalation anesthetic agents. N_2O is often used in conjunction with volatile anesthetics to reduce the amount of the latter needed. A muscle relaxant must also be given if needed. An interesting characteristic of N_2O is that it will rapidly diffuse out of the circulatory system and into a closed, air-filled cavity, such as the middle ear. The resulting increase in pressure can push against a newly placed tympanic membrane graft, so the surgeon may request that N_2O be turned off before graft placement during tympanoplasty.

 MAKE IT SIMPLE

To help to identify the category of an agent, use common word parts as hints. For example, if the name of an agent ends in "-ane," it is probably an inhalation anesthetic. Similarly, the names of local anesthetic agents usually end in "-caine."

The three most common volatile liquid anesthetics are isoflurane (Forane), desflurane (Suprane), and sevoflurane (Ultane). These agents are quite similar to previous volatile liquid

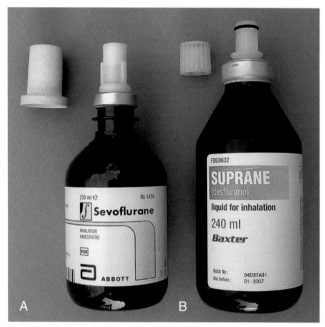

Fig. 14.9 (A) A sealed bottle of Abbott sevoflurane with its integral uniquely shaped filler (Quick-Fil). Note that the filler on the bottle is secured by a crimped metal seal. (B) Similarly, a sealed bottle of desflurane, with Saf-T-Fil system. The filler caps are shown alongside the bottles. As the contents are pressurized at ambient temperature, the glass bottle is encased in a plastic coat to prevent it exploding if damaged. (From Davey AJ and Diba A: *Ward's anaesthetic equipment*, ed 6, St Louis, 2012, Elsevier.)

anesthetic agents, except that they provide more precise control of maintenance and more rapid induction and emergence. Volatile agents are highly potent, and doses can be adjusted to provide some muscle relaxation and rapid emergence. Cardiac depression may be seen with higher doses, so the volatile agents are often used in combination with N_2O. See Table 14.2 for a list of inhalation anesthetic agents.

! **CAUTION**

Inhalation anesthetic agents (except for N_2O), either alone or in combination with succinylcholine (Anectine), have been identified as triggering agents of a rare but life-threatening condition called *malignant hyperthermia* (see Chapter 15).

TABLE 14.2 Inhalation Anesthetics

Generic Name	Trade Name
Gas	
nitrous oxide (N_2O)	N/A
Volatile Liquid (Vapor)	
isoflurane	Forane
desflurane	Suprane
sevoflurane	Ultane

N/A, Not applicable.

Neuromuscular Blocking Agents

Agents categorized as neuromuscular blockers are administered to relax skeletal muscles for intubation and surgery. Patients under general anesthesia may be unconscious, pain free, and memory free, but their skeletal muscles continue to respond to stimuli. To receive an ET tube, the patient must be adequately relaxed (i.e., the muscles must be relaxed). During some surgical procedures, especially in the abdomen, the patient's muscles must be relaxed to facilitate exposure of the surgical site.

Muscle Physiology Review

There are three types of muscle tissue: cardiac, smooth, and skeletal. Muscles function in circulation, labor and delivery, and intestinal movements, as well as in body movement. For a muscle to contract, it must be stimulated by a motor nerve. The neuromuscular junction is an area where the motor nerve axon is very near the muscle fiber (Fig. 14.10). The space between an axon and a muscle fiber is called a *synapse*. The neurotransmitter at the neuromuscular junction is acetylcholine (ACh). When ACh is released from the axon, it diffuses across the synapse (synaptic cleft) and binds to receptor sites on the cell membrane of the muscle fiber (the sarcolemma). ACh causes a wave of depolarization to spread across the muscle fiber to T-tubules, which conduct the wave of depolarization deep into the muscle fibers. As a result of the spreading wave of depolarization, calcium is released from its storage sites within the sarcoplasmic reticulum. The presence of calcium ions allows the contractile elements of the muscle, actin and myosin, to engage, resulting in muscle contraction. For muscle fibers to return to a resting state, ACh must diffuse away from the receptor sites at the neuromuscular junction and be broken down, or recycled, by an enzyme called *acetylcholinesterase*. This enzyme, which is present abundantly in extracellular fluid, breaks down ACh and terminates the contraction. Calcium ions are then transported back into the sarcoplasmic reticulum for storage and later release. Depolarizing muscle relaxants act like ACh; they bind with receptor sites and initiate a contraction (depolarization). Such contractions are observed as fasciculations, small involuntary muscle twitches just under the skin. Subsequent contractions are prevented as long as the depolarizing muscle relaxant stays on the binding sites. Nondepolarizing muscle relaxants act as ACh antagonists; they competitively block receptor sites and prevent ACh binding, thus preventing a contraction (see Fig. 1.17).

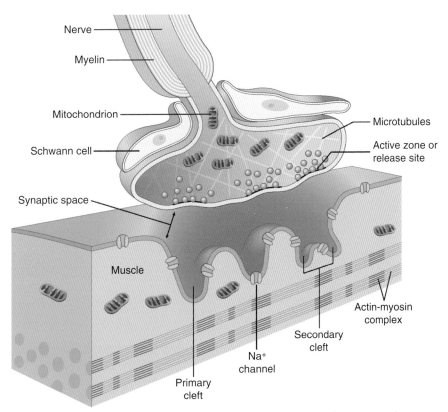

Fig. 14.10 Adult neuromuscular junction with the three cells that constitute the synapse: the motor neuron (i.e., nerve terminal), muscle fiber, and Schwann cell. The motor neuron from the ventral horn of the spinal cord innervates the muscle. Each fiber receives only one synapse. The motor nerve loses its myelin and terminates on the muscle fiber. The nerve terminal, covered by a Schwann cell, has vesicles clustered about the membrane thickenings, which are the active zones, toward its synaptic side and mitochondria and microtubules toward its other side. A synaptic gutter, made up of a primary and many secondary clefts, separates the nerve from the muscle. The muscle surface is corrugated, and dense areas on the shoulders of each fold contain acetylcholine receptors. Sodium channels are present at the clefts and throughout the muscle membrane. *Na+*, Sodium. (From Miller RD and Pardo M: *Basics of anesthesia*, ed 6, St Louis, 2011, Elsevier.)

There are two basic types of muscle relaxants, classified according to their action on the motor end plate: depolarizing and nondepolarizing. Examples of each type are listed with a brief description.

Succinylcholine (Anectine) is the only depolarizing muscle relaxant in use. Succinylcholine acts similarly to the neurotransmitter ACh, but its duration is longer. It causes persistent depolarization and produces fasciculations followed by flaccidity. Effects of succinylcholine are noted within 30 to 60 seconds after administration. Duration of effects is also short, usually only 5 to 10 minutes, but because no antagonist or reversal agent is currently available, succinylcholine must be allowed to wear off. Some adverse effects associated with administration of succinylcholine include increased intracranial pressure, increased intraocular pressure, increased intragastric pressure (which increases the potential for regurgitation), and muscle soreness postoperatively. Elevated serum potassium levels have been noted in burn patients receiving succinylcholine. Patients with pseudocholinesterase deficiency may experience prolonged neuromuscular blockade and respiratory paralysis because succinylcholine is not eliminated effectively without that enzyme. The US Food and Drug Administration warns against using succinylcholine in children because of cases of unrecognized muscular dystrophy that may lead to hyperkalemia and cardiac arrest. Succinylcholine may be used in children when emergency airway control is necessary (see Chapter 15).

! CAUTION

Succinylcholine has been identified as a triggering agent for malignant hyperthermia. See Chapter 15 for additional information.

There are several nondepolarizing muscle relaxants, categorized as long, intermediate, and short acting. These agents include pancuronium bromide, atracurium besylate, vecuronium bromide, cisatracurium besylate (Nimbex), rocuronium bromide, and mivacurium chloride. The first muscle relaxant, tubocurarine chloride (curare), is also

INSIGHT 14.7 First Muscle Relaxant

The earliest known muscle relaxant was curare. It is a toxin that is extracted from plants found in the rain forest. Indigenous peoples on three separate continents—South America, Africa, and Southeast Asia—used curare on the tips of darts to immobilize monkeys and other tree-dwelling animals. Once discovered by Western culture, curare was used in the experimental laboratory for various purposes. A German report in 1912 described the use of curare on humans, as an adjunct to anesthesia; however, the report was generally ignored. Not until 1942 was curare first used in surgery; it was used to relax abdominal muscles of a patient undergoing an appendectomy. Discovery of the benefits of curare radically changed anesthesia practice. Patients could now be routinely intubated, a sporadic practice before the use of curare. Since the introduction of curare, many agents have been developed to provide muscle relaxation.

nondepolarizing (Insight 14.7). Nondepolarizing muscle relaxants prevent muscle contractions by binding to cholinergic receptors, preventing ACh from binding to the receptor sites. Nondepolarizing muscle relaxants do not cause fasciculations and may be used before administration of succinylcholine to prevent fasciculations. The selection of a particular nondepolarizing muscle relaxant depends on its pharmacologic properties, such as onset and duration of effects, and side effects, such as those seen in the cardiovascular system. See Table 14.3 for a comparison of the duration of effects of neuromuscular blocking agents. Adverse effects of nondepolarizing muscle relaxants on the cardiovascular system include hypotension or hypertension, tachycardia, bradycardia, and arrhythmias. The dosage is variable, depending on onset time and depth of block required. Nondepolarizing muscle relaxants may be reversed, if necessary, with an antagonist, such as neostigmine. Neostigmine works by competing with ACh for attachment to acetylcholinesterase. This competition causes a buildup of ACh, which facilitates transmission of impulses across the neuromuscular junction. In addition, some reversal agents stimulate the presynaptic release of ACh, as well as binding to acetylcholinesterase.

Reversal Agents

Occasionally, the surgical procedure may be completed sooner than expected. An example of this situation is a radical hysterectomy. This procedure is expected to take several hours,

TABLE 14.3 Comparison of Duration of Neuromuscular Blocking Agents

Category	Generic Name	Trade Name	Duration (min)
Depolarizing	succinylcholine	Anectine	4–6
Nondepolarizing	mivacurium chloride	N/A	6–10
	atracurium besylate	N/A	20–35
	vecuronium bromide	N/A	25–30
	cisatracurium besylate	Nimbex	45–75
	rocuronium bromide	N/A	15–85
	pancuronium bromide	N/A	40–65

so several different long-acting anesthetic agents are administered. If unexpected metastases are discovered in the liver or scattered over the intestines, the procedure may be terminated without resection. This situation may require the administration of reversal agents to counteract specific anesthetic agents. Naloxone (Narcan), nalmefene, and naltrexone (Trexan) are used to reverse opioid analgesics, if necessary. Naloxone is administered intravenously to reverse respiratory depression caused by opioids. It has a short duration of action, 30 to 45 minutes. Nalmefene is a long-acting opioid antagonist. Benzodiazepines may be reversed with flumazenil (Mazicon). When indicated, nondepolarizing muscle relaxants may be reversed with an acetylcholinesterase inhibitor, such as neostigmine. See Table 14.4 for a list of reversal agents for various anesthetics.

TABLE 14.4 Reversal Agents for Anesthetics

Reversal Agent	Used to reverse
naloxone (Narcan)	Opioid analgesics
nalmefene (N/A)	Opioid analgesics
naltrexone (Trexan)	Opioid analgesics
flumazenil (Mazicon)	Benzodiazepines
neostigmine (N/A)	Nondepolarizing muscle relaxants

KEY CONCEPTS

- Safely providing anesthesia is an art, as well as a science. Various drugs and techniques have been used to achieve a state of anesthesia. Although several theories have been proposed, in some cases the exact mechanism of action of anesthetic drugs remains unclear.
- For some procedures it is important that the patient be under general anesthesia—unconscious, pain free, and immobile with no awareness of events. General anesthesia may be necessary because of patient factors or the naturN/urgical procedure.
- Four major components must be accomplished in general anesthesia: unconsciousness, analgesia, amnesia, and muscle relaxation.
- There are five phases of administration of a general anesthetic: preinduction, induction, maintenance, emergence, and recovery.
- The two methods or routes used to deliver general anesthetics are intravenous and inhalation.
- Intravenous induction agents include barbiturates, benzodiazepines, ketamine, etomidate, and propofol.
- Analgesics administered as an adjunct to general anesthesia are intravenous acetaminophen, fentanyl, alfentanil, sufentanil, and remifentanil.
- Common inhalation agents include the gas N_2O and volatile liquid anesthetics, such as isoflurane, desflurane, and sevoflurane.
- Muscle relaxants, given as an adjunct to general anesthesia, are categorized as depolarizing and nondepolarizing neuromuscular blockers.
- Agents that may be administered during emergence include naloxone, nalmefene, naltrexone, flumazenil, and neostigmine.
- Anesthesia is a complex physiologic state, often taken for granted by operating room personnel. To function effectively on the surgical team, the surgical technologist must understand the basic concepts of anesthesia and the names and purposes of common agents used.

LEARNING THE LANGUAGE (KEY TERMS)

Using your textbook or a standard medical dictionary, look up and write the definitions of each term.

anesthesia
emergence phase
endotracheal (ET) tube
extubation
fasciculation
induction phase
intubation

laryngeal masked airway (LMA)
maintenance phase
minimum alveolar concentration (MAC)
postanesthesia care unit (PACU)
preinduction phase
rapid sequence induction (RSI)

REVIEW QUESTIONS

1. What does the term *anesthesia* mean?
2. What are the indications for general anesthesia?
3. What is the surgical technologist in the scrub role doing during each phase of general anesthesia? What is the circulating surgical technologist doing?
4. What are the components of a general anesthetic?
5. Which categories of agents are used to accomplish general anesthesia?
6. Can you name an agent in each category?
7. How are depolarizing and nondepolarizing muscle relaxants alike? How are they different?
8. How should the potential for awareness under anesthesia impact the surgical technologist's practice?

CRITICAL THINKING

Scenario 1

Mrs. Diaz is a 45-year-old woman. She sustained a fractured wrist when she slipped on an icy sidewalk, exiting a restaurant. She has been admitted to surgery for closed reduction and cast application.

1. Which method of airway control do you think the anesthesia care provider will select for Mrs. Diaz? Justify your answer.

Scenario 2

Johnny Duncan is a 5-year-old boy. He sustained a greenstick fracture of the forearm when he fell from a park swing set. He has been admitted to surgery for a closed reduction and cast application.

1. Which method of anesthesia induction do you think the anesthesia care provider will select for Johnny? Justify your answer.

BIBLIOGRAPHY

Apfel CC, Turan A, Souza K, et al: Intravenous acetaminophen reduces postoperative nausea and vomiting: a systematic review and meta-analysis, *Pain* 154(5):677–689, 2013.

Bardal S, Waechter J, Martin D: *Applied pharmacology*, St Louis, 2011, Saunders/Elsevier.

Duke JC, Keech BM, editors: *Duke's anesthesia secrets*, ed 5, St Louis, 2016, Saunders/Elsevier.

Nagelhout J, Plaus K, editors: *Nurse anesthesia*, ed 5, St Louis, 2014, Saunders/Elsevier.

Vadivelu N, Mitra S, Schermer E, et al: Preventive analgesia for postoperative pain control: a broader concept, *Local Reg Anesth* 7:17–22, 2014.

INTERNET RESOURCES

Medscape, Drug & Diseases, Acetaminophen IV: http://reference.medscape.com/drug/ofirmev-acetaminophen-iv-999610.

Medscape, Transversus Abdominis Plane Block: https://emedicine.medscape.com/article/2000944-overview.

KEY TERMS

acupuncture
cryoanesthesia

hypnoanalgesia

According to its definition, the term *anesthesia* means "lack of sensation." How this effect is achieved may use many methods. In addition to the ones mentioned in the previous two chapters, the surgical first assistant should be familiar with some of these alternative anesthesia methodologies. Cryoanesthesia, or cryoanalgesia, is also known as *frost* or *refrigeration anesthesia*. It is defined as a local anesthesia produced by chilling a part of the body or peripheral nerves to near-freezing temperature to numb the area against pain. The application of cold to tissues creates a conduction block that is similar to a local anesthetic's effect. This technique uses an applicator (cryoprobe) or spray, such as Frigiderm (dichlorotetrafluoroethane). Cryotherapy is used in surgical specialties, such as dermatology for dermabrasion or removal of skin lesions and gynecology for endometrial cryoablation. In these procedures, the extreme cold freezes and destroys the targeted tissues. Another use for cryoanesthesia is spraying ethyl chloride (e.g., Gebauer's Ethyl Chloride) onto the skin as a topical anesthetic before injections or starting intravenous catheters or for venipuncture.

Hypnosis has long been associated with entertainment; however, there is a therapeutic hypnosis used in medical applications as well. Called *hypnoanalgesia*, it was approved by the American Medical Association in 1958 as an alternative form of medicine and has been used by dentists, obstetricians, and midwives in place of local anesthesia for many years. In 1996 a panel of the National Institutes of Health found hypnosis to be effective in easing pain caused by cancer. More recent studies have found it to be effective for relieving pain resulting from burns, cancer, and rheumatoid arthritis, and even for anxiety reduction associated with surgery. In a hypnotized state, a part of the central nervous system shows greater activity and influence on the patient's senses (as feeling and thoughts) and on the sensation of pain. When the mind is able to concentrate and focus, it can be used more powerfully. The person may experience physiologic changes, such as slowing of the pulse and respiration, and an increase in alpha brain waves. The person may also be more open to suggestions and goals, such as reducing pain.

However, this form of therapy can be unpredictable because its effect depends upon the patient's willingness and acceptance of the method and the fact that not everyone can be hypnotized.

Acupuncture originated in China more than 2000 years ago and is one of the oldest and most commonly used medical procedures worldwide. This group of procedures involves the stimulation of anatomic points of the body by varying methods. The most studied scientifically is the penetration of the skin with thin, metallic needles that are manipulated by hand or by an electrical stimulation (electroacupuncture). Acupuncture became better known to the American public after James Reston wrote an article for *The New York Times* about his experience in China in the 1970s. He had an emergency appendectomy, while visiting there, and acupuncture was used to help with his postoperative pain control. The first acupuncture clinic in the United States is claimed to have been opened by Dr. Yao Wu Lee in Washington, D.C. on July 9, 1972. The US Food and Drug Administration approved acupuncture needles for use by licensed practitioners in 1996. According to acupuncture theory, pain signals travel from the area of the injury to the spinal cord and brain. Acupuncture generates a stimulus that travels faster and crowds out the pain signals to effectively block and prevent them from reaching the brain. The result is that the patient never experiences the pain. Traditional Chinese medicine defines acupuncture theory as a technique to balance the flow of energy or life force (qi or chi) believed to flow through pathways in the body. Some believe the acupuncture points stimulate nerves, muscles, and connective tissue, and this stimulation boosts the body's natural painkillers and increases blood flow. In 2014 China issued 18 medical protocols for acupuncture and moxibustion to align these old traditional therapies with modern medicine. Moxibustion is the practice of burning the mugwort herb against the skin. Interesting to note, moxibustion has been successfully used to turn breech babies to normal head-down position before childbirth. Studies have shown moxibustion increases fetal movement in the uterus.

ADVANCED PRACTICES: REVIEW QUESTIONS

1. Describe how cryoanesthesia produces a local anesthetic effect.
2. Who has used hypnosis in the past to achieve an anesthetic effect?
3. How does hypnosis produce a local anesthetic effect?
4. Which alternative medical practice to achieve anesthesia is among the oldest and most widely used?
5. Describe one theory as to how acupuncture produces an anesthetic effect.

ADVANCED PRACTICES: BIBLIOGRAPHY

Lanfranco RC, Canales-Johnson A, Huepe D: Hypnoanalgesia and the study of pain experience: from Cajal to modern neuroscience, *Front Psychol* 5:1126, 2014.

Lewis DO: Hypnoanalgesia for chronic pain: the response to multiple inductions at one session and to separate single inductions, *J R Soc Med* 85(10):620–624, 1992.

Trescot AM: Cryoanalgesia in interventional pain management, *Pain Physician* 6(3):345–360, 2003.

ADVANCED PRACTICES: INTERNET RESOURCES

American Association of Acupuncture and Oriental Medicine: www.aaaomonline.org/.

Mayo Clinic, Acupuncture: www.mayoclinic.org/tests-procedures/acupuncture/basics/definition/prc-20020778?reDate=12082015.

National Acupuncture Foundation: https://nationalacupuncturefoundation.org/.

Reston J, *Now, let me tell you about my appendectomy in Peking…*, Acupuncture.com: www.acupuncture.com/testimonials/restonexp.htm.

RxList, Ethyl Chloride: www.rxlist.com/ethyl-chloride-drug.htm.

The Free Dictionary, Cryoanesthesia: http://medical-dictionary.thefreedictionary.com/cryoanesthesia.

WebMD, Feature, Hypnosis, Meditation, and Relaxation for Pain Treatment: www.webmd.com/balance/features/hypnosis-for-pain.

Emergency Situations

One goal of anesthesia is to maintain the patient in a stable physiological state throughout the course of anesthesia and surgery. However, surgery and anesthesia are complex processes that significantly impact the human physiological state. In addition, some patients requiring surgery are critically ill, and a few may have multiple organ system failure. The most common anesthesia emergency situations, which vary from mild to life-threatening, merit careful study by the surgical technologist. Emergency situations in the operating room may be caused by existing disease, trauma, the surgical procedure, anesthesia, or may be of unknown origin and may occur at any point during the patient's care. This chapter is specifically focused on selected anesthesia-associated emergencies that require pharmacological treatment. Two of the most pertinent to the surgical technologist—cardiac arrest and malignant hyperthermia (MH)—are discussed at length. The surgical technologist should be able to respond appropriately as a surgical team member to any patient emergency. To function in a competent manner, the surgical technologist must have a thorough knowledge of the medications frequently used in emergency situations.

RESPIRATORY EMERGENCIES

Intraoperative respiratory impairment or obstruction may be caused by a number of factors, including swelling from trauma or inflammation, allergic reactions, bronchospasm, or laryngospasm. In rare cases, surgical intervention (tracheotomy) may be indicated.

Allergic Reactions

Allergic reactions range from mild, with signs such as skin redness, hives, or raised skin patches, to life-threatening, with serious cardiovascular and respiratory problems, indicating anaphylaxis (a severe systemic allergic reaction). Respiratory symptoms include bronchospasm, dyspnea (labored breathing), tachypnea (rapid breathing), respiratory obstruction, and laryngeal edema. Signs of allergic reactions can occur in 2 to 20 minutes and persist for up to 36 hours.

If early signs of a mild allergic reaction appear, potentially triggering medications being administered are discontinued, 100% oxygen is administered, infusions of intravenous fluids are

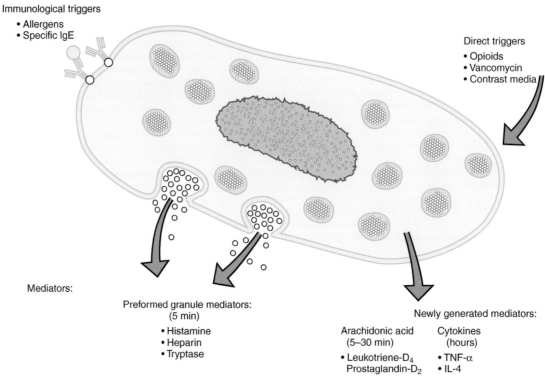

Immunological triggers
- Allergens
- Specific IgE

Direct triggers
- Opioids
- Vancomycin
- Contrast media

Mediators:

Preformed granule mediators:
(5 min)
- Histamine
- Heparin
- Tryptase

Newly generated mediators:

Arachidonic acid   Cytokines
(5–30 min)   (hours)
- Leukotriene-D$_4$ • TNF-α
  Prostaglandin-D$_2$ • IL-4

Fig. 15.1 Mast cells release prestored inflammatory mediators, such as histamine, which act rapidly. Other mediators, such as leukotrienes, are newly generated after their precursors are released and act more slowly. Some mediators are also produced by basophils. *IgE*, Immunoglobulin E; *IL-4*, interleukin-4; *TNF-α*, tumor necrosis factor α. (From Wecker L, Crespo L, Dunaway G, et al.: *Brody's human pharmacology*, ed 5, Philadelphia, 2010, Elsevier.)

increased, and a dose of epinephrine may be administered. In response to an allergen, the body releases a number of proteins including histamine (Fig. 15.1). Histamine causes significant vasodilation, which in turn causes hypotension. Two types of antihistamines are administered in surgery to counteract allergic histamine release: H1-receptor antagonists and H2-receptor antagonists.

QUICK QUESTION

What does an antagonist do? What is another name for a receptor antagonist? See the section on pharmacodynamics in Chapter 1 to check your answer.

Diphenhydramine (Benadryl) is a common antihistamine available as an over-the-counter medication, taken orally for mild allergies. In surgery, it is more specifically classified as an H1-receptor antagonist, and it is administered intravenously to treat allergic reactions. Diphenhydramine may be used alone or in combination with an H2-receptor antagonist when epinephrine and intravenous fluid replacement have not successfully reversed hypotension. An example of an H2-receptor antagonist used in this situation is famotidine.

QUICK QUESTION

Famotidine is classified as an H2-receptor antagonist. Which other drug category also describes these agents? What other condition may these drugs be used to treat? What is another indication to administer H2-receptor antagonists for surgery? See Chapter 12 to check your answers.

If conservative treatment is effective in treating a mild allergic reaction, surgery in progress may continue but without the use of the suspected agent. If conservative treatment is not effective, the allergic reaction may quickly progress to anaphylaxis.

Anaphylaxis

Anaphylaxis is a severe, systemic allergic reaction in a susceptible person, caused by a second exposure to a triggering agent. It is the most severe type of hypersensitivity reaction to medications, anesthetics, latex, or blood administered in surgery. Anaphylactic shock is a complete cardiovascular collapse, which occurs rapidly and may include cardiac and respiratory arrest. All patients receiving parenteral medications are at risk, especially those with a history of allergic reactions. Anaphylaxis is estimated to occur in 1 of every 4000 to 25,000 administrations of anesthetic agents. One of the most common causes of allergic reactions during anesthesia are the neuromuscular blocking agents (see Chapter 14), particularly succinylcholine.

NOTE: Medications that cause the most frequent allergic reactions include neuromuscular blockers (such as succinylcholine), antibiotics (such as penicillin and cephalosporins), iodine-based contrast media, morphine, and meperidine. Although rare, anaphylaxis associated with amide local anesthetic agents is thought to be attributed to the preservative methylparaben.

Anaphylaxis is characterized by the respiratory symptoms described earlier. Under general anesthesia, though, the first sign of anaphylaxis usually noted is hypotension. The first-line treatment for anaphylaxis in surgery is an intravenous bolus of epinephrine.

Epinephrine is a potent vasoconstrictor (see Chapter 8), so it is effective in counteracting vasodilation (and resulting hypotension) caused by histamine release. Because epinephrine is short acting, a repeat dose may be necessary. If circulatory collapse occurs, a larger dose of intravenous epinephrine may be administered as part of resuscitative efforts (see the section on cardiac arrest later in this chapter). Hypotension is also treated with increased infusion of intravenous fluids, as stated earlier. In addition, medications used to raise blood pressure (vasopressors and/or inotropic agents) are administered, as needed. Vasopressor agents include dopamine and phenylephrine. Agents such as vasopressin (antidiuretic hormone), norepinephrine, and milrinone may also be used to treat hypotension resulting from anaphylaxis.

Corticosteroids (see Chapter 8) are another class of medications that may be used to treat anaphylaxis in surgery. Although direct clinical evidence is not available to confirm the effectiveness of corticosteroids in treating anaphylaxis, agents such as methylprednisolone or hydrocortisone may be administered for acute anaphylaxis and to reduce the risk of a delayed anaphylactic reaction. See Table 15.1 for a summary of drugs used in respiratory emergencies.

Transfusion (Hemolytic) Reaction

Blood transfusion reaction is an infrequent but important type of intraoperative allergic reaction. Any adverse reaction to the administration of blood or blood products in surgery is a condition treated and managed by the anesthesia care provider. Transfusion reactions may be one of three types: febrile nonhemolytic, allergic, or hemolytic. Febrile nonhemolytic reaction is caused by antibodies binding to donor white blood cells or platelets and is rarely seen during surgery. It is characterized by a temperature increase of 1°C and is usually treated with antipyretic agents, such as acetaminophen. Allergic transfusion reaction is usually mild and caused by medications taken by the blood donor or additives used in blood product preparation. Mild allergic transfusion reaction is treated as any mild allergic reaction, previously discussed.

Hemolytic transfusion reaction occurs when ABO-type incompatible blood or blood products are administered (see Chapter 11). Mixing of incompatible donor red blood cell antigens and recipient antibodies causes hemolysis. Numerous safety precautions are taken during all phases of blood replacement to ensure that the patient receives only compatible blood, but errors can occur. Hemolytic transfusion reaction may be characterized by hypotension, hemoglobinuria (presence of hemoglobin in urine), anuria or oliguria, fever, and disseminated intravascular coagulopathy. Hemolytic transfusion reactions are first treated by discontinuation of blood products, followed by control of hypotension, as described previously. Diuretics, such as mannitol, may be administered to maintain kidney function.

Bronchospasm

Bronchospasm is defined as impaired breathing from constriction and inflammation of the bronchi. Severe bronchospasm could result in brain injury or death. Acute bronchospasm can be triggered by chemical or mechanical irritation, the most common of which is tracheal irritation caused during intubation (also known as *reflex bronchospasm*). Placement of a laryngeal masked airway (LMA) does not trigger bronchospasm. Other factors that place patients at greater risk for bronchospasm may include chronic obstructive pulmonary disease (COPD), mucosal edema, increased mucus production, and inflammation of the airway.

Bronchospasm associated with anaphylaxis is treated as previously discussed. When nonallergic bronchospasm occurs in surgery, it is *not* usually caused by an acute asthma event—especially when the asthma patient is asymptomatic at the time of surgery. If indicated, patients with symptomatic asthma may be treated preoperatively with oral or inhaled steroids. Preoperative breathing treatments may also include β-adrenergic agonists, such as albuterol.

Signs of bronchospasm may include wheezing, prolonged exhalation, decreased breath sounds, decreased oxygen saturation (called *desaturation*), increased airway pressures during positive pressure ventilation, and hypotension. When presented with these signs, the anesthesia care provider will look for

TABLE 15.1 Summary of Drugs Used for Respiratory Emergencies	
Generic Name	**Purpose**
epinephrine	Treat hypotension and relax bronchial smooth muscle
diphenhydramine	Block histamine release
albuterol	Relax bronchial smooth muscle
terbutaline	Relax bronchial smooth muscle
dopamine	Treat hypotension
dobutamine	Treat hypotension
norepinephrine	Treat hypotension
milrinone	Treat hypotension
vasopressin	Treat hypotension
doxapram	Stimulate respirations

mechanical causes, such as blockage of the endotracheal (ET) tube. The depth of anesthesia will also be assessed because it is critical to prevention of bronchospasm before and during airway management and intubation.

When intraoperative bronchospasm is diagnosed, 100% oxygen is administered, and the patient is ventilated manually. The underlying condition, such as a foreign body or secretions in the airway, incorrect ET tube placement, or inadequate depth of anesthesia is identified and corrected. Several different categories of medications may be used to treat bronchospasm. A group of drugs called *β-adrenergic agonists* are particularly effective.

> **? QUICK QUESTION**
> What is an agonist? See Chapter 1 to check your answer.

Albuterol may be aerosolized (nebulized) and administered via the ET tube. Another β-agonist, terbutaline, may be administered by inhalation or subcutaneously. Epinephrine is a hormone (see Chapter 8) that may be aerosolized through the ET tube or given subcutaneously to relax bronchial smooth muscle and relieve bronchospasm. Anticholinergics (see Chapter 12), such as atropine and ipratropium, may also be administered aerosolized through the ET tube to treat bronchospasm caused by COPD. If bronchospasm persists, corticosteroids (antiinflammatory agents; see Chapter 8), such as hydrocortisone or methylprednisolone, may be delivered in aerosolized form but are usually given intravenously.

Laryngospasm

Laryngospasm is an involuntary constriction of the vocal cords that may result in partial or complete closure. It may occur during intubation or shortly after extubation as a reaction to the ET tube. Patients are most at risk for laryngospasm if they are lightly anesthetized at the time of extubation. Laryngospasm is seen more frequently in children and infants and is characterized by a high-pitched "crowing" sound (called *stridor*) on inspiration. The risk is increased for infants aged 0 to 3 months and significantly increased for those with asthma or upper respiratory infection.

Positive airway pressure is administered by masked ventilation with chin-lift, in an effort to break a partial spasm, but may make a complete spasm worse. If the spasm does not respond to positive pressure ventilation and pulse oximetry shows oxygen desaturation, a dose of the depolarizing muscle relaxant, succinylcholine, will be administered intravenously. (For further discussion of succinylcholine, see Chapter 14.) In general, small doses of succinylcholine will achieve reasonable vocal cord relaxation and allow adequate mask ventilation. Larger doses of succinylcholine can be used to relax muscles to allow reintubation, which may be necessary to achieve adequate ventilation and oxygenation. Atropine may be administered in pediatric patients to treat bradycardia caused by hypoxemia.

> **? QUICK QUESTION**
> Atropine is classified under which drug category? How does atropine work to treat bradycardia? See Chapter 12 to check your answer.

CARDIAC ARREST

Cardiac arrest is the sudden, unexpected loss of cardiac function, breathing, and consciousness. Cardiac arrest may occur at any time before, during, or after an anesthetic. Cardiac arrest may be attributed to several causes. For example, some anesthetic agents can cause cardiac irritability or arrhythmias; in other cases, the patient may have an existing condition, such as cardiac disease, low serum potassium, or hypovolemia that might precipitate a cardiac arrest. Cardiac or respiratory arrest in surgery is called a *code blue*. When cardiac arrest occurs in other departments of the hospital, an announcement is usually made throughout the hospital, over the public address system, to notify members of the code blue team (including an emergency physician and designated members of the anesthesia and respiratory care departments) to report to the location of the arrest. Most surgery departments do not announce the code blue to the entire hospital, though, because the surgical team is its own code blue team.

All surgical technologists must be certified in American Heart Association Basic Life Support (BLS) at the healthcare-provider level. Surgical technologists should know exactly what must be done to treat cardiac arrest in the operating room. Cardiac arrest in surgery could occur in any number of possible scenarios, so it is helpful to use critical thinking techniques to analyze each situation. The surgical technologist must be familiar with the roles of various team members and understand the functions performed by each team member during cardiac resuscitation. Usually, it is the anesthesia care provider who makes the diagnosis, officially calls the code blue, and initiates treatment.

Cardiac arrest occurring in surgery is distinct from that occurring in a nonhealthcare setting; for example, the patient may be under anesthesia and already unresponsive. It is not necessary to activate the Emergency Management System and get an automated external defibrillator because the surgical team is the emergency response team, and a cardiac defibrillator is readily available. It is rarely necessary to check the pulse manually because electrocardiogram leads are connected to the patient soon after admission to the operating room and the pulse can be heard audibly. If there is no pulse, effective chest compressions are initiated immediately by a member of the surgical team and the patient is defibrillated when indicated.

> **NOTE:** American Heart Association BLS guidelines are continuously evaluated and periodically updated. Required recertification in BLS will provide the surgical technologist with the most up-to-date information, which is also available on the American Heart Association website.

An intravenous line is usually initiated in the preoperative area, before patient transport to the operating room (except in young children). If intravenous access is not established or additional lines are needed and circulatory collapse prevents placement of an intravenous catheter, intraosseous access may be performed (Insight 15.1).

The anesthesia care provider manages the airway and breathing. If the ET tube has not been placed when the cardiac

During emergency situations in surgery, additional intravenous access may be necessary. If the patient is experiencing circulatory collapse, traditional methods used for intravenous access may not be successful. An alternative is to establish intraosseous (IO) vascular access. This method is simpler and faster than placing a central line. Because bone marrow has excellent venous drainage, medications and fluids administered by this route can be delivered into central circulation within seconds. A battery-operated drill with a specialized needle/cannula combination is used to drill through the cortex of a long bone to access bone marrow. The drill and needle are removed, leaving the cannula in place. Standard infusion tubing is connected to the IO cannula to deliver fluids and medications. IO access may remain in place for up to 24 hours, if needed.

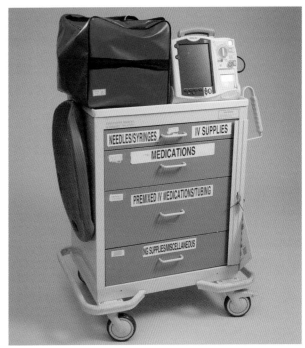

Fig. 15.2 A crash cart. (Courtesy Frank Pronesti T/A heirloomstudio.com.)

arrest occurs, succinylcholine (see Chapter 14) is administered, an immediate laryngoscopy is performed, the ET tube is placed, and mechanical ventilation is initiated. If the patient has been intubated before the cardiac arrest, mechanical ventilation continues. Cardiac compressions may be initiated by any member of the surgical team trained in cardiac pulmonary resuscitation, depending on the situation. For example, if the operation has not yet begun, any member of the team may begin compressions. If the operation is in progress, the surgeon, surgical first assistant, or surgical technologist may administer cardiac compressions from the sterile field. Alternatively, the circulator may perform cardiac compressions under the sterile drapes. The effectiveness of cardiac compressions is monitored by capnography (see Chapter 13). Vasopressors and antiarrhythmic drugs, such as epinephrine, vasopressin, and amiodarone, are administered by the anesthesia care provider or the circulating nurse, as needed. A designated team member calls for or goes to get the crash cart (Fig. 15.2), which contains emergency medications and a cardiac defibrillator. The defibrillator is brought into the operating room and prepared for use. Defibrillator electrodes are placed on the patient's chest by the surgeon, surgical first assistant, or registered nurse. The electrodes are connected to the defibrillator and used to deliver electric shocks to the patient's heart to reinstate normal cardiac rhythm. If the thoracic cavity is open, sterile internal defibrillator paddles are opened, connected to the defibrillator, and placed by the surgeon into direct contact with the heart muscle.

Several factors influence the tasks the surgical technologist performs in resuscitation efforts. These factors may be identified by answering key questions, such as the following:
- Did the arrest occur before administration of general anesthesia?
- The surgical technologist may be able to break scrub to help.
- Did the arrest occur after the surgical incision has been made?
- The surgical technologist may be required to stay scrubbed to protect the surgical site.
- Did the arrest occur during the regular surgery schedule day?
- More personnel are usually available to come to the room and help.

- Did the arrest occur in an on-call situation?
- The basic surgical team members may be the only personnel available.

In addition, the resuscitation tasks performed by the surgical technologist may vary depending on the role the surgical technologist is performing on the surgical team: scrub role, second assistant, surgical first assistant, or circulator. In the scrub role, the surgical technologist may remain sterile to cover the surgical site if necessary or to prepare the internal defibrillator paddles for use. If an additional surgical technologist is scrubbed in as a second assistant, that surgical technologist may be asked to break scrub to obtain the crash cart. If necessary, the second assistant may be designated as the official record keeper, documenting all medications given, dosages, and times of events on a special cardiac resuscitation form, provided on the crash cart. A surgical technologist in the surgical first assistant role may perform cardiac compressions, close the surgical incision if needed, or serve as record keeper. In the circulating role, the surgical technologist may notify appropriate personnel of the situation, bring in or call for the crash cart, assist the anesthesia care provider, perform cardiac compressions, or serve as record keeper.

Cardiac Resuscitation Medications

Regardless of the role or tasks performed during resuscitation, it is vital that the surgical technologist be familiar with medications given during a cardiac emergency and their purposes. The following is a brief synopsis of drugs frequently used for cardiac resuscitation (Table 15.2).

The first-line pharmacological treatment for cardiac arrest (also known as *asystole*—the absence of a heartbeat) is epinephrine. Epinephrine is a hormone (see Chapter 8) that acts as a vasopressor (causes vasoconstriction and raises blood pressure) and inotrope to strengthen the force and rate of myocardial

TABLE 15.2 Summary of Cardiac Resuscitation Drugs

Condition	Generic Name
Cardiac arrest	epinephrine
	vasopressin
	amiodarone
Bradycardia	epinephrine
	atropine
	dopamine
Tachycardia	adenosine
	amiodarone
	diltiazem
Ventricular fibrillation and/or ventricular tachycardia	epinephrine and vasopressin

contractions (to improve coronary perfusion pressure and myocardial blood flow). Administered intravenously, epinephrine is a short-acting agent and often requires additional dosing during resuscitation. Another first-line drug, vasopressin may be given to replace the first or second dose of epinephrine in adults, but is given only once because of its longer duration of action. Vasopressin causes intense peripheral vasoconstriction to support myocardial blood flow during a cardiac event. Other vasopressors, such as dopamine, phenylephrine, norepinephrine, or milrinone, may be used to raise blood pressure, as previously described for anaphylaxis.

Certain types of cardiac dysrhythmias may lead to cardiac arrest, so treatment is initiated with specific pharmacological agents. These agents are used to restore normal cardiac rhythm. Bradycardia (slow heart rate, usually fewer than 60 beats per minute) may be treated with epinephrine, atropine, or dopamine. Tachycardia (rapid heart rate) may be treated with various agents, depending upon the type of tachycardia. For example, antiarrhythmic agents, such as adenosine or amiodarone, and calcium-channel blockers, such as diltiazem, are used for supraventricular tachycardia (SVT). The first-line treatment for ventricular fibrillation and/or ventricular tachycardia (called *V-fib/V-tach*) is epinephrine and vasopressin. If these drugs fail to convert the patient to normal cardiac rhythm, cardiac defibrillation is administered. If these arrhythmias persist, amiodarone may be administered. Lidocaine is used only if amiodarone is not effective.

 TECH TIP

Many different drugs may be used during a cardiac emergency, and only the most common are introduced here. It is strongly suggested that the surgical technology student review an actual crash cart, at a local clinical facility, to further study the medications used to treat cardiac arrest.

Miscellaneous Cardiovascular Drugs

There are a huge number of cardiovascular drugs, only a few of which are of concern to the routine practice of surgical technology.

INSIGHT 15.2 Agonists/Antagonists and the Autonomic Nervous System

Many drugs are agonists or antagonists (see Chapter 1). Recall that agonists are drugs that bind to or have an affinity for (attraction to) a receptor, causing a particular response. Hence antagonists are drugs that bind to a receptor and prevent a response, also called *receptor blockers*. Many types of drugs affect the autonomic nervous system: adrenergic agents affect the sympathetic system, and cholinergic agents affect the parasympathetic system. Recall from physiology class that neurotransmitters are natural chemicals that cause responses in the autonomic nervous system. The sympathetic (adrenergic) neurotransmitters are epinephrine and norepinephrine, and the majority of the miscellaneous cardiovascular medications discussed in this text affect the sympathetic system. The major parasympathetic neurotransmitter is acetylcholine (ACh).

- Adrenergic agonists are agents that mimic the effect of epinephrine and norepinephrine (sympathomimetics).
- Adrenergic antagonists block the effects of epinephrine and norepinephrine (sympatholytics).
- Cholinergic agonists mimic the effects of ACh (parasympathomimetics).
- Cholinergic antagonists (called *anticholinergics*; see Chapter 12) block the effects of ACh (parasympatholytics).

The surgical patient may be taking various cardiovascular medications to manage chronic heart problems, such as angina or congestive heart failure (CHF). In addition, some cardiovascular medications may be administered during the course of anesthesia and surgery. Many of these agents affect the autonomic nervous system and are classified in several categories (Insight 15.2). Only the most common agents are discussed in this chapter.

Adrenergic Agonists

Adrenergic agonists, also called *sympathomimetics*, are agents that mimic the effect of epinephrine and norepinephrine.

- Dopamine is an adrenergic agonist and antiarrhythmic agent used to increase blood pressure and cardiac output. It may be given to treat bradycardia.
- Phenylephrine is an α-adrenergic agonist used to treat cardiac arrhythmias and to treat hypotension by causing peripheral vasoconstriction.
- Dobutamine is a β-adrenergic agonist and positive inotropic agent used to treat cardiac failure (medically, for chronic conditions) and hypotension (intraoperatively, for acute situations).
- Isoproterenol hydrochloride is a β-adrenergic agonist and positive inotropic agent administered to increase the rate and force of myocardial contractions. It is also used to treat bradyarrhythmias and serves as a bronchodilator.
- Norepinephrine is a β-1 adrenergic agonist and potent peripheral vasoconstrictor used to raise blood pressure, subsequently increasing coronary artery blood flow.
- Albuterol and terbutaline are selective β-2 adrenergic agonists used to treat bronchospasm, as earlier described for respiratory emergencies.

Adrenergic Antagonists

Adrenergic antagonists, also called *sympatholytics*, are agents that block the effects of epinephrine and norepinephrine. These agents are also categorized more specifically as β-adrenergic antagonists and are referred to by the more common name of *β-blockers*. β-blockers, such as atenolol, metoprolol, and labetalol, are used to slow the heart rate. Also classified as Class II antiarrhythmic drugs, they are used to treat tachyarrhythmias and hypertension.

Cholinergic Agonists and Antagonists

Cholinergic agonists, also called *parasympathomimetics*, are agents that mimic the effects of acetylcholine (ACh). Cholinergic agonists are *not* used in the treatment of cardiac conditions and are presented here for comparison only. Cholinergic agonists include pilocarpine (used in ophthalmology for miosis and treatment of open-angle glaucoma; see Chapter 10) and neostigmine (used to reverse nondepolarizing muscle relaxants; see Chapter 14).

Cholinergic antagonists, also called *anticholinergics* or *parasympatholytics*, are agents that block the effects of ACh. Atropine sulfate is a cholinergic antagonist used to block the effects of the vagus nerve on the sinoatrial node of the heart. As part of the parasympathetic nervous system, the vagus nerve helps to slow the heart rate—so atropine is used to treat bradycardia and raise the heart rate when needed. Blocking the effects of the vagus nerve also prevents bradycardia, resulting from a stimulus, such as stretching the peritoneum during a laparotomy or placing traction on eye muscles during retinal procedures. Recall that atropine or a similar drug, glycopyrrolate, may be given preoperatively (see Chapter 12) to dry oral secretions (antisialagogue). This is an example of a systemic effect (see Chapter 1) in which some types of agents exert effects throughout the body.

Antiarrhythmic Agents

Antiarrhythmics are agents used to prevent or treat irregularities in the force or rhythm of the heart. Most of these agents are grouped in Classes I through IV.

- Class I antiarrhythmics are sodium-channel blockers and include procainamide and lidocaine. These agents were used as second-line agents to treat ventricular fibrillation and ventricular tachycardia but have been replaced by amiodarone, a Class III antiarrhythmic.
- Class II antiarrhythmic agents are the β-blockers (adrenergic antagonists discussed previously), including atenolol and metoprolol, which are used to treat tachyarrhythmias.
- Class III antiarrhythmic agents are potassium-channel blockers, the most common of which is amiodarone.
- Class IV antiarrhythmic agents are calcium-channel blockers and include diltiazem and verapamil. Calcium-channel blockers are agents that reduce the flow of calcium into cells of the heart and blood vessels, resulting in relaxation of the blood vessels (vasodilation).
- Adenosine is an antiarrhythmic agent not classified in Classes I through IV. It is a naturally occurring nucleotide (part of the adenosine triphosphate [ATP] molecule), and it is used in the diagnosis and treatment of SVT.

Various types of antiarrhythmic agents may be used to treat cardiac dysrhythmias, such as atrial fibrillation, atrial flutter, SVT, and paroxysmal supraventricular tachycardia (PSVT).

> **NOTE:** PSVT is a rapid heart rate that begins and ends suddenly. PSVT can be so rapid that it prevents the heart chambers from filling completely, which can reduce blood flow to the rest of the body.

Vasodilators

Vasodilators are agents that relax smooth muscle cells in blood vessel walls, reducing blood pressure and enabling less-restricted blood flow to vital tissues. Nitroglycerine and nitroprusside are nitrovasodilators used to treat angina, acute myocardial infarction, and CHF.

> **❓ QUICK QUESTION**
> What does the acronym CHF stand for? See Chapter 7 to check your answer.

Nicardipine and nifedipine are calcium-channel blockers and arterial vasodilators used to treat stable angina and some types of tachycardia.

Inotropes and Vasopressors

Drugs classified as inotropes and/or vasopressors are administered to increase blood pressure. Inotropic agents are drugs that increase the force of cardiac muscle contraction, such as dobutamine, which increases blood pressure. Vasopressors, such as phenylephrine and norepinephrine, cause vasoconstriction, which increases blood pressure. Dopamine and epinephrine are drugs that are both inotropics and vasopressors.

Inotropic agents change the force of cardiac muscle contractions. Related medical terms are used to classify other cardiac drugs by their action on the heart. Dromotropic agents increase the conductivity of cardiac nerve or muscle fibers. Chronotropic agents influence the rate of cardiac contractions. See Box 15.1 for a summary of miscellaneous cardiac drugs.

MALIGNANT HYPERTHERMIA

MH is a rare but life-threatening reaction triggered in susceptible individuals by administration of certain anesthetic agents. MH is an inherited muscle condition that causes a hypermetabolic state in patients exposed to those specific trigger agents. It is estimated to occur in 1 in 15,000 children and 1 in 50,000 adults. More than 50% of cases are seen in patients younger than 15 years. When trigger agents are administered, huge amounts of calcium accumulate in muscle cells, causing sustained contractions. At first the patient's metabolism is aerobic, causing increased oxygen consumption, an increase in end-tidal carbon dioxide (CO_2, hypercarbia), respiratory acidosis, and heat production. As ATP is used up, metabolism becomes anaerobic, resulting in lactic acid production, metabolic acidosis, and more heat production. Muscle cell membranes become stressed and break down (rhabdomyolysis), releasing potassium, myoglobin (a muscle cell protein), and creatine kinase.

If untreated, mortality is nearly 80%. Agents known to trigger this disease are succinylcholine and all inhalation anesthetics, except nitrous oxide. Although the condition is rare, it is crucial that the surgical technologist understand the signs,

BOX 15.1 Summary of Miscellaneous Cardiac Drugs

Category: Adrenergic Agonist
dopamine
phenylephrine
dobutamine
isoproterenol
norepinephrine
albuterol
terbutaline

Category: Adrenergic Antagonist (β-Blockers)
atenolol
metoprolol
labetalol

Category: Antiarrhythmics
Class I procainamide, lidocaine
Class II atenolol, metoprolol, labetalol
Class III amiodarone
Class IV diltiazem, verapamil
adenosine

Category: Vasodilators
nitroglycerine
nitroprusside
nicardipine
nifedipine

Category: Inotropes
dobutamine
dopamine
epinephrine

Category: Vasopressors
phenylephrine
norepinephrine
dopamine
epinephrine

treatment, and pharmacology involved in such a crisis to provide competent assistance to the anesthesia team. It is important to realize that patients who are identified preoperatively as susceptible to MH should not be at risk for an intraoperative MH episode, because a number of precautions are taken to prevent exposure to trigger agents. The anesthesia delivery system is cleared of trace inhalation agents by changing breathing circuits and soda lime canisters, and the machine is flushed with oxygen or air for at least 20 minutes. Vaporizers are inactivated or removed from the machine to prevent administration of those trigger agents. In addition, succinylcholine will *not* be administered to MH-susceptible patients during the course of general anesthesia.

! CAUTION

Once MH has been triggered, the patient can die in as short a time as 15 minutes, so prompt diagnosis and treatment are vital.

Clinical Signs of Malignant Hyperthermia

In some patients, the onset of MH may be subtle with only mild signs noted at first, but MH may also manifest as an immediate and exaggerated physiological response. The administration of succinylcholine (in combination with volatile inhalation agents) is thought to speed the onset of this condition and increase the magnitude of its signs. Clinical signs of MH may be evident shortly after induction or may not appear until several hours later. The term *hyperthermia* may appear to indicate otherwise, but pyrexia (rapid increase in body temperature) is *not* an early indicator of MH. A significant rise in patient temperature indicates that a full crisis is in effect.

> **NOTE:** For assistance in the detection of a sudden rise in patient temperature, it is recommended that a core temperature monitor be used for patients expected to be under general anesthesia for more than 30 minutes. Core temperature may be assessed from the esophagus, nasopharynx, tympanic membrane, bladder, or pulmonary artery.

The earliest sign usually presented is an increase in end-tidal CO_2. An increase of even 5 mm Hg could be significant. End-tidal CO_2 can increase for several reasons other than MH, but when other possibilities have been ruled out, the anesthesia care provider may begin to alert the operating room staff that potential exists for an MH crisis.

Additional early signs include tachycardia and tachypnea. These conditions may have other causes, but in combination with the signs described here, tachycardia and tachypnea are classic symptoms of MH. Both tachycardia and tachypnea are means the body uses to eliminate the excess CO_2 that is accumulating because of the hypermetabolic crisis.

Muscle rigidity, especially masseter muscle rigidity (MMR), can be an early warning of MH, but there are other, benign causes of MMR. Opinions vary on the correlation here, but if MMR is present, the patient should be closely monitored for MH. In combination with signs described previously, MMR is considered a classic sign of MH, and it is noted in approximately 75% of cases. In addition, the patient may exhibit an unstable blood pressure, arrhythmias, cyanosis, diaphoresis (profuse sweating), and pyrexia. Temperatures of higher than 42°C have been reported. Other late signs include skin mottling, myoglobinuria (seen as cola-colored urine), and hyperkalemia. See Box 15.2 for a list of the major clinical signs of MH.

🏃 TECH TIP

Regardless of how busy the surgical technologist may be during a surgical procedure, we must always be aware of (sometimes subtle) signs indicating that our patient's condition may be changing. We must learn to be aware of what is going on with our patient "behind the curtain." If we do not know the signs and significance of MH, we are not able to recognize or understand this crisis. If we are not paying attention to what these signs mean, we are not able to react quickly and efficiently to assist the surgical team in resolving the crisis.

BOX 15.2   Clinical Signs of Malignant Hyperthermia

Increase in end-tidal carbon dioxide
Tachycardia
Tachypnea
Masseter muscle rigidity
Unstable blood pressure
Arrhythmias
Cyanosis
Diaphoresis
Pyrexia

Malignant Hyperthermia Treatment Protocol

Once MH has been identified, the surgical procedure is stopped, if possible, and all triggering agents are discontinued. The patient is hyperventilated with 100% oxygen to help eliminate the excess CO_2 that accumulates in the blood. An MH cart (Fig. 15.3), stocked with items to treat the crisis (Box 15.3), is brought into the operating room. Dantrolene sodium (Dantrium, Revonto), a skeletal muscle relaxant developed specifically to treat MH, is administered intravenously. The initial dosage is a bolus of 2.5 mg/kg. Dantrolene is packaged in 70-mL vials of lyophilized powder containing 20 mg of dantrolene and 3000 mg of mannitol, which must be reconstituted with 60 mL of sterile water. In an adult patient weighing 80 kg (176 lb), 200 mg of dantrolene (10 vials) is required to begin treatment. Dosages may reach 10 mg/kg, so in this case, 800 mg (40 vials) of dantrolene might need to be reconstituted. If additional help is not available (as seen when doing emergency on-call procedures), it may become necessary for the scrubbed surgical technologist to break scrub and help reconstitute dantrolene, as directed by the anesthesia care provider.

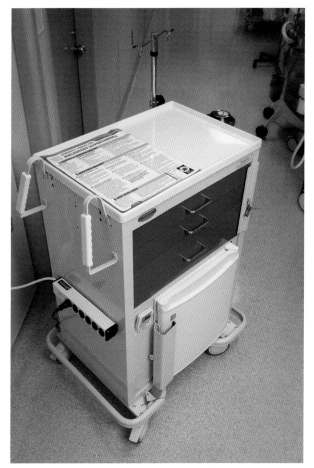

Fig. 15.3 A malignant hyperthermia cart. (Courtesy Frank Pronesti T/A heirloomstudio.com.)

TECH TIP

Surgical technologists are trained to read medication labels, draw up, and reconstitute medications in a sterile manner. These tasks are a routine part of a surgical technologist's scope of practice. A skilled surgical technologist can be exceptionally helpful in an emergency, such as MH, particularly in an on-call situation when few other personnel are available to help.

BOX 15.3   Medications Typically Stocked on a Malignant Hyperthermia Cart

Dantrium/Revonto/Ryanodex
Sodium bicarbonate
Dextrose 50%
Calcium chloride 10%

Once sterile water has been injected into the vial, the mixture must be shaken vigorously until the solution becomes clear yellow, indicating complete reconstitution. Dantrolene may be repeated in a dose of 2 mg/kg every 5 minutes, then 1 to 2 mg/kg/h and is administered until symptoms disappear. MH may also be seen in children, so the number of vials reconstituted is adjusted accordingly by patient weight.

In 2014 the US Food and Drug Administration approved a new formulation of dantrolene called *Ryanodex*. Each 20-mL vial of Ryanodex contains 250 mg of dantrolene. Ryanodex is a sterile lyophilized powder that must be reconstituted with 5 mL of sterile water for injection (without bacteriostatic agent). Reconstituted, it becomes an orange-colored suspension that is ready for injection in less than 30 seconds and can be administered in less than 1 minute. The initial dose of this form of dantrolene remains at 2.5 mg/kg, but a volume of only 4 mL (200 mg) is required for a full initial dose in an adult patient weighing 80 kg. If symptoms continue, additional doses up to 10 mg/kg may be administered.

MH causes sustained skeletal muscle contractions, which eventually lead to destruction of those muscle cells. When muscle cells are destroyed, a number of substances are released, including large amounts of potassium (K+), which leads to hyperkalemia. Several steps are taken to treat hyperkalemia during an MH crisis, including intravenous administration of sodium bicarbonate. Sodium bicarbonate is also used to treat severe metabolic acidosis that may result from high concentrations of lactate in the blood. Blood gases are monitored frequently to assess acidosis.

The patient's temperature must be reduced rapidly to prevent brain damage. Ice packs are applied to the groin, neck, and axilla—places where large blood vessels pass close to the skin. Iced lavage of the stomach, rectum, or bladder may be performed to help cool the patient's core temperature.

Another substance released as muscle cells are destroyed is myoglobin (a protein). Myoglobin tends to accumulate in the kidneys, which may obstruct normal flow. For the kidneys to be kept functioning properly, diuretics, such as 20% mannitol or furosemide (see Chapter 7), are given intravenously. Diuresis also helps to eliminate excessive potassium and treat hypokalemia.

Insulin is another agent used to treat hyperkalemia. Insulin enables cells to take in glucose, and glucose also carries potassium into those cells, thus reducing the amount of potassium in the blood. Glucose is administered with insulin to prevent hypoglycemia.

The combination of acidosis, hyperkalemia, and hyperthermia causes unstable blood pressure, cardiac irritability, and arrhythmias. These physiological disturbances may lead to cardiac arrest. Cardiac arrhythmias are treated with antiarrhythmic agents, as previously described, with the exception of Class IV agents, which are calcium-channel blockers. In addition, calcium chloride may be administered to reduce the risk of ventricular fibrillation caused by hyperkalemia.

All these treatment steps are taken virtually simultaneously, but they are arranged in an order to help the student remember key points. Basic treatment steps for an MH crisis are summarized in Box 15.4.

❓ MAKE IT SIMPLE

The treatment steps for MH are easier to learn if you formulate an easy-to-remember acronym, such as "How do surgical technologists do it?" or HDSTDI.

- H for hyperventilate
- D for dantrolene
- S for sodium bicarbonate
- T for temperature management
- D for diuretics
- I for insulin

All patient vital functions are monitored closely to determine response to treatment. Continuous monitoring of expired CO_2 (capnography) is crucial, as are establishment of arterial lines, frequent blood gas assessment, and accurate temperature measurement. A Foley catheter should be in place to measure urine output.

Treatment can be considered successful when vital signs and blood gases return to within normal limits. Elective surgery is discontinued. Surgery for a life-threatening condition

BOX 15.4 Malignant Hyperthermia Treatment Steps

Hyperventilate—with 100% oxygen
Dantrolene—administer 2.5 mg/kg, up to 10 mg/kg intravenously
Sodium bicarbonate—administer intravenously to treat metabolic acidosis
Temperature management—treat with ice packs and lavage
Diuretics—administer mannitol or furosemide intravenously
Insulin—treat hyperkalemia

is resumed, but with different anesthetic agents and a different anesthesia machine (cleared as previously described) to prevent residual inhalation agent from triggering a second crisis. On cancellation or completion of the surgical procedure, the patient is transported to the intensive care unit or postanesthesia care unit, accompanied with the replenished MH cart, because another episode could yet occur. Always consult and follow individual institution policies covering an MH crisis. The surgical technologist should become familiar with all institutional policies covering any emergency situation, including MH. In addition, the surgical technologist should be familiar with the signs, treatment, and pharmacology of MH to provide competent assistance during an MH crisis, as directed by the anesthesia care provider.

For additional information, visit the Malignant Hyperthermia Association of the United States website at www.mhaus.org. A 24-hour hotline staffed by volunteer physicians has been established to assist with information and support during an MH crisis: 1-800-MH HYPER (1-800-644-9737).

KEY CONCEPTS

- A number of emergency situations arise associated with anesthesia, including respiratory conditions, cardiac arrest, and MH.
- Although not common in surgery, these situations merit careful study and continuing education. As an allied health professional, the surgical technologist must attain and maintain the proficiency required to function effectively in these emergency situations.
- Drugs used to treat cardiac arrest include epinephrine, vasopressin, and amiodarone.
- Numerous miscellaneous cardiovascular drugs are also administered in surgery to treat various conditions.
- MH is a hypermetabolic crisis triggered by some anesthetic agents. Signs of an MH crisis include tachycardia, tachypnea, MMR, unstable blood pressure, arrhythmias, cyanosis, diaphoresis, and pyrexia.
- Basic treatment steps for MH include hyperventilation with 100% oxygen, intravenous injection of dantrolene and sodium bicarbonate, temperature management, and administration of diuretics and insulin.

▌LEARNING THE LANGUAGE (KEY TERMS)

Using your textbook or a standard medical dictionary, look up and write the definitions of each term.

anaphylaxis
asystole
bradycardia
bronchospasm

diaphoresis
pyrexia
tachycardia
tachypnea

REVIEW QUESTIONS

1. What are some complications that can occur during anesthesia?
2. Which medications may be used to treat those complications?
3. Can you name some drugs used to treat cardiac arrest? What is the purpose of each of those agents?
4. What are the signs of MH?
5. What are the basic treatment steps for MH?
6. Which tasks might the surgical technologist perform during a cardiac emergency?
7. Which tasks might the surgical technologist perform during an MH crisis?

CRITICAL THINKING

Scenario 1

You have just finished first scrubbing for a tonsillectomy. While you are cleaning up, the patient is extubated and begins emitting a high-pitched "crowing" sound, indicating that the patient is experiencing laryngospasm.
1. What steps do you take?
2. What steps does the anesthesia care provider take?

Scenario 2

You are scheduled to scrub an abdominal aortic aneurysm repair on a 63-year-old man who has been identified as susceptible for MH.

1. What additional preparations must be made for this patient and why?

Scenario 3

It is 8 a.m., and you have just scrubbed in to retract (second scrub role, not first scrub) on an open colon resection. The patient is draped, but no incision has been made, when the anesthesia care provider calls a "code blue." The patient is in cardiac arrest.
1. Which basic duties must be performed?
2. What is each team member doing as part of the resuscitation?
3. What duties might you be required to perform?

BIBLIOGRAPHY

Bardal S, Waechter J, Martin D: *Applied pharmacology*, St Louis, 2011, Saunders/Elsevier.
Duke JC, Keech BM, editors: *Duke's anesthesia secrets*, St Louis, 2016, Saunders/Elsevier.
Nagelhout JJ, Plaus KL, editors: *Handbook of anesthesia*, St Louis, 2013, Saunders/Elsevier.
Nagelhout JJ, Plaus KL, editors: *Nurse anesthesia*, St Louis, 2014, Saunders/Elsevier.

INTERNET RESOURCES

ACLS Training Center, Anesthesia ACLS Algorithms: www.acls.net/aclsalg.htm.
American Heart Association: www.heart.org/en.

Compton SJ, Ventricular Tachycardia, Medscape: http://emedicine.medscape.com/article/159075-overview.
Garth D, Hyperkalemia in Emergency Medicine, Medscape: http://emedicine.medscape.com/article/766479-overview.
Gluckman W, Forti RJ, Intraosseous Cannulation, Medscape: http://emedicine.medscape.com/article/908610-overview.
Gugneja M, Kraft PL, Paroxysmal Supraventricular Tachycardia, Medscape: http://emedicine.medscape.com/article/156670-overview.
Malignant Hyperthermia Association of the United States: www.mhaus.org/.
Revonto: www.revonto.com/.
Ryanodex: www.ryanodex.com/.
Tay ET, Hafeez W, Intraosseous Access, Medscape, http://reference.medscape.com/article/80431-overview#a01.

absorption: Process by which a drug is taken into the body and moves from the site of administration into the blood.

acute renal failure (ARF): Kidney failure resulting from a dosage-related toxic injury to the renal tubules.

adverse effect: Undesired, potentially harmful side effects of drugs.

agglutination: Clumping of particles, such as red blood cells.

agonist: Drug molecule that binds to a receptor and causes a response.

AHFS: American Hospital Formulary Service, a reference published by the American Society of Health-System Pharmacists; provides accurate information on almost all prescription medications marketed in the United States.

alternative medicine: Practices based on a philosophy different from Western medicine, such as folk healthcare and acupuncture.

amnestic: Pertaining to amnesia, loss of memory.

analgesia: Pain relief; literally "without pain."

anaphylaxis: Severe, systemic allergic reaction.

anaplastic: Term referring to cells that revert to more primitive or undifferentiated forms.

androgen: Hormones produced primarily by the adrenal glands, which include testosterone.

anesthesia: The absence of sensation.

antagonist: Drug that binds to specific receptor sites and prevents other medications from binding to these same sites, reversing or not allowing them to have an effect.

anterograde: From a point forward.

antibiotic resistance: Ability of some strains of pathogenic microbes (bacteria) to prevent or withstand the activity of antimicrobial agents.

antibody: A protein produced by the immune system when it detects harmful substances called *antigens*.

anticholinergic: Agents that block the action of the neurotransmitter acetylcholine.

anticoagulants: Agents that inhibit or prevent blood clotting.

anticoagulation therapy: Treating specific conditions, such as pulmonary embolism and deep vein thrombosis, with anticoagulants.

antigen: Substance that stimulates an immune response.

antisialagogue: Agent that inhibits mucous secretions of the respiratory and digestive tract.

anxiolysis: Relief of anxiety.

aPTT: Activated partial thromboplastin time. A test that measures the activity of the intrinsic and extrinsic pathways in coagulation and determines the correct dosage of medications, such as heparin.

arrhythmia: An irregular heartbeat or abnormal heart rhythm.

aspiration: Condition in which gastric contents enter the lungs.

asystole: Absence of a heartbeat.

auscultation: Listening to the sounds of the chest.

autologous: In blood transfusion, when the recipient and donor are the same person.

autotransfusion: Reinfusion of the patient's own blood.

bactericidal: Characteristic of an antibiotic that kills bacteria.

bacteriostatic: Characteristic of an antibiotic that inhibits bacterial growth.

benign: Condition of cells that are not cancerous.

benzodiazepine: Chemical classification of drugs used to control anxiety.

bioavailability: The extent to which an administered amount of a drug reaches the site of action and is available to produce its effects.

biomedicine: Name given to clinical medicine based on principles of natural sciences, such as biology and chemistry.

biotechnology: Concepts of genetic engineering and recombinant deoxyribonucleic acid (DNA) technology.

biotransformation: Process of changing the chemical composition of a drug from lipid-soluble molecules into water-soluble molecules that can be more easily excreted; usually takes place in the liver; also known as *drug metabolism*.

blood pressure: Measure of the force of blood against the vessel walls.

bolus: Entire dose of medication given all at once.

bovine: Referring to cows or cattle.

brachytherapy: Form of radiotherapy in which isotopes are placed directly into the tumor.

bradycardia: Condition of slow heart rate, usually fewer than 60 beats/min.

bronchospasm: Constriction of the bronchi.

cancer: Group of diseases involving abnormal cell growth with the potential to invade and spread.

capnometry: Measurement of carbon dioxide (CO_2) exhaled by the patient.

carcinogen: Substance directly involved in causing cancer.

carpule: Glass tube containing a drug; the tube has a rubber cap that is penetrated by a special needle attached to a Tubex syringe.

CDC: Centers for Disease Control and Prevention. Agency under the US Department of Health and Human Services that protects the health and safety of people by providing credible information to enhance health decisions.

Celsius scale: Measurement scale for temperature using the boiling point of water as 100°C and its freezing point as 0°C.

central line: Special catheter placed inside a large vein, such as the subclavian, to deliver intravenous fluids.

civilian time: Method of expressing time using a 24-hour scale with a.m. designating morning and p.m. evening.

clotting cascade: Complicated body process initiated by blood loss and resulting in a clot.

coagulants: Agents that enhance or promote blood clotting.

colloid: Solution similar to crystalloids but have the added component of a colloid substance that does not freely diffuse across a semipermeable membrane.

congestive heart failure (CHF): Condition in which the heart muscle is too weak to pump effectively.

constrict: To make an opening smaller.

contraindication: Condition when the use of a given medication should be avoided.

controlled substance: Medication with the potential to be misused or abused, controlled by the Drug Enforcement Administration, and given a classification/schedule.

Controlled Substances Act: Federal act passed in 1970 that designated certain medications as controlled substances.

crystalloid: Solution of predominantly sterile water with electrolytes to approximate the mineral content of human plasma.

culture and sensitivity (C&S): Process of growing microbes in culture to determine the infecting pathogen and exposure of the pathogen to various antibiotics to determine which agent will best inhibit the pathogen's growth.

cycloplegics: Paralytic agents that dilate the pupil.

cytotoxic: Substance toxic to cells.

DEA: Drug Enforcement Administration, part of the Department of Justice, established to enforce the Controlled Substances Act.

decimal point: Point, signified with a dot, that separates the whole number part from the fraction part of a number.

diaphoresis: Excessive perspiration or sweating.

differentiation: Term for development from one to another, change.

dilate: To make an opening larger.

diluent: Inert fluid (such as saline) used to make a drug formulation thinner or less concentrated.

distribution: Process in which the circulatory system transports a drug throughout the body and drug molecules eventually diffuse out of the bloodstream to the site of action.

diuresis: Excretion of large amounts of dilute urine.

diuretic: Medication administered to reduce body fluids by preventing reabsorption of sodium and water by the kidneys.

drug dependence: Term currently used to indicate drug addiction or habituation.

duration: Time between onset and disappearance of drug effects.

DVT: Deep vein thrombosis. Blood clot (thrombus) in a deep vein—usually in the legs.

dye: Solution that colors or marks tissue for identification.

efferent arteriole: The arteriole that carries blood away from the glomerulus.

efficacy (of a drug): Degree to which a drug is able to produce its desired effects.

electrocardiography: Process of recording the electrical impulses of the heart.

electrolyte: Mineral in blood or body fluids made up of electrically charged particles held together by ionic bonds, which helps the body to maintain homeostasis.

emergence phase: Phase of the process of general anesthesia that begins as the surgical procedure concludes and ends when the patient is transported to the PACU.

emulsion: Medication contained in a mixture of water and oil bound together with an emulsifier.

endocrine system: Collection of glands that produce hormones that regulate body functions.

endogenous: Pertaining to a source of bacteria within the patient.

endometriosis: Condition in which the endometrial lining grows outside the uterus.

endotracheal (ET) tube: Tube placed inside the patient's trachea to facilitate ventilation.

enteral: Pertaining to the intestinal tract.

epidemiology: Science that studies factors that determine and influence the frequency, distribution, and cause of disease.

epidural: Pertaining to above or upon the dura; an injection into the space surrounding the dura mater.

etiology: Cause of disease.

eukaryotes: Multicellular organisms, including fungi, plants, and animals; cells possess a nucleus.

euthyroid: State of normal thyroid gland functioning.

excretion: Process of elimination of drug molecules from the body; usually by the urinary system.

exogenous: Pertaining to a source of bacteria from outside the patient.

exponent: Shortcut to showing multiplication of a number times itself.

exsanguination: Draining of blood.

extracapsular: Technique for cataract extraction in which the lens is removed, while the back of the capsule is left in place to allow implantation of an intraocular lens.

extrinsic pathway: Blood clot formation initiated by factors outside the blood.

extubation: Removal of an endotracheal tube.

Facts and Comparisons: Reference containing prescription and over-the-counter medications with comparison charts and tables.

Fahrenheit scale: Measurement scale for temperature using the boiling point of water as 212°F and the freezing point as 32°F.

fasciculation: Small involuntary muscle twitches just under the skin.

FDA: US Food and Drug Administration. Agency within the Department of Health and Human Services that regulates the pharmaceutical industry.

fibrocystic breast changes: Alterations in breast tissue that cause noncancerous lumps.

fraction: Number that represents one or more equal parts of a whole.

generic: Nonproprietary or official name of a medication, listed in lowercase letters on the label.

glaucoma: Term used to describe a group of conditions characterized by an increase in intraocular pressure.

Gram staining: Rapid identification test that assists the physician in prescribing an initial course of antibiotic therapy based on the probable pathogen causing the infection; method to distinguish types of bacteria using a series of staining agents.

H&P: History and Physical. Medical document prepared by the physician that gives concise information about the patient's history and examination findings at the time of admission.

HAI: Healthcare-associated infection. Infection that was not present or incubating at the time of patient admission.

half-life: Time it takes for 50% of a drug to be cleared from the bloodstream.

hematocrit: Proportion of total blood volume that is composed of red blood cells.

hemoglobin: Protein in red blood cells that carries oxygen.

hemolysis: Breakdown of red blood cells.

hemostatics: Agents used to arrest bleeding.

heparin lock (Hep-Lock): Small tube inserted into the arm or other site for injection of medications that keeps the vein accessible. Heparin is used to flush the site.

homologous: In blood transfusion, when blood is removed from a donor and given to another person.

hormones: Chemical substance produced by the body that controls and regulates body functions.

hydration: Drinking the proper amount of fluids for homeostasis.

hypercalcemia: Condition of too much calcium in the blood (>12 mg/dL).

hyperkalemia: Condition of too much potassium in the blood (>5.5 mEq/L).

hypernatremia: Condition of too much sodium in the blood (>150 mEq/L).

hypersensitivity: Allergic response resulting from previous exposure to a drug or a similar drug; a type of adverse effect to a drug.

hypertension: High blood pressure.

hypertonic: Condition of fluid on the outside of the cell membrane having greater tonicity and osmotic pull than fluid on the inside of the cell membrane.

hypocalcemia: Condition of too little calcium in the blood (<8.5 mg/dL).

hypokalemia: Condition of too little potassium in the blood (<2.5 mEq/L).

hyponatremia: Condition of too little sodium in the blood (<135 mEq/L).

hypotonic: Condition of fluid on the outside of the cell membrane having a lesser tonicity and osmotic pull than fluid on the inside of the cell membrane.

hypovolemia: Condition of low circulating blood volume.

idiosyncratic effect: Rare and unpredictable adverse effects of some drugs on individuals, in which the mechanism of the effect may not be known or clearly understood.

in situ: Term for in its original place or confined to its original site.

indication: Reason a medication is used to treat a condition.

induction phase: Phase of the process of general anesthesia that begins when medications are administered to initiate general anesthesia and concludes when an adequate depth of anesthesia is reached and the patient's airway is secured.

INR: International normalized ratio. Laboratory measurement used to determine the effectiveness of oral coagulants, such as warfarin.

intracameral: Type of administration of a substance by direct injection into the chamber of the eye.

intracapsular: Technique for cataract extraction, in which the lens is completely removed within its capsule and left without a lens.

intrathecal: Pertaining to an injection through the dura mater into the subarachnoid space and cerebrospinal fluid in the lumbar area of the spine.

intravenous: Within a vein.

intrinsic pathway: Blood clot formation initiated by substances contained in the blood.

intubation: Process of placing an endotracheal tube.

iodinated: Agent that contains iodine.

IOP: Intraocular pressure. Fluid pressure inside the eye.

isotonic: Solution in which the solute and solvent are equally distributed so the cell neither expands nor shrinks.

laryngeal masked airway (LMA): Supraglottic airway positioned in the laryngopharynx to cover the epiglottis and larynx.

LMWHs: Low-molecular-weight heparins. Newer class of anticoagulants derived from unfractionated heparin that can be self-injected by the patient.

local anesthesia: Parenteral administration of an anesthetic agent to nerve endings in the immediate surgical site.

local effect: Medication acts at the site of application.

maintenance fluids: Fluids used to sustain normal fluid and electrolyte balance.

maintenance phase: Phase of the process of general anesthesia that begins as the patient's airway is established and secured and continues until the surgical procedure has been completed.

malignant: Condition that tends to become worse and end in death.

metabolic acidosis: Condition of excess acid in body fluids.

metastasis: Spread of a cancer or disease from one part or organ of the body to another.

methicillin-resistant *Staphylococcus aureus* (MRSA): Strain of *S. aureus* that has developed a resistance to methicillin.

metric system: International standard of weights and measurements used by scientists and engineers.

military time: Precise method of expressing time using a 24-hour scale without a.m. or p.m. designations.

minimum alveolar concentration (MAC): Measure of the potency of an inhalation agent that at one atmosphere of pressure stops the motor response to incision in 50% of patients.

miotics: Agents that constrict the pupil by stimulating the sphincter muscle of the iris.

monitored anesthesia care (MAC): Specific anesthesia service for a diagnostic or therapeutic procedure that includes all aspects of anesthesia care—before, during, and after the procedure.

morphology: Study of shapes; usually in reference to bacteria.

mydriatics: Paralytic agents that dilate the pupil by paralyzing the sphincter muscle of the iris.

nanometer: Term for measurement designating one billionth of a meter.

narcotics: Term for a controlled substance that depresses the central nervous system for pain control and has the potential to become habit-forming.

National Patient Safety Goals: Set of goals established by The Joint Commission that are reviewed annually and address current health and safety issues.

neoplasm: Abnormal growth, or tumor.

nephron: Microscopic filtering unit in the kidney that removes water and waste solutes.

NPO: *Nil per os*; nothing by mouth.

NSAIDs: Nonsteroidal antiinflammatory drugs used to treat inflammation, mild-to-moderate pain, and fever.

onset: Time between administration of a drug and the first appearance of effects.

opioid: All drugs, natural, semisynthetic, or synthetic, having morphine-like actions.

OSHA: Occupational Safety and Health Administration. Agency within the US Department of Labor whose mission is to ensure the safety and health of American workers by setting and enforcing standards.

osmolarity: Measure of solute concentration in solution.

osmosis: Passage of water through a semipermeable membrane from an area with a lower concentration of solutes to an area of higher concentration.

OTC: Term used for over-the-counter medication that does not require a prescription.

PACU: Postanesthesia care unit.

palliatives: Medications or treatments to alleviate the symptoms without curing the disease.

parenteral: Pertaining to any drug administration route other than the intestinal tract.

patent: Pharmaceutic company's exclusive right to market a medication it developed, for a period of 20 years.

PDR: *Physicians' Desk Reference.* Reference that provides information on medications used in medical and surgical practice.

PE: Pulmonary embolism. Blocking of a major blood vessel in the lung, usually by a blood clot.

percentage: Fractions that mean "per every one hundred," where the denominator is understood to be 100, and is shown by the % symbol.

peribulbar: Area above and below the orbit of the eye.

peripheral line: Small, short catheter used to administer intravenous fluids into a peripheral vein.

phacoemulsification: Surgical procedure for extracapsular cataract extraction using ultrasonic vibrations that break up the lens.

pharmacodynamics: Study of how drug actions affect the body.

pharmacogenetics: Study of genetic factors in predicting a medication's action and how it could vary from its intended response.

pharmacogenomics: General study of genes and genetic technology that determine medication behavior.

pharmacokinetics: Study of how the body processes drugs.

PICC line: Peripherally inserted central catheter. Form of intravenous access that can be left for a prolonged period of time.

plasma protein binding: Process in which some drug molecules attach to proteins (albumins and globulins) contained in blood plasma.

platelet aggregation: Clumping together of platelets.

polymicrobic infections: Infections caused by several different microbes (bacteria).

porcine: Referring to pigs.

potency (of a drug): Relative concentration required to produce an effect; how much of the drug is needed.

potentiation: Situation that occurs when two drugs are taken together and their effect is greater than the effect of either given alone.

preinduction phase: Phase of the process of general anesthesia that begins as the patient is admitted to the preoperative holding area and continues up to the point of administration of anesthetic agents.

prescription drugs: Medications that require a physician's order before they can be dispensed.

primary site: Original site of a tumor.

prokaryotes: One-celled organisms that do not have a fully developed nucleus; bacteria are prokaryotes.

proliferate: Term for rapid reproduction of a cell, part, or organism.

proportion: Statement of equality between ratios, such as $a/b = cd$.

PT: Prothrombin time. Blood test that measures the time it takes the liquid plasma of the blood to clot.

PTT: Partial prothromboplastin time. Blood test that determines how long it takes the blood to clot; normal clotting should occur in 25 to 35 seconds.

pulse oximetry: Noninvasive measure of the oxygen saturation of blood.

Pure Food and Drug Act: Federal regulation act passed in 1906 that set standards for quality and required proper labeling of medications.

pyrexia: Rapid increase in body temperature.

radioisotope: A version of a chemical element that has an unstable nucleus and emits radiation as it decays.

radiopaque: Characteristic of contrast media in which the substance does not permit x-rays to pass through.

radiopaque contrast media (ROCM): Agent used in certain diagnostic radiographic tests to enable pathologic conditions, such as tumors, stones, or blockages, to become visible on an x-ray; high-density pharmacologic agents used to visualize low-contrast body tissues that include vascular structures, the urinary bladder, kidneys, the gastrointestinal tract, and the biliary tree.

rapid sequence induction (RSI): Process used to secure and control the airway quickly.

ratio: Comparison of two numbers, as a and b, expressed as *a:b* or *a/b*.

reconstituted: Mixing a powder with a liquid to form a solution.

regional anesthesia: Technique used to accomplish both sensory and motor block to an entire area of the body.

relative value: Determination of a number's value by looking at the spaces it holds to the left of the decimal point.

remission: State of disease symptoms being abated or arrested.

replacement fluids: Fluids used to replenish losses caused by hemorrhage, vomiting, and diarrhea.

retrobulbar: Area behind the eyeball (the muscle cone) used as the injection site of regional anesthetic agents.

secondary site: Site where cancer has spread beyond the initial cancer.

selective toxicity: Ability of an antibiotic to act against pathogenic microorganisms without harming host cells.

sepsis: Whole-body condition, caused by an infection, that is potentially life-threatening.

side effect: Predictable but unintended effect of a drug.

solubility: Characteristic indicating how easily a drug can be dissolved in a fluid.

solutes: Dissolved substance in a solution.

solution: Mixture of drug particles fully dissolved in a liquid.

solvent: Substance that dissolves a solute resulting in a solution.

SSI: Surgical site infection.

staining agent: Solution that is used in surgery to help to differentiate abnormal cells from normal cells.

steroid: Hormone produced by the adrenal cortex divided into two categories: glucocorticoids and mineralocorticoids.

superbug: Strains of bacteria that are resistant to several types of antibiotics and can be potentially life-threatening.

superinfection: Additional infection that appears during the course of antibiotic treatment of a primary infection.

suspension: Mixture of undissolved drug particles floating in a liquid.

synergist: Drug that enhances the effect of another drug.

systemic effect: Medication acts throughout the body.

tachycardia: Condition of rapid heart rate.

tachyphylaxis: Unique situation in which the body has a decreased responsiveness to a drug after only one or two doses.

tachypnea: Rapid breathing.

teletherapy: Form of radiotherapy delivered by an external source (machine) pointed at a specific part of the body.

teratogenic: Any agent that can cause developmental malformations of the embryo or fetus.

The Joint Commission: Organization that evaluates and accredits healthcare organizations and programs in the United States.

therapeutic levels: Range in which a drug in the bloodstream is effective without causing serious side effects.

thrombocytopenia: Condition of low levels of blood platelets (thrombocytes).

thrombolytics: Agents used to speed the breakdown of existing blood clots.

tolerance: Term for when the body has decreased responsiveness to a medication through repeated exposure to the agent.

topical: Pertaining to a surface; drug administration route applied to the skin or a mucous membrane–lined cavity.

tumor: Another name for neoplasm; abnormal mass of tissue.

urticaria: Hives; a skin rash with pale red, raised, and itchy bumps.

USP-NF: *United States Pharmacopeia* and *National Formulary*. Two different official national lists of approved medications.

vagolysis: To block receptors on the vagus nerve.

vancomycin-resistant enterococci (VRE):   Group of enteric (digestive tract) bacteria that has developed resistance to vancomycin.

WHO: World Health Organization. Specialized agency of the United Nations that acts as an international authority on public health.

INDEX

Note: Page numbers followed by "f" indicate figures, "t" indicate tables, and "b" indicate boxes.